浙江省百项档案编研精品

英文文献中的
"温州"资料汇编（1876-1949年）
THE COMPILATION OF MATERIALS ON WENZHOU
IN ENGLISH LITERATURE (1876-1949)

【第一辑】

近代温州
疾病及医疗概况

瓯海关《医报》译编

A PROFILE OF DISEASES AND MEDICINE
IN MODERN WENZHOU

译编　温州市档案局（馆）

社会科学文献出版社
SOCIAL SCIENCES ACADEMIC PRESS (CHINA)

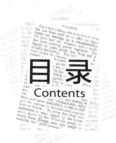

目 录
Contents

第二部分　英文文献

瓯海关 《医报》 简介

　　《海关医报》（*Medical Reports*）是清朝末年中国海关关册《海关公报》（*Customs Gazette*）的一部分，原则上每半年（从每年的4月1日到9月30日，再从10月1日到下一年的3月31日）出版一次，目的在于记录中国各通商口岸的疾病情况，包括疾病的种类和数量等，并将它们置于当地气候、地理和民间生活习俗上加以分析。从事记录工作的人员都是驻当地的医员，他们不仅负责海关职员及其家属的疾病治疗工作，还要对当地的医疗事宜进行调查，资料汇总后汇报给海关稽查统计处（The Statistical Office of the Inspectorate General of Customs）出版。《海关医报》从1871年出版第1期到1910年9月为止，本应出版80期，但自1904年3月第67期刊行之后便中断，直到1910年9月出版第68期又续刊，此后便完全停刊。但需要注意的是，《海关医报》虽然在1910年停刊，但各商埠海关医官仍在撰写海关医报，并在《博医会报》（*The China Medical Journal*）上继续发表，一直持续到1932年《博医会报》停刊。

　　作为《海关医报》的一部分，瓯海关《医报》从1878年3月发行第一期起，到1919年止，共有29期。负责记录的医官和记录年份分别为：梅威令（W. W. Myers）医生（1877 年 9 月至 1879 年 9 月）、玛高温（D. J. Macgowan）医生（1881 年 3 月至 1884 年 4 月）、劳里（J. H. Lowry）医生（1891 年 3 月至 1895 年 3 月）、霍厚福（Alfred Hogg）医生（1895 年 3 月至 1899 年 9 月）、鲍理茂（W. E. Plummer，包莅茂）医生（1901 年 9 月至 1903 年 9 月）、斯默登（E. W. Smerdon）医生（1910 年 3 月至 1910 年 9 月）、安格司（W. B. G. Angus）医生（1913 年 9 月至 1914 年 4 月）与施德福（E. T. A. Stedeford）医生（1914 年 6 月至 1919 年）。

导读: 近代外国人在温州的医疗活动

——以海关和传教士为中心

杨祥银　王少阳

一　近代温州的医疗环境与背景

温州地处中国东南沿海的浙江省南部,东临东海,北靠瓯江,气候温暖湿润,平均年降雨量约 1800 毫米,既是全省降水资源最丰富的地区,又是我国多雨地带,与世界同纬度地区相比雨量之多尤为突出,又因该地区多瘴气,这为致病微生物的滋生提供了便利条件,每年夏、秋两季常遭强台风袭击,造成大量人畜死亡,霍乱病流行。近代温州医疗卫生条件较差,一旦疾病流行,一般疾病患者不是看中医,就是求助于神明,即使在西医传入之后,仍有相当多的人相信神力之医疗效。1878 年 8 月、9 月,温州地区霍乱肆虐,蔓延迅猛,整个城市陷入恐慌。单就城里华人聚居之区,每日被夺走生命者 15~20 人之多。另有一群多达 360 名的乞丐,一天之内竟死 80 余名。有一洋人女性得病后,24 小时内就死了。海关中有 2 名华员,分别于 12 小时内、33 小时内死去。此疫流行时,城内居民惶惶不可终日。他们连续几天在城市的主要干道路口摆出桌子,上面摆满了祭品。此外还有人抬着神像,后面跟着和尚、道士到处巡游,走到祭桌前时,就念咒驱鬼,口中念念有词,借以平息鬼神之怒,妄想以己之苦来感动上苍和瘟神。此类疫情至 9 月底也就自然减弱消失了,入秋后又会卷土重来,这与温州的水井大多浑浊不洁是分不开的。① 类似情形在苏慧廉②之妻苏路熙写的《乐往中国》一书中也有记载。在第 13 章中,她写道:"温州人相信疾病是因为鬼神,他们

---

① 杭州海关译编《近代浙江通商口岸经济社会概况——浙海关、瓯海关、杭州关贸易报告集成》,浙江人民出版社,2003,第 477~478 页。

② 苏慧廉(William Edward Soothill, 1861—1935),英国哈利法克斯(Halifax)城人,英国偕我会(后改名为偕我公会)传教士,是把西方医学传入温州第一人。

有一套理论。霍乱和伤寒是由最恶劣的瘟神引起，每年都要失控流行。成百上千的人死去，死讯不断，让人悲伤。有时候棺材匠都忙不过来，女人们在墓地旁棺材边痛哭，劝都没有用。霍乱一般在秋天流行，人们相信霍乱是因为瘟神进了城，于是要献上祭品举办典礼来安慰瘟神。"①

　　在旧时的温州，无论是政府，还是民间团体和个人，慈善义举和活动都有着悠久的历史。早在 1747 年，温州民间便创办了育婴堂（晚清时称温州府育婴堂），其日常运营经费主要来自民众的捐款和政府划拨土地的租金收益，所收孩童的数目一度达到两三百人。民国初年，时任瓯海道尹的黄庆澜整顿育婴堂，创建广济院，委派钱振勋负责管理，使家乡穷苦百姓"冻馁者得所养，疾病者得所治"，免受"号寒啼饥""疾病呻吟"之苦。② 此外，北洋政府在其统治时期，忙于筹款征税，无视人民健康和福利事业。劳动人民生活困苦，如患重病，无力就医，迷信无知者，就去求神保佑，贫病交迫而自杀者屡有所闻。鉴于此，1923 年秋，工商界开明人士蔡冠夫等人，关心贫民医疗事业与社会卫生，特发起筹款创立"普安施医施药局"。局内常驻医生 4 人，杂工 3 人，管理及财会人员皆为义务兼职。诊病给药，概不收费。病家感激，群众赞扬，名医乐于任事。③

　　在医院建设方面，1885 年，清末著名改良派思想家、造诣深厚的中医学大师陈虬于瑞安县城创立利济医院，招收学徒，聘请讲师，培训医士，利济医院是浙南最早的一所医院，也是我国最早的中医院之一。同年陈虬还创办了利济医学堂，堪称我国第一所中医学校。④ 1895 年，温处道宗源瀚资助 200 银圆，陈等又在郡城设立利济分院。同年创办利济医学堂。1919 年，杨玉生等人创办瓯海医院。开诊后，当时社会上霍乱流行，群情惶恐，院里挤满了病人。由于治愈率很高，结果医院声誉大振，进院求诊

---

① 苏路熙（Lucy Soothill）著《乐往中国》（A Passport to China），吴慧译，非正式出版物，2007，第 106 页。
② 方韶毅主编《瓯风新刊》（第三集），黄山书社，2011，第 167~168 页。
③ 蔡仲瑜：《永嘉普安施医施药局纪要》，温州市政协文史资料委员会编《温州文史精选集》（一），2001，第 282~283 页。
④ 俞天舒：《利济医学堂和医学报》，温州市政协文史资料委员会编《温州文史精选集》（一），2001，第 26 页。

者络绎不绝。1922 年 6 月，医院迁至新址，为民众治疗各种疾病，解除了
民众的痛苦。①

二　传教士在近代温州的医疗传教活动

（一）医疗传教活动概述

　　医疗传教（medical missionary）最早是由来华新教传教士郭实腊在实
际宣教活动中总结出来的以医务活动作为传教手段的一种方法。他在《中
国沿海三次航行记》中反复强调在华人中行医送药的效果和他们对西医的
渴求。郭实腊认为，中国人对行医的传教士有好感就意味着传教机会的存
在。② 19 世纪基督教传教呈现全球化现象。鸦片战争后，英国内地会③和
偕我公会④传教士相继来温州传教，开创了基督教新教在温州的历史。为
了扩大教会影响，更有效地开展传教工作，他们兴办新式学校和医院，一
定程度上为当时正处于社会转型期的晚清温州迈向近代文明起了推动
作用。

---

① 潘长江：《创办瓯海医院史略》，温州市政协文史资料委员会编《温州文史精选集》
　　（一），2001，第 291 ~ 292 页。
② 方韶毅主编《瓯风新刊》（第三集），黄山书社，2011，第 172 页。
③ 内地会（China Inland Mission）成立于 1865 年，1872 年在上海设立总部，创始人
　　为戴德生。内地会严格意义上说不是一种宗派，而是跨宗派的传教团体。但是，
　　由于它对中国基督教的影响很深，规模也很大，所以其存在意义已远远超出了一
　　般团体的范围。内地会的传教士不受宗派、国别的限制，来自很多国家。内地会
　　传教的方式被称为"戴德生模式"，这种模式以传授福音为主，而以教育和医
　　务为辅助手段，不太注重大规模建立学校和医院。他们甘心吃苦，即使遇到中
　　国政府或民间的迫害，也不向本国政府上诉，而且拒绝赔偿，这一点与其他团
　　体有很大差别。所以，他们在中国的上层没有大的影响，但是在社会下层的影
　　响很大。
④ 偕我公会（Methodist Church）是基督教新教卫理宗教会之一。18 世纪产生于英国。
　　指卫理宗教会在英国的部分，以及 1851 年由英国传入中国的该宗教会。当时在温
　　州传教的是英国偕我公会的分支 United Methodist Free Churches，时称圣道公会，也
　　称偕我会，1934 年并入偕我公会。

　　1867 年 11 月和 1883 年 1 月，内地会传教士曹雅直①和偕我会传教士苏慧廉先后来到温州。由于在鸦片战争前中国采取闭关锁国政策，以天朝上国自居，对西方文明几乎一无所知且带鄙夷态度，被迫开关后，对武力入侵的西方列强自然带有强烈的敌对情绪，温州也是如此。在晚清温州，他们无疑就是西方的代表，同时他们所宣扬的基督教教义和中国传统文化存在很大隔阂，因此在传教过程中遭遇的文化障碍是可想而知的。②曹雅直在初到温州的 3 个月时间里和同伴蔡文才③先生生活在一间客栈里。当地人都惧怕他们，没有人愿意将自己的房间租给可恶的外国人。后来，当地有一位较有影响力的人因为自己陷在鸦片毒瘾和赌博中无法自拔，从而愿意提供一间房子给曹雅直。但是第二天，消息传遍了那一带，当地愤怒的人群聚集门前，强迫曹雅直搬出去。他们砸烂了曹家的大门，在房间里大肆破坏。④苏慧廉来温的头两年，生活孤苦，当他在桥下传教时，那里的人对他很粗暴，还差点将他的妻子扔进河里。1884 年，甲申教案⑤爆发，当地人用火烧了苏慧廉的住宅，苏路熙在《乐往中国》中这样写道：“周六的一天，二三十个基督徒在苏慧廉家旁的房间里举行礼拜。开场的赞美诗还没有唱完，苏慧廉的家里就遭到了袭击，一群暴徒聚集在那里，因为前门很坚固，他们就转而攻击后门，结果成功了。很快，石头砸进门和窗户，后门被他们合力推倒，混乱中，这群人涌进了院子。……他们拿着棍子，还扔石头。用洋油灯的油点燃木质的楼板，燃起熊熊大火。这群

---

① 曹雅直（George Scott，1835—1889），苏格兰人，内地会传教士，1867 年 11 月来温宣教，晚年因病返回英国，后死于法国，是新教在温开教第一人。

② 方韶毅主编《瓯风新刊》（第二集），黄山书社，2011，第 45 页。

③ 蔡文才（J. A. Jackson，? —1909），全名为“Josiah Alexander Jackson”，内地会传教士，1866 年 9 月 30 日来华，主要在浙江台州传教。19 世纪 70 年代一度来温协助曹雅直宣教，1875 年赴处州（丽水）传教，遭当地官府和民众排斥，于 1878 年赴沪经商，其妻病逝于温州。

④ 苏慧廉著《晚清温州纪事》（*A Mission in China*），张永芳、李新德译，宁波出版社，2011，第 13 页。

⑤ 1884 年 8 月 16 日，温州民众一夜间焚毁城西基督教堂、花园巷耶稣堂（今花园巷教堂），周宅祠巷天主堂等 6 所教堂。结果清官府赔偿新教 27641 银圆，因是年干支为甲申，故史称“甲申教案”。

人看着滔天火势，洋洋自得。"①

　　苏慧廉为赢得当地人的好感，削减他们对自己的敌对情绪，开始尝试开办一所男童寄膳寄宿学校。后来又觉得单一设学传教，不如双管齐下，治病给药。1880年，他在温州五马街开设了一家西式医院，规定开诊前先听讲道，前来看病者医药费全免。② 苏慧廉当年只是一个无多大医疗能力的青年传教士，随身携带点奎宁、阿司匹林等家常用药，可能西药功效比较明显，有不少人前来求医，甚至要求苏为他们做些小手术，③ 苏在给他们施药前必先进行讲道。后来，苏发现人们对西医的需求与日俱增，非专业人士不能满足人们的需求。于是他多次写信给英国的偕我公会差会，要求派遣专业的医务人员前来开展医疗工作。1890年，海和德④从宁波携药来温，苏慧廉同他在城西教堂附近建立了一家医务室，聘请在瓯海关任职的劳里医生担任门诊大夫。1893年，基督教差会派霍厚福⑤医生来温协助苏慧廉开展医疗工作。1894年2月，在教堂后面建立诊所，病房借用苏慧廉之前搭建的鸦片诊疗所，霍厚福作为专职医生应诊。开诊后由于病员日益增多，病房不足，必须建造新医院才能满足越来越多的医疗需求。1897年，英人约翰·定理⑥来温，由他捐资，苏慧廉等人购地，在杨柳巷建造

---

① 苏路熙（Lucy Soothill）著《乐往中国》（*A Passport To China*），吴慧译，第10页。
② 胡珠生：《温州近代史》，辽宁人民出版社，2000，第214页。
③ 苏慧廉在《晚清温州纪事》（*A Mission in China*）中提到，他曾先后两次尝试做手术，一次为一个年轻人拔虎牙，一次为一位老人做睑内翻小手术，术后老人很快康复，视力也比以前好多了。出于感激，老人在村里建了一间教堂。
④ 海和德（R. J. W. Heywood），英国人，偕我会传教士，1883年从宁波来温，在城西教堂设医务室施诊，协助苏慧廉筹办教会学校"艺文学堂"。1907~1927年为偕我公会温州教区主要负责人之一，在温传教40余年，1927年离温。
⑤ 霍厚福（Alfred Hogg）1893年年底来温，在城西教堂医务室任专职医生，1897~1902年任定理医院院长，1902年离温回国。
⑥ 约翰·定理（John Dingley），英国人，传教士、建筑师，1896年来温，捐资在温州城区杨柳巷创建温州第一所西医院——定理医院。该院与下文所讲的白累德医院就是今日温州市第二人民医院的前身。在温州市第二人民医院的门诊大楼后面，立着当年定理医院的院碑石刻。正中有楷书"定理医院"四个大字，左边文字是"光绪二十三年"，右边为"耶稣降世一千八百九十七年"。

了一家小型医院，这就是定理医院，设男女病房、门诊部、药房和厕所。鲍理茂医生每次出诊的时候，身边都会跟着五六个基督徒身份的医学生，负责分发圣诗单，上面印有一首四行赞美诗、《圣经》经文和一篇短小的祷告以及门诊时间、收费标准。读解了赞美诗之后，医生用风琴奏乐。接下来是简短的布道，最后以祷告结束整个礼拜过程，时间严格控制在 15 分钟之内。① 定理医院历时九年，共接待门诊病人 7 万余人次，住院病人 4000 余人次，这里面有一半的人在来医院前从未听到过赞美上帝的圣歌，甚至也不曾听过有上帝的存在。后来，虽然医院不断扩张，医疗资源仍是不够使用，必须建造新医院。苏慧廉利用在英国休假的机会四处筹款，他特意走访了约翰·定理的朋友亨利·白累德先生，后者欣然同意承担新医院的建设费用。1905 年，亨利·白累德出资 1650 英镑为定理医院在大简巷建造了一座新医务大楼，这就是后来的白累德医院，医院由英国人设计，浓郁的西洋风格和高大宽敞的楼层成为当时温州标志性建筑之一。1905 年 1 月，苏慧廉主持开业典礼，温州主要官员悉数出席，不少本地士绅也有参加。新医院设有多个手术室、男女独立病房、药房等，每日上午门诊，下午手术，没有专职护士，30 多名工友兼任病房护理。白累德医院的建立对当时温州人民来说不啻为福音，开业后一年内就有 12285 人前来求医，住院病人达 923 人，手术 321 例。② 医院为住院病人每天都举行礼拜，参加者总是认真地听讲。"我们并没有强迫每个病人都那样做，但很久以前他们就心甘情愿地跪下来敬拜他们每天所听到的全能的上帝。她们中的一些人非常虔诚，以至于等到祷告结束后她们才去服药。"③ 此外，温州天主教会于 1908 年在岑山寺购地兴建董若望医院，1913 年建成，同年 9 月 13 日开诊，内设男女病房、门诊部、住院部、姆姆（女医务人员）住房等，有病床 28 张，并在城区东、南、西三个分堂设门诊点。上海仁爱会总会派遣法籍修女娄斯·戴卡莱担任首任院长，医务人员除修女外，另聘请男医生 1 名、护士 28 名。医院服务态度良好，规模不断扩大，至 19 世

---

① 苏慧廉著《晚清温州纪事》，张永芳、李新德译，宁波出版社，2011，第 118 ~ 119 页。

② 方韶毅主编《瓯风新刊》（第二集），黄山书社，2011，第 51 ~ 52 页。

③ 苏慧廉著《晚清温州纪事》，张永芳、李新德译，宁波出版社，2011，第 121 页。

纪 40 年代发展到每天接待 200 多个病人，病床增加到 230 张，姆姆由 4 名
增至 10 名。① "很难想象，还有什么事能比我们医院的工作更像耶稣的
所为，因为是耶稣基督把天国福音的传布与医治病人结合在一起。我们
医院的信条就是：差遣他们去宣传上帝的道，医治病人"。② 这些教会医
院的设立，解除了部分受诊者的病痛，在客观上促进了温州医疗的近
代化。

（二）对医疗传教效果的讨论

近代西方传教士在温州的医疗活动，目的在于振兴教会事业，广传福
音，扩大教会影响。而要想在一个外国人不曾居住的国家或地区开辟传教
区，没有比开办一个诊所更能尽快赢得当地人的信任和好感了。③ 苏慧廉
说："从事医疗工作的传教士到中国并不是要做神迹的创造者，甚至很难
说是出于同情受难的人类。事实上，他们是被差遣的，而非自己要来，因
为在背后有着和使徒背后一样的力量在支撑着他们，这种神的力量是一贯
的。"④ "当我巡回布道时，这些药物当然能帮我吸引更多的听众；病人在
接受一定量的药物之前得听讲道，而且尽可能多听些讲道的内容；这种想
法是可行的，如果不能一石二鸟，至少可用布道与治疗这两张网抓住一
只。"⑤ 事实上，传教士在给温州百姓施药治病的同时，不失时机地对他们
进行宣讲布道，在医院有了一定规模后，传教事业也得到了较快速的
发展。

对于医疗传教的效果，苏慧廉是持肯定态度的。他在《晚清温州纪
事》中提到这样一个例子：在两个礼拜前，一个要求洗礼的男子告诉我，
十多年前他就是在这间小诊所里首次被吸引来认识基督教的。他曾经把他
那患皮肤病的妻子带来，在海和德医生给他们治疗一段时间之后，他自己
就能够在家里给妻子治疗了。影响他的，不仅仅是治疗疾病，还有海和德

---

① 方韶毅主编《瓯风新刊》（第三集），黄山书社，2011，第 173 ~ 174 页。
② 苏慧廉著《晚清温州纪事》，张永芳、李新德译，宁波出版社，2011，第 122 页。
③ 爱德华·V. 吉利克（Edward V. Gulick）著《伯驾与中国的开放》，董少新译，广
西师范大学出版社，2008，第 73 页。
④ 苏慧廉著《晚清温州纪事》，张永芳、李新德译，宁波出版社，2011，第 113 页。
⑤ 苏慧廉著《晚清温州纪事》，张永芳、李新德译，宁波出版社，2011，第 115 页。

想他们之所想，提供给他们来回旅费的花销。这事给他们留下了深刻的印象，外国医生不仅善良，投入时间和药品给他们看病，而且希望他们平安回家。他已经参加周日礼拜好多年了，现在要求受洗。① 另外一个例子是：一个患了麻风病的40岁的男人，已经被折磨得不成人样了，他来诊所哀求给他医治，诊所接受了他。几个月后，他被送给回家时变成了一个新人，他的皮肤经过治疗变得干净，浑身也有了力量，尽管手脚还有些麻木，但他能够回到自己的家，自己放牧山羊了。"他很快被我们救主的大能所吸引，回到家后不久，他就召集一些亲朋好友，建立了一个教会。"② 这样的例子还有很多，似乎充分证明了医疗传教是成功的。

然而，有些传教士对医疗传教的效果却持一种怀疑的态度。首先，他们认为，很多贫穷的温州下层人民，患病以后没钱医治，听说教会医院可以提供免费或低价治疗，迫不得已才会去那里碰碰运气。他们加入基督教并非出于真正的信仰，而是因为西医传教士的善举帮助他们解除了身体上的病痛，出于感激才会花钱建立教堂和加入教会，其实他们对基督教教义并不了解。其次，在传教之外又肩负起医疗重任的传教士们，由于医院工作繁忙，便很少有时间和精力去干预传福音事业，医疗成了他们履行传教使命的负担。再次，传教士在传教过程中难免要受到温州本土文化的冲击，他们很担心病人会把自身疾病的治愈完全归功于西方现代医学的成功，而非宗教信仰所致，从而对医学效果产生依赖，最终失去对基督教教义的认识机会。这样的例子在苏慧廉的《晚清温州纪事》中也可窥见一二："有一位剃头的，在第一次康复后，好几年一直是诊所的常客，并宣誓跟随基督，然而他的婚姻安排不允许他接受洗礼，因此他从未真正'认识过'基督。后来，他又退出了教会的活动。"③ 1884年甲申教案的发生也反映了温州民教矛盾之尖锐，实为医疗传教所难以化解。

---

① 苏慧廉著《晚清温州纪事》，张永芳、李新德译，宁波出版社，2011，第116页。
② 苏慧廉著《晚清温州纪事》，张永芳、李新德译，宁波出版社，2011，第116页。
③ 苏慧廉著《晚清温州纪事》，张永芳、李新德译，宁波出版社，2011，第121页。

对医疗传教意义的理解，并不在于治疗疾病本身，而在于它的社会意义。诚如人类学家 Mary Douglas 所说："人体对于所有人而言都是一样的，只有我们的社会条件是不同的。建立在人体基础上的各种象征被用来表达不同的社会体验。"① 也就是说，身体在某种意义上是缩小了的社会，而社会则是放大了的身体。那些因患疾病而被社会淘汰的人，在精神上遭受的痛苦并不亚于身体。传教士对病人疾病的治疗，体现了教会对人的尊重。② 然而，我们必须看到，在近代西方入侵东方的历史大背景下，医疗传教某种程度上也充当了医学殖民的角色，是殖民主义者为扩大在华权益、消除华人抵抗情绪而采取的一种策略。他们妄图通过小恩小惠，收买人心，改变中国人的信仰，最终达到灭亡中国的目的。③

三　海关在近代温州的医疗活动

（一）温州开埠与瓯海关的设立

温州地理位置优越，是一个天然良港，英国等西方列强从鸦片战争爆发后就已开始觊觎温州。英国曾于 1843 年派军舰测量温州港口南北水道，绘制海图，掌握了进港航道。另据《瓯海关十年报告：1882—1891 年》记载："然而人所周知的事实，在尚未开埠而太平军未进入台州以前，已有各国外洋船只进入本口岸停靠。在 1859 年有 17 艘船舶在'坛子尖'（Jar Point）地方下锚，又在 1862 年，四艘外国船只在该处为英国炮舰所掳获，以在未开放口岸贸易罪名押往福州，扣押好几个月之后，方才释放。次年直至开埠，据报告有许多船只停靠温州，但贸易因被太平军驱散，以后始终未恢复。"④

---

① 转引自约翰·克罗桑《耶稣传》，高师宁、段琦泽，中国社会科学出版社，1997，第 100 页。
② 文庸编著《耶稣》，辽海出版社，1998，第 65~66 页。
③ 胡珠生：《温州近代史》，辽宁人民出版社，2000，第 216 页。
④ 杭州海关译编《近代浙江通商口岸经济社会概况——浙海关、瓯海关、杭州关贸易报告集成》，浙江人民出版社，2003，第 409 页。

　　1842 年，《中英南京条约》签订后，中国被迫开放的五个通商口岸的贸易状况并不像英国人想象的那样乐观。据 1844 年升任英驻华大使的德庇时①在《战时和缔和后的中国》中记载，五个通商口岸在 1844～1847 年的贸易中，广州有所下降，厦门有所波动，福州最为糟糕，宁波毫无起色，上海显著增长。鉴于福州和宁波两港贸易的失败，他主张裁撤宁波领事馆，并反对在福州建立领事馆，想通过谈判获得中国沿海的一个或两个港口以替换福州和宁波。经过再三考虑，最终决定以位于上海和厦门中间位置的温州来取代福州。1854 年，英、美两国驻华大使为扩大既得利益，共同提出修约要求。他们要求开放中国全境，至少要开放温州等港。由于修约要求缺乏合理依据，加上未使用武力，被清政府拒绝。1868 年，正值《中英天津条约》10 年期满，英驻华公使阿利国在美驻华公使劳文罗斯配合下，再次向清政府提出开放温州等 10 个城市为商埠的修约要求。经过交涉和谈判，于 1869 年 10 月签订《中英新修条约》，把开放温州列为主要内容之一。尽管清政府已经同意，但英国当局因修约所得权益未能满足本国商人的贪求，未予批准。1875 年，英国又以"马嘉理（A. R. Margary）事件"②为借口，用断交、战争手段相要挟，逼迫清朝政府于 1876 年 9 月 13 日在烟台签订了《中英烟台条约》，其中明文载明："随由中国议准，在湖北武昌、安徽芜湖、浙江温州、广东北海四处添开通商口岸，作为领事官驻扎处所。"从此，温州的大门被英国殖民者打开，温州继宁波后成为列强侵略浙江的又一个重要基地。1877 年 1 月，海关总税务司赫德委派

---

① 德庇时（John Francis Davis, 1795—1890），英国人。他是一位中国通，18 岁就到了广州，在东印度公司任职。1816 年作为英国使团随员到过北京。1833 年英国成立驻华商务监督署，被任命为商务监督。1844 年 5 月 7 日抵港，5 月 8 日就职第二任香港总督，并兼任英国驻华公使，直至 1848 年 3 月 21 日，任期 4 年。晚年，他隐居布里斯特尔，潜心中国历史文化的研究。1876 年获英国牛津大学荣誉博士学位。1890 年去世，终年 95 岁，是享年最高的一位港督。

② 英法等国在打开中国沿海门户及长江后，又想打开内陆的"后门"，从 19 世纪 60 年代起，不断探测从缅甸、越南进入云南的通路。1874 年，英国再次派出以柏郎上校为首的探路队，在近 200 人的武装士兵护送下，探查缅滇陆路交通。英驻华公使派出翻译马嘉理南下迎接。1875 年 1 月，马嘉理到缅甸八莫与柏郎会合后，向云南边境进发。2 月 21 日，在云南腾越地区的蛮允附近与当地的少数民族发生冲突，马嘉理与数名随行人员被打死。这即"马嘉理事件"，或称"滇案"。

英籍税务司好博逊筹设温州海关。1877 年 4 月 1 日，温州海关建立，温州港正式对外开放，好博逊为首任税务司。半年后，海关总税务司署指令改温海关名称为瓯海关。①

（二）海关医员与温州医疗史

近代外国人通过不平等条约攫取中国海关管理权后，开始陆续出版一些海关关册，其中《海关医报》是清朝末年中国海关关册《海关公报》的一部分，原则上每半年（从每年的 4 月 1 日到 9 月 30 日，再从 10 月 1 日到下一年的 3 月 31 日）出版一次，目的在于记录中国各通商口岸的疾病情况，包括疾病的种类和数量等，并将它们置于当地气候、地理和民间生活习俗上加以分析。从事记录工作的人员都是驻当地的医员，他们不仅负责海关职员及其家属的疾病治疗工作，还要对当地的医疗事宜进行调查，资料汇总后汇报给海关稽查统计处出版。医报从 1871 年出版第 1 期到 1910 年 9 月为止，本应出版 80 期，但自 1904 年 3 月第 67 期刊行之后便中断，直到 1910 年 9 月又续刊出版第 68 期，此后便完全停刊。② 兹将《海关医报》中有关温州的资料整理如表 1 所示。

表 1 《海关医报》中有关温州资料整理

报告期间（医报期数）	报告口岸	负责撰写医员
1877. 10. 01 ~ 1878. 03. 31	温州	Dr. W. W. Myers
1878. 10. 01 ~ 1879. 03. 31	温州	Dr. W. W. Myers
1881. 04. 01 ~ 1881. 09. 30	温州	Dr. D. J. Macgowan
1881. 10. 01 ~ 1882. 09. 30	温州	Dr. D. J. Macgowan
1883. 04. 01 ~ 1883. 09. 30	温州	Dr. D. J. Macgowan
1883. 10. 01 ~ 1884. 03. 31	温州	Dr. D. J. Macgowan
1891. 04. 01 ~ 1891. 09. 30	温州	Dr. J. H. Lowry
1891. 10. 01 ~ 1892. 03. 31	温州	Dr. J. H. Lowry
1892. 04. 01 ~ 1892. 09. 30	温州	Dr. J. H. Lowry

---

① 胡珠生：《温州近代史》，辽宁人民出版社，2000，第 85 ~ 88 页。
② 戴文锋：《〈海关医报〉与清末台湾开港地区的疾病》，《思与言》第 33 卷第 2 期，1995 年 6 月，第 159 ~ 160 页。

续表

报告期间（医报期数）	报告口岸	负责撰写医员
1892. 10. 01 ~ 1893. 03. 31	温州	Dr. J. H. Lowry
1893. 04. 01 ~ 1893. 09. 30	温州	Dr. J. H. Lowry
1893. 10. 01 ~ 1894. 03. 31	温州	Dr. J. H. Lowry
1894. 04. 01 ~ 1894. 09. 30	温州	Dr. J. H. Lowry
1894. 10. 01 ~ 1895. 03. 31	温州	Dr. J. H. Lowry
1895. 04. 01 ~ 1895. 09. 30	温州	Dr. Alfred Hogg
1895. 10. 01 ~ 1896. 03. 31	温州	Dr. Alfred Hogg
1896. 04. 01 ~ 1896. 09. 30	温州	Dr. Alfred Hogg
1896. 04. 01 ~ 1897. 09. 30	温州	Dr. Alfred Hogg
1897. 10. 01 ~ 1898. 09. 30	温州	Dr. Alfred Hogg
1898. 10. 01 ~ 1899. 09. 30	温州	Dr. Alfred Hogg
1901. 10. 01 ~ 1902. 03. 31	温州	Dr. W. E. Plummer
1902. 04. 01 ~ 1902. 09. 30	温州	Dr. W. E. Plummer
1903. 04. 01 ~ 1903. 09. 30	温州	Dr. W. E. Plummer
1910. 04. 01 ~ 1910. 09. 30	温州	Dr. E. Wilmot Smerdon

　　报告的内容大体可分为三个部分，分别介绍温州的地理位置与自然环境；月平均气温、降雨量等天气状况；有关医疗卫生事宜的记述。其中对前两部分内容的记载，是因为医员们认为它们是导致温州地区疾病的重要因素。例如，1895年夏天，尽管平均气温不是很高，但大部分时间空气非常干燥，外国居民感到十分闷热，精神萎靡，水井几近干涸，当地居民便纷纷去河里取水。这为传染病的传播提供了机会，霍乱导致多人死亡。在外国人居住区，有两个人死亡，其中一名女士已在温州居住了大约四年时间，她在去上海的船上中暑而死；另外死亡的是一名传教士刚出生的儿子，他因为消化不良被父亲送往市区医治，病情一度好转，但后来突然出现严重腹泻、腹痛，在20小时内便死掉了。① 1897年秋天的气温变化突然

───────────

① "Dr. Alfred Hogg's Reports on the Health of Wenchow for the Half-year ended 30th September 1895," *Medical Reports*, Shanghai: Statistical Department of the Inspectorate General of Customs, p. 30.

变得很不正常，温差一度超过 10℃。这样的天气下，儿童最易得痢疾等症。这年 9 月有两个人死亡，其中一名是一个 14 个月大的女婴，她连续一两天出现轻微腹泻，第三天症状依然持续，身体更加虚弱。父母带她去看医生，当晚拒绝吃饭，两个小时后遭受急腹痛沉重打击，体温升高至 108℉，第二天早上便死了。① 第三部分内容是报告的主题，包括疾病的种类、患病人数统计、疾病症状、病因与治疗情况等。由于报告中涉及的疾病种类很多，参考同时期台湾府医员戴维·曼森在 1872 年第 4 期《海关医报》中的分类法，大致可以分为沼气性疾病、外因性疾病、体质性疾病、神经系统疾病、循环系统疾病、呼吸系统疾病、消化系统疾病、泌尿系统疾病、生殖系统疾病、运动系统疾病、外皮肤疾病、眼类疾病、耳鼻类疾病、毒瘾类疾病、剧烈官能伤害等。兹将《海关医报》之温州报告中的疾病种类统计如表 2 所示。

表 2　《海关医报》之温州报告中疾病种类统计（1877~1910）

疾病种类	英文名称
1. 沼气性疾病	Miasmatic Diseases
疟疾热	Malarial Fever
间歇热	Intermittent Fever
弛张热	Remittent Fever
疟疾	Ague/Malaria
霍乱	Cholera
2. 外因性（传染性）疾病	Enthetic（Zymotic）Diseases
梅毒	Syphilis
天花	Small-pox
痘疮	Variola
水痘	Chicken-pox
淋巴腺肿	Bubo

① "Dr. Alfred Hogg's Reports on the Health of Wenchow for the year ended 30th September 1897," *Medical Reports*, Shanghai: Statistical Department of the Inspectorate General of Customs, p. 30.

续表

疾病种类	英文名称
3. 体质性疾病	Constitutional Diseases
风湿病	Rheumatism
肌肉风湿症	Muscular Rheumatism
清热	Febricula
溃疡性狼疮	Lupus Exedens
伤寒	Typhoid
肠热病	Enteric Fever
贫血	Anemia
淋巴腺炎	Lymphadenitis
败血症	Blood – Poisoning
流行性感冒	Influenza
肺结核	Phthisis
4. 神经系统疾病	Diseases of Nervous System
神经痛	Neuralgia
晕厥	Syncope
神经应激性和虚脱	Nervous Irritability and
失眠症	Prostration
子痫、惊厥	Insomnia
神经衰弱	Puerperal Eclampsia
5. 循环系统疾病	Nerve prostration
心脏脂肪变性	Diseases of Circulatory System
心力衰竭	Fatty Degeneration of Heart
脑出血	Cardiac Failure
心悸	Cerebral Congestion
6. 呼吸系统疾病	Cardiac Palpitation
黏膜炎	Diseases of Respiratory System
支气管卡他	Catarrh
喉炎	Bronchial Catarrh
哮喘	Laryngitis

续表

疾病种类	英文名称
咯血	Asthma
胸膜炎	Hemoptysis
肺充血	Pleuritis
百日咳	Pulmonary Congestion/Congestion of lungs
7. 消化系统疾病	
	Whooping-Cough　肝淤血
腹泻/痢疾	Diseases of the Digestive System
口炎性腹泻	Congestion of the Liver
消化不良	Diarrhea
蛔虫	Sprue/Psilosis
蠕虫	Dyspepsia
便秘	Ascarides
肠炎	Vermes
痔疮	Constipation
胃炎	Enteritis
口腔炎	Hemorrhoids
咽炎	Gastritis
扁桃腺炎	Stomatitis
脱肛	Pharyngitis
内寄生虫	Tonsillitis
肠虫病	Prolapsus Ani
腹泻性贝毒	Entozoa
胆紊乱	Worms
疝气	Shell-fish Poisoning
油漆中毒	Biliary Derangement
8. 泌尿系统疾病	Hernia
肾、输尿管绞痛	Varnish Poisoning
血尿症	Diseases of the Urinary System
尿酸结石	Renal Colic
淋病	Hematuria

续表

疾病种类	英文名称
9. 生殖系统疾病	Uric Acid Caleulus
闭经	Gonorrhea
妊娠	Diseases of Generative System
月经困难	Dysmenorrhea
卵巢炎	Amenorrhea
白带	Pregnancy/Uterine Vomiting
子宫癌	Ovaritis
10. 运动系统疾病	Leucorrhea
痛风	Carcinoma of Womb
萎缩性关节炎	Diseases of Locomotiva System
腰痛	Podagra/Gout
网球员腿病	Rheumatic Gout
11. 外皮肤疾病	Lumbago
疥癣	Lawn-tennis Leg
象皮病	Diseases of Integumentary
慢性荨麻疹	Scabies
麻疹	Elephantiasis
生疖	Chronic Urticaria
牛皮癣	Measles/Rubeola
瘙痒症	Boils
冻伤	Psoriasis
掌脓肿	Pruritus
红斑	Frostbites
湿疹	Palmar Abscess
疱疹	Carbuncle
12. 眼类疾病	Eczema
眼炎	Herpes
虹膜炎	Diseases of the Eye
结膜炎	Ophthalmia

续表

疾病种类	英文名称
基质性角膜炎	Iritis
眼角膜破裂	Conjunctivitis
结膜瘀斑	Interstitial Keratitis
13. 耳鼻类疾病	Rupture of Cornea
耳液溢	Ecchymosis of Conjunctiva
中耳炎	Diseases of the Ear and the Nose
耳膜炎	Otorrhea
14. 毒瘾类疾病	Otitis
鸦片	Aural Catarrh
15. 剧烈官能伤害	Poisons
比目鱼肌破裂	Opium
臂肌、腰方肌扭伤	Lesions Violence
锁骨/颅骨骨折	Rupture of Soleus
手臂有创骨折	Sprain of Gluteus and Quadratus
手掌/拇指创伤	Lumborum
踝关节/肩部扭伤	Fracture of Clavicle/Skull
手部烧伤	Compound Fracture of Arm
手指切除	Incised Wound of Palm/Thumb
脸部和后背创伤	Sprain of Ankle/Shoulder
意外枪伤	Burns of Hands
肩关节/腕关节脱臼	Amputation of Fingers
	Stabbing Wound of Face and Back
	Gunshot Accident
	Dislocation of Shoulder – joint/ Wrist – joint

　　由于篇幅所限，接下来，我将结合医员在报告中对霍乱疾病的记载进行分析。霍乱在近代温州，乃至整个中国的历史上都很活跃。医员们在报告中对年内霍乱暴发事件的记载很多，略举两例如下：1877年夏天，温州经历了一场霍乱，时间持续10~14天，死亡率很高。当地人很少或没有采取治疗措施，感染者先是腹泻，后来出现虚脱、体寒、轻微痉挛等症状，很少呕吐，通常会在6~24小时内突然死亡。尤其是鸦片吸食者，大多数必死无疑。当地的医生很快辨别出了这场疾病的病症，当地官府出面料理已死的和垂死的病人。这场霍乱并未蔓延至全城，仅局限在几条街道，要统计确切的死亡数据是不可能的，但可以肯定的是，平均每天至少死亡10人，有两天这一数字还一度达到了35人。之后，人们开始尝试做一些诸如清扫房间、焚烧床和死人的衣服等消毒措施。尸体被迅速掩埋或运到城墙以外很远的地方进行处理。梅威令医生当时对3人进行了治疗，其中1人死亡。他发现把水合氯醛和摩擦、加热等治疗方法混合使用效果很好，而戊烷基的亚硝酸盐却达不到这样的效果。有一个吸食鸦片成瘾的人，在这次霍乱中遭受了致命打击。梅威令医生在报告中写道："他如此固执，在我离开的短暂时间内，也坚持要拿一杆烟枪。但我并没有发现他身上有什么不良症状，体温保持在99°F左右。我大概3点钟离开，8点钟的时候有一个送信的人过来告诉我，他的病已经完全好了。我很想亲自去看看他，然而，当我和送信人再次到他家的时候，发现他刚刚死掉了。他曾起床喝了些牛奶，再躺床上的时候就突然死了。他的亲戚都一再坚持让我确定他的死亡，因为他是如此了不起的一个鸦片吸食者。他们是否想通过乘我不在的时候给他提供无限制的鸦片来证明他们的预言，我并不确定；即使他们那样做了，也并非想要得到诚挚的告诫或强烈的承诺，拒绝病人提供鸦片。"[1] 1902年7月中旬，一场霍乱开始肆虐温州，而平阳在两三个月前就已开始受其侵袭。此疫传播速度极快，两周内即已传遍全城。7月底死亡人数最多，8~9月逐渐减少。夏季出现异乎寻常的干旱少雨，水源极度缺乏，所有的东

---

[1] "Dr. W. W. Myer's Reports on the Sanitary Condition of Wenchow for the Half-year ended 31st March 1878," *Medical Reports*, Shanghai: Statistical Department of the Inspectorate General of Customs, pp. 9 – 10.

西都干了。9月15日夜突降大雨，巧合的是，霍乱死亡人数也随之剧增，并表现出另一种流行方式，严重程度远大于上次霍乱。据估计，全城死于此次霍乱的人口在5000~6000人，全府至少死亡30000人。① 可以看出，霍乱在干旱季节应为不同于水型传播的另一种传播方式，推测为通过陆路进行的交往接触传播。另外，报告中提到，同年8~9月间疟疾在全府流行，那些以前因在山区而表现出对霍乱有一定免疫力的人，也同平原地区的人们一样饱受疟疾之苦，死亡人数非常多。据此可知，霍乱流行需要有特定的条件。居住在山地的人一般较少受到侵害，因为这里人口密度小，无法满足传染病流行的高人口密度条件，另外，他们与外地联系较少，客观上阻碍了霍乱病菌的传入。山区水流通畅不淤积，不利于病菌再次滋生。②

玛高温医生③对霍乱颇有研究，他在提交的《1881年3月至9月温州健康报告》中写道："温州已经饱受霍乱蹂躏之苦，对相关数据的研究无法给病理学家提供有用的信息，但它作为中国历史上众多流行病的一种，却是很有意义的"。④ 权威界人士论证说，霍乱最早起源于1813年印度的Gangetic Delta地区。也有人对此提出质疑，认为霍乱在此之前就已开始流行于东方的其他地方。更多时候，这些反对者的观点认为，霍乱不仅在印度流行，在欧洲和美国也很流行，人们为控制霍乱的蔓延采取了许多不同措施。普遍的说法是，霍乱通过病人排泄物里的细菌从一个人传到另一个人身上，水是霍乱病毒传播的途径。反对者则认为，霍乱不是通过人与人传播，而是由空气传播的，遵循一定的规律，受大气和地球环境的影响，水里并不能产生它的特殊病菌。马六甲一

---

① "Dr. W. E. Plummer's Reports on the Health of Wenchow for the half-year ended 30th September 1902," *Medical Reports*, Shanghai: Statistical Department of the Inspectorate General of Customs, p. 37.

② 单丽：《1902年霍乱在中国的流行》，中国海洋大学出版社，2008，第30页。

③ 美国基督浸礼会传教士马高温于1843年在宁波兴办华美医院（现宁波市第二医院），是我国最早建立的西医医院之一。

④ "Dr. D. J. Macgowan's Reports on the Sanitary Condition of Wenchow for the Half-year ended 30th September 1881," *Medical Reports*, Shanghai: Statistical Department of the Inspectorate General of Customs, p. 46.

带的中国人是最先遭受印度霍乱侵袭的华人群体，早在 1819 年它就通过泰国陆路到达那里了，同年 5~6 月出现在温州，差不多同时出现在宁波。据宁波的一位 70 多岁的老人回忆，这场霍乱（时称"蟹爪病"）在当时造成了很大伤亡，很多人正走在大街上就死去了，因而一位法国病理学家称其为"旋即死"。关于这场霍乱，Chiahsing 市的一名医生说，它最先于 1821 年在 Chiahsing 市爆发，时称"脚筋吊"或"吊脚痧"，医生们把它当成普通霍乱来医治，结果没有治好一个病人。普通霍乱一般由积热引起，需要用冷却食物疗法治疗，这名医生却持相反的观点，他认为一般霍乱是由积冷引起的。在接下来的两年时间里，它反复出现，毒性不减。从那以后，它便经常肆虐于这个国家的土地上，特别是 1860 年发生在浙江的那一次。中国几乎每年夏天都会发生霍乱疫情，后来它被认为是一种地方性疾病。在中国部分地区，典型的"干燥霍乱"在炎热的天气里也很普遍，被称为"痧"，袭击人体时很突然。在广州，它比其他地方发生得更加频繁，广州市民承认"痧"从很久以前就已经开始在他们中间流行了。1880 年冬，上海浦东地区暴发了印度霍乱，持续 3 天时间。中国人对这次疫情的解释是，长时间的干旱以及河水遭到污染（本地人承认当气候异常湿润时，也会暴发一些疾病）。毫无疑问，印度霍乱在中国北方被视为一种新的疾病。然而，它也可能是在沉寂了一段时间后重新暴发的一种固有疾病。有一篇很知名的医学论文把肌腱收缩视为普通霍乱中的一种偶然症状。而吴有性①医生则认为，尽管两者有一个相似之处，但它们仍然是两种不同的疾病。他或许已经证实了那个时候没有人会认为"突然呕吐和便秘症"是可以在人与人之间传播的。这种新型疾病被认为具有传染性。然而，也有很多人认为它只是感冒或疟疾。玛高温医生最后得出结论说："通过以上我搜集的信息可以说明，印度霍乱对中国而言是一种新型疾病，它不是通过人与人传播，而是通过空气细菌传播的；它受大气和地球环境的影响，为防止移动微生物病菌的侵袭而采取的隔离管制措施是

---

① 吴有性，字又可，江苏震泽人，生活于明代末期 1582~1652 年间。其生活时代正值明末战乱，饥荒流行，致使疫病流行。他潜心钻研，认真总结，提出了一套新的认识，为温病学说的形成与发展做出了贡献，著有《瘟疫论》。

没有用的。"①

对霍乱疾病的治疗，前文中提到，当地人往往会求助于传统中医或神明。起初，他们对西医并不信任。梅威令医生就曾在 1878 年的报告中写道："尽管我很努力地想在当地开展医疗救治工作，但很难说我实现了自己的愿望。中国人似乎羞于让外国医生给他们医治，对于西医的功效，他们感到既奇怪又矛盾。一方面，他们似乎认为很多死亡病例都是外国人造成的；另一方面，他们对传统中医的权威充满信任，在那里病人的表情不会显得那么失望。"② 然而，随着西医疗法治好的病人越来越多，其效果有目共睹，很多人开始慢慢接受西医和吃西药，西医逐渐变得普遍起来。当地一些江湖郎中便开始打着西医的名号行骗，造成了不少的医疗事故。大清律例规定："凡庸医为人用药针刺，误不如本方因而至死者，责令别医辨验药饵穴道，如无故害之情者，以过失杀人论，依律收赎给付其家，不许行医。若故违本方，乃以诈心疗人疾病而增轻作重乘危以取财物者，计赃准盗窃论，因而致死及因事私有所谋害，故用反症之药杀人者，斩监候。"③ 尽管如此，仍旧不能断绝庸医的出现，这可能与当地官府执法不力有关，也从另一个方面说明了西医西药一定程度上得到了当地百姓的认可。

四 传教士与海关在近代温州医疗史上的角色与贡献

(一) 温州传教士与海关的医疗互动与合作

初来温州的传教士及他们的家属由于对当地的气候环境不适应，常会

① "Dr. D. J. Macgowan's Reports on the Sanitary Condition of Wenchow for the Half-year ended 30th September 1881," *Medical Reports*, Shanghai: Statistical Department of the Inspectorate General of Customs, pp. 46 – 48.
② "Dr. W. W. Myers's Reports on the Sanitary Condition of Wenchow for the Half-year ended 31st March 1878," *Medical Reports*, Shanghai: Statistical Department of the Inspectorate General of Customs, p. 9.
③ 姚雨芗原篆《大清律例会通新篆》(4)，胡仰山增辑，文海出版社，1964，第 2587 页。

患上一些疾病，甚至会因此死去。例如，1894 年 12 月到 1895 年 3 月间，温州暴发了一场天花，死亡率非常高。开始主要在儿童中流行，后来成年人也开始受到感染。一名天主教遣使会的牧师在照顾他患病的同事的时候感染上了天花，并最终死去。① 1895 年夏天，温州气候干燥，传染病盛行，一名传教士的儿子因为消化不良和腹泻而死去。② 另外有一名传教士感染上霍乱，四天内死去。他的妻子也因感染霍乱，在 40 小时内就死了。③

　　由于起初来温的传教士数量不多，而懂医学的人更是少之又少，开展医疗传教工作显得力不从心，在这种情况下，驻温的海关医员们除了服务于海关的工作人员及其家属以外，也积极参与当地的医疗救治工作。前文中提到的劳里、霍厚福和鲍理茂三位海关医员就曾先后在城西教堂医务室、定理医院和白累德医院担任医生。劳里于 1890 年来到海和德和苏慧廉开办的诊所任职。苏慧廉说："当时，在温州海关工作的劳里医生也自愿在空闲时间来帮忙。或在诊所里面工作，或协助我们宣教。作为一个传教团，我们非常感激他的热心与高超的医术。"④ 霍厚福医生在 1893 年被教会派往温州协助苏慧廉，1897 ~ 1902 年间任定理医院院长，鲍理茂医生在 1902 ~ 1917 年间先后担任定理医院和白累德医院院长。玛高温医生出生在美国马萨诸塞州，是北爱尔兰移民的后代，后来他作为南部浸礼会的一名医学传教士来到中国，在温州海关担任医官。他是在华时间最长的美国居民，去世时享年 78 岁。⑤ 另外，因为传教士在温州民间传道的时候，可以

---

① "Dr. J. H. Lowry's Reports on the Health of Wenchow for the Half-year ended 31st March 1895," *Medical Reports*, No. 49, Shanghai: Statistical Department of the Inspectorate General of Customs, p. 3.

② "Dr. Alfred Hogg's Reports on the Health of Wenchow for the Half-year ended 30th September 1895," *Medical Reports*, Shanghai: Statistical Department of the Inspectorate General of Customs, p. 30.

③ "Dr. Alfred Hogg's Reports on the Health of Wenchow for the Half-year ended 31st March 1896," *Medical Reports*, Shanghai: Statistical Department of the Inspectorate General of Customs, p. 92.

④ 苏慧廉著《晚清温州纪事》，张永芳、李新德译，宁波出版社，2011，第 116 页。

⑤ *New York Medical Journal*, Vol. 83, 1893, p. 355.

有机会看到本地人的一些患病情况，海关医员便委托他们中的一些人采集相关研究资料，是为双方医疗合作的另一种情形。例如，苏慧廉不是医生，但他经常携带药品在民间进行传道。鉴于医疗传道的良好效果，他建议：任何想到缺医少药之地宣教的人，先接受几个月的医疗培训及简单的外科手术训练。假如他不能做到这一点，那就带上一箱子的简单药品吧。①后来在他的努力下建立起来的白累德医院，其日常病历采用大本笔记簿，病史以罗马字母拼写的温州方言记载，② 这些病历成为海关医员研究温州地区疾病的绝好资料。在医学教育方面，白累德医院建立后，不但设有手术室、独立病房和药房等，还设有培训本地学生的教室，由医院医生担任教职，在当地推广西医教育，培养本土西医医生。海关医员鲍理茂在任院长期间，不但给本地西医学生上课，讲授西医理论知识，还在出诊时带他们到医院病房进行临床实践考察。

由上文可知，海关医员为医疗人力不足的传教士们提供了有力支持，同时也依靠他们搜集一些研究本地疾病情况的资料，双方共同致力于西医教育，培养本土西医医生。他们当时同属在温的少数外国人，其中不少人来自同一国家，具有相同的宗教信仰，或是出于治病救人的职业道德，或都对医学研究和医学教育怀有热情，这可能是彼此合作的原因。

（二）对温州社会的贡献

西方教会在温创办医院，初衷是为了振兴教会事业，扩大西方文化的影响，客观上也为温州地方培养了一大批本土西医人才，如陈梅豪③、张德辉、何其美、郑求是、郑济时等当时温州著名医生，均出自教会医院。另外，白累德医院于1926年创办高级护士、助产护士学校，二十年共培养毕业生150多名，形成了一支护理队伍。近代外国人在温州开展的医疗救助活动，带有强烈的人道主义色彩，一定程度上赢得了温州社会各界人士

---

① 苏慧廉著《晚清温州纪事》，张永芳、李新德译，宁波出版社，2011，第115页。

② 胡珠生：《温州近代史》，辽宁人民出版社，2000，第215页。

③ 陈梅豪，1895年5月出生，1912年被保送到当时由英国教会创办的白累德医院（温二医前身）学医，学成后留校执教和从事临床医学研究。其间，被任命为白累德妇产科学校的校长。新中国成立后，白累德医院被政府接收，改名为温州市第二人民医院，陈梅豪出任医院副院长兼任妇产科主任。

的支持与同情。西方传教士通过办医院、兴医学，将西医教育引入温州，在治病救人的同时，也加快了温州的近代化进程。①

驻温的海关医员是医疗兼研究的医生，他们对近代温州的医疗与医学研究做出了实质性贡献。除了尽一名医生救死扶伤的职责外，举凡他们对温州的疾病、民俗、气候、地理的记录，说明他们对温州居民产生了职业以外的兴趣，对当时的温州社会颇有观察。他们的报告不仅对研究近代温州的医疗卫生史具有重要意义，甚至在某种程度上可以被视为业余的人类学报告，给我们提供了一个看待和解读温州近代历史的新视角。

总之，传教士与海关医员在近代温州医疗史上扮演着重要角色，他们为温州带来西式医疗和医学教育，培养本地学生，弥补教会医疗人力的不足，有益于传教事业的发展，也为温州医疗市场增添了一项就医选择。此外，他们尝试改变本地人对洋人的态度，积极投身当地医疗慈善事业，对当时的温州有一定贡献。

---

① 方韶毅主编《瓯风新刊》（第三集），黄山书社，2011，第 174 ~ 175 页。

第一部分

中文
翻译

n-Chê sea coast, it seems that th
of Fukien and T'aichow are sti
merous and as savage as ever.
and its consort bound from Ningpo
w laden with rice and sundries wer
y attacked near Wênchow by a c[...]
pirates, who boarded the merchant
[h]aving ransacked everything of valu
[t]he latter, left them with twenty-six
[...] seriously wounded Sir[...]
have been issued by the Governo[r]
[...], T'an, for the capture of the pirate
[...]ite a large fleet of war junks is no[w]
[...]t it seems to be the universal opinio[n]
[...] most will be unsuccessful

[...] xpression, spread himself out over th[e]
[w]hole subject of the health, pestilence
[f]amines, and topography of the place
[T]hirty-six closely printed pages hav[e]
[n]ot sufficed to relieve him of his whol[e]
[b]urden of knowledge, for at the begin
[n]ing of his paper he says that he reserve[s]
[t]he medical [...] [oc]casion; but
[...] f which he h[...]
[...]lly have th[...]
[...]hat we sho[...]
[...]uch a trifle
[...]ply [...] He begins [...]
[...] [d]istrict in wl
[...]e gr[...] [a]nd passing
[...]
[...]

[ca]l Report
[...] Americau
[...]rt of the most influential
[a]fter trip with improved [...]
[r]esults, seems now to have
[...] that point where if more
[...] of necessity become m
[...] superfluity. As has bee[n]
[...] the impetus given by
y means of shipment has [...]
nt export of a[ll]
[...]spects for tea

During a fierce gale which raged at Wen
[c]how about a fortnight ago, several seriou[s]
[d]isasters occurred, attended in many case
with loss of life. Four large junks, lade[n]
with poles, were upset and many other
[d]ragged anchor or sustained other injuries
whilst a great number of small fishing craf[t]
[s]uffered a worse fate. The villagers on th[e]
[c]oast showed great barbarism. Instead o[f]
[a]ffording succour, they busied themselve[s]
with picking up wreckage thrown ashore
[I]n the worst cases they even wrested th[e]
[p]oles away from the shipwrecked people
who in their exhausted state were made t[o]
[y]ield the logs to the merciless people
[O]wing to the unusually cold weather a[t]
[W]enchow there is considerable suffering
[a]mongst the poorer classes, who are no[t]
[p]rovided with extensive wardrobes, and
[e]specially amongst those who have a pre
[...]

(FROM A CORRESP[...]
Notice to mariners, also
[...]d to feminine sphere-
[r]emarkable Peak on the
[n]avigators see on their [...]
[W]enchow, having only
[...]nd never named, has no
[...]e denizens of Wêncho[w]
[...] Hart's Peak," in recogni
[...]ices which the Inspecto[r]
[I]mperial Maritime Custo[m]
[...]y illuminating the coas[t]
[...]ormal recognition of th[e]
[...]y the Wênchowese, in pic-nic assembled
[...]n the 22nd March, and that being th[e]
[b]irthday of the Emperor of Germany, hea[...]
[...] celebration of the Queen's Jubilee
[...]nd within measurable distance of th[e]
[n]atal day of President Cleveland, th[e]
[h]ealth of those estimable rulers was drun[k]

RIOT AT WENCHOW.

[th]e Yungning, from Wen[c]
[...]d here on Saturday, b[rings]
[...]ulars of a riot which had
[...]how on the night of the
[...]rst intimation of this ri[ot]
[...]ed up from Ningpo from information
[...]ied by the Yungning on arrival a[t]
[...]port, though efforts had been made b[y]
[E]. H. Parker, British Consul, and als[o]

Parker taking leave on a new de-
[s]ure, having first secured the last instal-
t of the indemnity that the authorities
ed to pay for losses sustained by
[fore]igners in the recent disturbances. To
[...]be Mr. E H. Parker's success in giving
[gene]ral satisfaction to foreigners and native
[auth]orities in regard to the questions raised
[th]e riot to good luck, would be unjust to
accomplished officer. It was tact that
[effec]ted an amicable settlement

[...]ay-[...], running as she [...]
[...]rt of the most influential

[d]evastation that met ou[r]
[th]e river of Wênchow wa[s]
[mi]les and miles the countr[y]
vast expanse of wate[r]
[s]teads and graves, an[d]
[mou]nds crowded with cattl[e]
[...] frowning background [...]
[...] most depressing an[d]
We passed too quickl[y]
by the pen. Women an[d]
[g]roups doubtless talkin[g]
[...]sses, while the men wer[e]
[bu]sy in their boats. In some places wher[e]
[t]he bridges were still standing only th[e]
[u]pper portion of their arches was visibl[e]
[l]ooking like mirages—water above, belo[w]
[a]nd around them! Great indeed mus[t]
[h]ave been the downpour to have caused suc[h]
[a]n inundation. It was a comforting chang[e]
[t]o turn one's gaze from the immense
[c]ountry to the numberless fishermen pu[r]
[s]uing their calling as if no such thing [...]
[s]ome troubles existed. The flooded cou[ntry]
[...] passed it was pleasing to note th[...]

[...]which a reference to Mr. Do[n]
[...]'s table on the opposite page rend[...]
[...]ent. My views elsewhere publi[shed]

[...]tants of the so-called [...]
[a]re put away their store-cl[...]
[a]r. The rejoicings were co[...]
[qu]ietness and decorum, the
[...] of nastiness was eaten,
[a]mount of tomtomming and [...]
[indu]lged in ; in fact, everyth[ing]
[...] accordance with "olo c[...]
[...] Year's Eve most of the
[pri]ncipal thoroughfares were
[...]ted with coloured lamps, [...]
[...]re lighted in nearly all th[...]
[...]ty and suburbs. That thi[s]
[amu]sement did not result in [...]
[c]onflagration is simply miraculous,
[com]munity is by all right-thinking
[...]tributed to the special interve[ntion]
[T]ien Tien Ta Ti, the great Lord of
[H]eaven, or some other benevole[nt]
[t]hough here, as elsewhere, scoffers
[fo]und who point to the saturated con[dition]
[ev]erything or to some other such [...]

To the Editor of the
NORTH-CHINA DAILY NEWS.

[S]IR,—Although the subject of r[...]
[C]hina was ably discussed at a late
[...] of the Shanghai Literary and D[...]
[Soc]iety the question was not so exha[usted]
[t]reated as to preclude me from c[...]
[sm]all contribution, assuming that
[...] be unacceptable to those who
[...]ry (but not

[...]ically, it m[...]
[...] think the
[...]mature, tha[t]
[...]where it m[...]
[...] needed ; f[...]
[no]rthern Ch[...]
[...]courses, and [...]
[...] is doubtful
[su]ccessfully c[...]
It was urge[d]
[...]yed by an i[...]
[...] of China,

[...] OWN CORRES[P]
[...]ing, on enter
[...]d some straggl[ing]
[s]trawropes, the

that were d[...]
[...]ent the enemy'[s]
[...]ng. [Had] they resisted the[y]
would have been as useless
A proposition that was made
[...] channel has been abandoned
[...] a panic was created by a p[...]
[re]quiring every family to brin[g]
[man]darins a basket of stones.
[...] as secure as if they had a[...]
[...] protection; the authorities
[...] solicitous for their safety. S[...]
[...] threw missiles, and others cr[...]
[...] but they were bamboozed [...]

[...]e sent to Ta-ch[...]
[Y]o-ching-hsien
[...] pirate-robbers
[c]aused considerat[...]
[...]ies of both this [...]
[c]how. Some tim[...]
[d]oes plundered two
[...] the Yu H'uan Bay
[...]e) which caused the
[...] to order one of his
[...] against them. On [a]
[...] of the bay the office
[...] vessel decided to an[...]
[...]ed a party of soldier[s]

Macgowa[n]
[...]ow recen[tly]
put down
[ass]umption
[S]outhwaite
[...]ld be tra[...]

瓯海关《医报》（1877.10.01—1878.03.31）

梅威令医生有关温州卫生状况的报告

温州城坐标为北纬 $27°18'4''0'''$，东经 $120°38'28''50'''$，地处江阔水深的瓯江南岸，离出海口大约 20 英里。

瓯江自西向东奔流入海，瓯江南北则为大片山岭。

温州城的卫生状况表明，中国人对卫生知识的掌握程度，似乎已经远超卫生法规的初级认识阶段。无论是在北京还是在其他城市，中国传统卫生知识长期处于失落状态，公共卫生设施也处于崩坏和没落之中，但温州的情况却截然相反。温州街道井然有序，铺设细密，道路从中间向两边倾斜形成坡度，并与水沟相连，水沟又在拐弯处和遍布全城的水渠连接。街道每隔一百码可以看到公共厕所和小便池，它们会在每天早上的特定时间被清理干净。上述设施供水情况良好，保证秽物不会因为长久滞留而出现腐败，其自成系统，可谓卫生科学方面值得称道的进步。清晨，清洁夫开始工作，他们会清洁街道和两旁的水沟，清理各家各户前晚的马桶，并收集垃圾与废物。垃圾会被烧掉，粪秽则会用来肥田。通常来讲，水渠的水量总是相当丰沛，即便是在旱季蒸发量很大的情况下，也足以维持充足供水。各处水渠彼此连通，汇聚成片，注入小湖；这个缓慢却稳定的循环系统一直在发挥作用。水渠不断被疏浚，疏浚过程中，人们会小心收拾河道两旁的蔬菜或其他杂物（以防污染水渠）。可以想象，没有感受到因各种有机物腐坏而产生的恶臭，是温州与中国其他大部分城市显著的差别。这里的居民，从整体上来说，生活富足，大部分家庭能住上比较宽敞和通风的房屋。这些房子被一堵堵高墙隔开，并且大部分情况下都有宽敞的院子。我从未在温州见过拥挤的人潮，由此判断，我认为温州人口并未出现过剩，住房足以供给当地需要；另外，温州人往往居住得相当分散。

　　温州被恰如其分地称为"教堂之城"：展现在人们面前的，是众多壮丽的寺院，无数神父和修女①沉浸在他们引人注目的虔诚精神世界。寺庙遍布的好处是，其大量绿化和开阔的空间，普遍使得空气流通状况和清洁程度得到极大改善，往往能吸引各地的俗人、老人和年轻人聚集于此，他们能够在寺庙里呼吸新鲜空气并感到愉悦。

　　温州人看起来对饮用水非常仔细小心，水井往往被挖在离他们住处尽可能远的地方。井口四面砌墙，以避免水井被地表水污染。据我所观察到的情况，井水仅做饮用，而洗涤等则会用渠水。因此，在其他地方常见的饮用水被船只污染或遭到其他方式污染的现象，在温州即便不能说完全被禁绝，也可以说得免其弊。除极少例外，温州人不会在城内安葬亡者，且正如前文所述的缘故，几乎看不到腐败的蔬菜或动物尸体，水质相当不错。在此我可以高兴地讲，在我能够携带显微镜到温州后，立刻对当地水质进行了化学与显微镜检测，结果证实了这一点。

　　去年整个华南都异常潮湿，温州的潮湿情况也不无类似，我会在后文附上湿度一览表。温州每月实际降雨天数并没有我之前预想的那么多，雨天和晴天异常交错。我们记录下雨天大气与南北山岭的湿度，在这种情况下，当我们去回顾这些记录时意外发现，雨天如此之少。潮湿天气会从6月一直持续到下一年1月，几乎从不间断。遇上晴天是最令人愉悦的事情，夏季炎热难耐，偶有清新海风穿过斗状山谷直入城中，可惜鲜有此福。我在7月、8月来温州路上途经上海和宁波，就我个人经验来说，与这两地相比，温州的体感温度更令人舒适。

　　城里完善的排水系统避免了潮湿天气所带来的诸多不利影响；城市对面的征服岛（即江心屿）居民并不多，气象设备设置在岛上，岛上湿气更重。尽管如此，我还是坦率地指出，温州的大多数上游地区，在相当程度上总会让人感到沮丧和抱怨；另一方面，多亏了随时准备迎接我们的海风，常能让我们感到爽快和凉意，大大缓解了我们在其他地方的不适。当然，根据我一年来的观察——这意味着我有发言的资格，但有一点除外——谈论温州的气候可能为时尚早；但我希望自己的结

―――――――――――

①　按照上下文，这里应指僧侣和尼姑，前文所说的"教堂"也应包含庙观。——译者注

论足够公道，并且在某种程度上，我相信温州能够兼具沿海城市的优点，又能避免多数沿海定居点的缺憾。毫无疑问，定居点最终会扩张至河口地带，届时温州港将成为滨海城市；关于这个话题，我会进一步详谈。

温州为低矮群山环抱，城墙跨山越岭，依山而建。地势则高出瓯江许多，因此洪灾在温州闻所未闻。山谷南面是高大山岭，平原顺山势延展，直抵城墙。平原大量种植水稻，无数水渠起到灌溉与运输的作用。农业区与城区分离，我在城内没有遇到和找到疟疾或类似病例。整个城内，有很多漂亮的双层仓库，这些仓库如果略加修饰（如安装玻璃窗、更多地板等），立刻就能变成舒适又健康的住所。温州的另一个好处是房租相当低廉，我相信当地人不久就会发现，这个问题需要充分考虑。

我们抵达温州后，对牛肉的需求十分强烈，但市场上销售的牛肉十分倒人胃口，要么是些病死牛肉，要么是占卜活动的祭肉。不久之后，外国居民与一名中国买办达成协议，由他定期屠宰供应，牛和屠宰后的肉类都会经过检疫。由此我们总算能够获取过得去或者说还算健康的肉类；最近屠夫不时会宰只羊，总之我们感到情况似乎比最开始要好得多。天冷时我们能够吃到山羊肉；对其他人而言，这是个不错的替代品，菜谱的变化令人高兴。鹅肉、禽肉、蛋类、鸭肉与蔬菜的供应很充足；温州的猪通常是圈养，并受到精心饲养和照料，如果能放下固有偏见，温州的猪肉其实相当不错。

上面我提到的食品价格都很便宜，可以想见，当地粮食供应不会太糟糕。

从医学观点看，我只能说外国居民的总体健康状况还算不错，我还没有遇到改变现状的重大事件，当然我的工作经历还太短。当然，也应该提到如下事实，即在 1877 年 12 月 31 日，这里有 26 位外国居民；但截止到 1878 年 3 月 31 日，只剩下 23 位外国居民，其中包括 5 位女性和 3 个小孩，在这些孩子中，最小的只有 18 个月，最大的是 4.5 岁。

虽然尽了最大努力，希望自己能成为一名真正的本土医生，但结果实在不尽如人意。中国人在接受外国治疗时非常羞怯，同时他们还会持有一些极端奇怪和自相矛盾的观点。一方面，他们开始认为洋人的医术可以针对某些疾病起死回生；另一方面，他们坚信只要尚未病入膏肓，中医治疗就更为优越。

我偶尔会遇到农村地区过来的疟疾患者。眼炎，事实上包括多数眼科疾病，在当地很常见，尤其是黏膜炎和角膜翳。当地居民尚未接受天花种痘，但天花病例没有想象中那么多。去年夏天，与中国大部分地区一样，霍乱肆虐过一段时间，持续了 10 天到两个星期。针对霍乱的治疗手段则几乎为零。患者在染病初期会排泄一次或两次洗米水状粪便，随后病人开始出现衰竭，体温下降，轻微痉挛，常常无法小便，没有或仅有少许呕吐。6～24 小时后，病人会突然死亡。吸食大烟的患者几乎必死无疑。这些症状从外部观察十分隐蔽，许多病人往往出现恢复迹象，却又出人意料的突然死亡。如前文所述，除非在有限范围内，当地人很少会采取灌肠或催吐疗法；一旦患上霍乱，死亡率非常高。我强烈地意识到，如果能够采取合理治疗，结果会大不相同，起码能够挽救更多患者；但当地人似乎并未做任何尝试。当地医生在做出诊断后就会离开，随后家人开始准备丧事。

此次霍乱并未扩散至全城，却被证实在某些街道，尤其是在某一街区肆虐。我无法获取到相关的精确统计数字，但每天的死亡率在初期不会低于 10%，有 2 天甚至攀升至 35%，接着又跌落到 10%，随后不久这位不受欢迎的"访客"终于离去。此次霍乱传染危害有限，我认为应毫不犹豫地归功于当地良好的卫生状况；我很高兴地看到当地人会采取一些消毒措施，如清扫死者房间、焚烧床上用品和衣物。随后，尸体会很快入殓，并被运送到偏远地区，通常是在城外。我治疗了 3 名霍乱患者，其中有一人死亡。我发现皮下注射水合氯醛，再结合按摩、热敷等其他治疗手段，疗效最为显著。另外据我观察，使用戊基亚硝酸盐并不能取得效果。死亡的患者后来被证实有烟瘾，他的烟瘾如此之大，在病情有所恢复、趁我短暂离开期间，马上迫不及待地拿起烟枪过瘾。凌晨 3 点离开之前，我没有在他身上发现任何危险的症状，病人体温保持在 99℉。第二天早上 8 点，有人向我报告说病人情况良好。因为想要亲自查看，所以我与来人一同前往其家中，结果发现病人已经死亡。据其家人称，当时他准备起身喝些牛奶，突然倒下。病人亲属坚持要我确定他是否真死了，因为病人烟瘾太大。我不能确定在我离开期间，其家人是否让病人无节制地吸食了大量毒品，但如果事实果真如此，我可以说，我并不是没有给他们劝告，他们也曾向我保证会避免病人吸烟。

我曾经见过一两次象皮病，但目前还没办法对其发病率、病因或其他相关问题谈太多。当地皮肤病相当普遍，其中疥疮最为常见。外因性皮肤病很多；当地众多庵堂似乎助长了皮肤病的传播，许多尼姑实际上不过是妓女，她们成为染病的主因。尽管相较而言价格不菲，且民众大多知道染病风险，但这些尼姑仍旧大受欢迎。大约有40座庵堂，公然蓄有妓女，这表明当地道德水平极低，许多已婚妇女因行迹放荡而声名狼藉。为何梅毒会在温州传播，在这里能够轻易找到答案。

鸦片中毒的病例在一年中的某段时期非常普遍，偶尔几次人们来找我帮忙时，病人往往已经处于无意识状态。通过使用阿托品、士的宁和冷水洗胃疗法，我能让大部分病人恢复清醒。针对治疗鸦片中毒，当地一些土法非常流行：首先会让病人就近服用夜壶或厕所里的尿液；然后喝下新鲜的温热血液，血液取自绵羊、山羊或者家禽被割开的喉咙。后一种治疗方法暂且不说，前一种方法除了让人惊恐外，实际并不能让胃部排出多少东西。这种土法看起来实在莫名其妙，上述催吐剂的效果也往往不尽如人意。

也许我能就温州外国租借地的卫生状况说上几句。其备选如下：（a）城东的一块土地，由达文波特先生提议；（b）温州城对岸的宝塔山一带，由好博逊先生提议；（c）停泊锚地外或瓯海关下游附近地区。

我相信温州城对岸的江心屿会被选为租借地。江心屿地处瓯江中流，岛上有一座巨大的寺庙和两座宝塔；但我估计这些寺庙、宝塔马上就会被拆除。假如一座港口有利可图，值得建立永久租借地或定居点（settlement），那么任何一个普通商人（但买下当地寺庙，夷平它，然后在原址上建立自己的货栈，这样做是否应当呢）都会不惜代价让自己能在当地过得尽量舒适。又或者货栈虽然建在别处，但拆毁古建筑也能为两三栋住宅提供空间。这种想法并不仅仅是某种可能，而是确实发生的，中国人需要放弃备受尊崇的庙宇，江心屿上的宝塔因为前述的荒谬歪理而被拆除。港口的发展，或者说温州的规模与地位的重要性，使得有必要在此建立租借地。

如果温州与宁波类似，只有沼泽地可供选择，又或者我们必须要将临近温州城作为首要考虑条件，那么也许——不要指望能踩在坚硬的泥土上——我们会选择第一个方案建租借地；如果选择了这个方案，那么我们需要无数的木桩和碎石去建造厚实的地基，以承载房屋的重量，这个工程可能需要耗费一两年时间。地基即便打得再高，潮水一来，浓稠如烂泥的泥土立刻会被冲走。这个方案缺点如此之多，即便这是温州唯一能够提供的土地，我还是看不出有什么理由在这里建租借地。我还意识到，这块土地即便不是全部，也有相当部分属于一两名官员所有；但这条理由并不充分，不足以让外国居民支付金钱在此建立定居点，为了清除瘴疫需要花费太多时间，医疗与埋葬费用也应纳入考虑。诚然，在邻近城市的地区兴建优良疗养所能够解决医疗问题，但长久来看，虽或有节省，但总账必定不菲。如果必须在河对岸的低平土地上建租借地，那么选址也应更靠后，地基至少应在最高水位线以上；外国居民没必要选这块有害健康的土地建租借地，选一些地势相对高的土地，能很容易规避上述缺点。

宝塔山方案（b）由好博逊先生提议，从卫生角度来看，这个方案几乎能够满足所有卫生要求。夏季时宝塔山位于海风风向上，冬季又能有所遮蔽。至少从三个方向来看，其视野都极其开阔，因为地基都是干燥的沙砾，因此能够建起优良的房屋。唯一的缺憾是离温州城太远，宝塔山在江对岸（北面），江阔 0.5 ~ 0.75 英里。另外，轮船和帆船只能停泊在靠近温州城的一侧，另一侧并不适合做锚地。

上述两个方案之所以被提出，是基于这样一个假定，即外国定居点必须尽可能靠近城市。靠近城市是为了方便接触商人和商行，但这条理由目前在温州并不适用，简而言之，目前温州城内几乎没有什么商人和商行。温州的大部分贸易都是针对内地农村地区的，温州出口茶叶等货物，进口货物为布匹、鸦片、煤油等。大部分温州城里人，不会进行大宗货品贸易或从事商业投机，由此带来的结果是，遍布河网与海岸的舢板船，反而成为消费主力军。不可否认，外国人来到温州建立起轮船航线，并催生其他形式的贸易，使得温

州得以成为且必将成为贸易网中的重要一点；但当地的本土中间商
几乎全是外地人，他们之所以会居住在温州，是因为外国人在这里
创造了商业需求。这些外地中间商的人数并不比外国人数少，此外，
他们的活动往往十分依靠外国人。最近一段时期，货物贩运至内地，
尤其是船运出口（茶叶最为典型），许多情况下船只进入温州后根本
不会停靠在锚地，外国人出现在哪里，贸易地点就集中在哪里。商
人们想要尽量靠近贸易点，因此希望把租借地建在河口，选择一处
地势较高的地点，就能完全避免停泊不利的麻烦。我常听说福州的
租借地选址是个错误，其地势的高低实在是各种麻烦的根源。我相
信为了贸易便利，并没有靠近城市建租借地的必要，牛庄下游数英
里远的营口①即明证。

在河口地带建立租借地，对于贸易来讲具有无可比拟的优势，同时其
卫生条件也极为有利。从卫生观点看，河口有山岭靠近水岸，河口南岸背
山靠水，且形成一定坡度。这里有一两个小一点的山丘，它们介于众山之
间、河岸之后，与那些没有很好位置来建造房屋的地方相比，这里可以建
造优良、干燥、卫生状况良好的房屋。河岸前，能够建最高水位标记，此
处建货栈非常完美，100 码的河岸足以停泊最大的船只。由于靠近大海，
此处租借地必能发展成为海滨胜地；山岭荫蔽与邻近海洋的地形，也必能
使此地冬暖夏凉。此处拥有深水航道，通往农村腹地的道路也四通八达，
距离温州城 8～10 英里，因此卸货、航行、运输量一定非比寻常。上述条
件使得有可能在这里建立起华南最卫生的租借地，这一点使人印象深刻。
附近山岭和无数山谷，构成美丽的风景，漫步其中让人身心沉醉。总而言
之，温州商业地位由地理位置决定，而将外国定居点建在河口则能够满足
所有要求。

另附上瓯海关气象观测记录表（1877.04.01—1878.02.28），如图 1～
图 4 所示。

---

① 英文原文是指"Yingtze"（扬子江），而根据文意，这里应该是指营口
（Yingkow）。——译者注

ABSTRACT of METEOROLOGICAL OBSERVATIONS taken by the Customs

Latitude 27° 18′ 41″ 0″ North

DATE.	BAROMETER.		THERMOMETERS.				HYGROMETER.					
			Dry Bulb.		Wet Bulb.		Temperature of Dew-point computed.		Elastic force of Vapour.		Humidity 0—1.	
	9.30 A.M.	3.30 P.M.	9.30 A.M.	3.30 P.M.	9.30 A.M.	3.30 P.M.	9.30 A.M.	3.30 P.M.	9.30 A.M.	3.30 P.M.	9.30 A.M.	3.30 P.M.
APRIL:—	inches.	inches.	°F.	°F.	°F.	°F.	°F.	°F.				
Max......	30·07	29·95	75·	79·	73·	74·	71.6	70·5	·774	·745	·965	·882
Mean.....	29·91	29·89	69·90	71·8	68·5	69·63	67·4	67·84	·670	·680	·917	·873
Min.......	29·79	29·75	65·	67·	64·	65·	64·	63·4	·596	·583	·889	·752
MAY:—												
Max......	30·08	30·05	78·	78·	72·	74·	67·8	71·2	·680	·763	·874	·896
Mean.....	29·93	29·92	71·64	72·3	68·7	69·2	66·34	66·72	·645	·654	·834	·829
Min...	29·79	29·78	64·	65·	62·	63·	60·2	61·4	·575	·544	·709	·796
JUNE:—												
Max......	30·04	29·97	84·	89·	81·	81·	78·9	76·2	·987	·902	·992	·882
Mean.....	29·85	29·84	77·4	78·2	74·3	74·7	72·13	72·25	·787	·789	·839	·818
Min.......	29·67	29·68	68·	69·	67·	67·	66·2	65·4	·643	·625	·838	·660
JULY:—												
Max......	30·00	29·98	88·	91·	82·	83·	78·4	78·2	·970	·964	·941	·942
Mean.....	29·72	29·79	82·2	82·6	79·1	78·87	76·93	76·25	·924	·902	·838	·810
Min.......	29·64	29·59	77·	75·	75·	74·	73·6	73·3	·827	·819	·828	·662
AUGUST:—												
Max......	30·07	30·05	85·	90·	82·	85·	79·9	82·0	1·019	1·092	·847	·775
Mean.....	29·85	29·82	80·8	83·6	77·7	79·2	75·53	76·12	1·222	·899	·840	·681
Min.......	29·62	29·62	76·	76·	73·	74·	70·9	72·6	·755	·800	·820	·480
SEPTEMBER:—												
Max......	30·19	30·15	84·	86·	79·	81·	75·5	77·5	·882	·942	·939	·828
Mean.....	30·05	29·99	75·43	76·87	73·	74·07	71·29	72·01	·763	·784	·868	·851
Min.......	29·90	29·85	67·	68·	66·	65·	65·2	62·6	·621	·567	·757	·758
OCTOBER:—												
Max......	30·44	30·39	75·	80·	71·	74·	68·2	69·8	·689	·728	·794	·711
Mean.....	30·21	30·16	67·2	72·9	62·2	66·3	58·20	61·22	·485	·540	·728	·686
Min.......	30·06	29·95	56·	62·	48·	52·	40.0	43·0	·247	·277	·550	·497

图 1　瓯海关气象观测记录表（1）

ΝΝCHOW, for the ELEVEN MONTHS ended 28th February 1878.

ongitude 120° 38′ 28″ 50‴ East.

SELF-REGISTERING THERMOMETERS.		RAIN IN 24 HOURS.	WIND.				CLOUDS.		No. of days in each month on which no rain or snow fell
Maximum in Air.	Minimum in Air.		Force as per Naval Scale.		Summary of Direction.		0—10.		
9.30 A.M.	9.30 A.M.	Inches.	9.30 A.M.	3.30 P.M.	9.30 A.M.	3.30 P.M.	9.30 A.M.	3.30 P.M.	
°F.	°F.								
83°	73°		2·	2·					
75·17	67·04	·8	1·090						6
68°	57°	·000	·000						
84°	73°		4·	4·					
74·98	68·29	·758	1·111						21
67°	59°	·000	·000						
91°	83°		2·5	3·					
75·6	74·05	·425	·783						16
69°	66°	·000	·000						
94°	88°		7·	3·					
85·64	79·24	·427	·895						21
76°	74°	·000	·000						
90°	88°		2·	3·					
87·63	77·79	·580	·870						21
76°	70°	·000	·000						
93°	79°	2·	2·	2·					
81·60	71·80	1·272	·4	·566					17
71°	66°	·000	·000						
86°	70°	1·1	2·	4·					
77·26	62·13	·475	·838	1·					25
67°	50°	·000	·000	·000					

(In default of a Rain-gauge no observations were taken.)

图 2 瓯海关气象观测记录表（2）

DATE.	BAROMETER.		THERMOMETER.				HYGROMETER.					
			Dry Bulb.		Wet Bulb.		Temperature of Dew-point computed.		Elastic force of Vapour.		Humidity o—1.	
	9.30 A.M.	3.30 P.M.	9.30 A.M.	3.30 P.M.	9.30 A.M.	3.30 P.M.	9.30 A.M.	3.30 P.M.	9.30 A.M.	3-30 P.M.	9.30 A.M.	3-30 P.M.
NOVEMBER:—	inches.	inches.	° F.	° F.	° F.	° F.	° F.	° F.				
Max......	30·57	30·44	69·	77·	67·	73·	65·4	70·2	·625	·733	·882	·796
Mean.....	30·29	30·21	60·7	64·3	58·	61·1	55·57	58·22	·441	·485	·830	·805
Min.......	30·01	29·92	49·	52·	46·	49·	42·7	46·0	·274	·310	789	799
DECEMBER:—												
Max......	30·44	30·50	62·	71·	61·	69·	60·1	67·4	·519	·670	·935	·881
Mean.....	30·21	30·20	52·2	56·7	50·1	54·2	48·	51·70	·335	·384	·856	·834
Min......	29·99	29·86	41·	43·	38·	41·	34·1	38·6	·196	·234	760	·844
1878.												
JANUARY:—												
Max.....	30·62	30·53	53·3	62·	53·	58·	52·70	54·4	·402	·423	·987	·850
Mean.....	30·70	30·57	40·45	44·79	38·54	41·98	31·45	38·60	·176	·234	701	790
Min......	29·99	29·79	29·	32·	28·	31·	24·4	28·7	·126	·154	738	762
FEBRUARY:—												
Max......	30·57	30·51	53·	56·	52·	55·	51·	54·	·374	·417	·930	·928
Mean.....	30·33	30·29	43·27	45·94	41·88	43·63	40·21	40·85	·249	·255	·896	·805
Min......	30·07	29·99	36·	39·	33·	37·	28·5	34·4	·153	·199	721	·642

Instruments placed in verandah facing S. on Conquest Island.

REMARKS.

Dew-point, Elastic force of Vapour, and Humidity computed from the Greenwich factors published in 1856.

The readings for April commenced on the afternoon of the 19th, those for February ceased for all the instruments except Barometer on the 18th, and those of the latter on the 13th when it was unfortunately broken.

The following record of observations made during the typhoon of the 3rd July 1877, may be of interest:—

At 9.30 A.M. the force of wind was estimated at 7 of the Naval Scale, from which hour the storm increased up to some time between 11 and 12 o'clock noon, when it began to moderate, and by 3.30 P.M. had quite abated. The wind, which kept steadily at East during continuance of the gale, had come round to South at 3.30 P.M. The following is the note made for the day:—"Forenoon blowing terrifically and rain coming down in torrents; about noon began to moderate and clear off, afterwards gentle breeze with drizzling rain."

Readings of Barometer, July 3rd 1877.

	Inches.		Inches.		Inches.		Inches.
6 A.M.	29·65	10 A.M.	29·34	1 P.M.	29·40	5 P.M.	29·55
7 "	29·61	11 "	29·20	2 "	29·45	6 "	29·64
8 "	29·55	11.30 "	29·10	3 "	29·50	7 "	29·70
9 "	29·47	Noon	29·22	4 "	29·52	8 "	29·75

图 3　瓯海关气象观测记录表（3）

SELF-REGISTERING THERMOMETERS.		RAIN IN 24 HOURS.	WIND.				CLOUDS.		No. of days in each month on which no rain or snow fell.
Maximum in Air.	Minimum in Air.		Force as per Naval Scale.		Summary of Direction.		0—10.		
9.30 A.M.	9.30 A.M.	Inches.	9.30 A.M.	3.30 P.M.	9.30 A.M.	3.30 P.M.	9.30 A.M.	3.30 P.M.	
°F.	°F.								
82'	66'	'3	4'	4'			13 at 10	16 at 10	
67'57	56'57	'18	1'333	1'366					17
52'	48'	'000	'000	'000					
73'	59'	1'1	5'	5'			11 at 10	13 at 10	
57'47	47'10	'428	1'310	1'379					19
47'5	36'	'000	'000	'000					
54'	51'5	'5	4'	4'			12 at 10	17 at 10	
44'48	36'88	'242	1'709	1'903					22
35'	27'	'000	'000	'000					
68'	46'5	'9	4'	4'			15 at 10	14 at 10	
48'47	38'91	'46	'875	1'125					16
41'5	35'	'000	'000	'000					

Rain Guage 4 feet above ground.

Naval Scale for estimating force of wind, from Col. Sir H. JAMES's *Instructions*; app. p. 31.

			Pressure in lb. per sq. ft.
0	Denotes calm.		
1	Light air just sufficient to give steerage way.		¼
2	Light breeze	with which a well-conditioned man-of-war under all sail and clean full would go in smooth water from	1 to 2 knots 1
3	Gentle breeze		3 to 4 knots 2¼
4	Moderate breeze		5 to 6 knots 4
5	Fresh breeze	in which the same ship could just carry close hauled	Royals, etc. 6¼
6	Strong breeze		Single-reefs and top-gallant sails 9
7	Moderate gale		Double-reefs, jib, etc. 12¼
8	Fresh gale		Triple-reefs, courses, etc. 16
9	Strong gale		Close-reefs and courses 20¼
10	Whole gale	with which she could only bear	Close-reefed main topsail and reefed foresail. ...{ 25
11	Storm	with which she would be reduced to	Storm stay-sails 30¼
12	Hurricane	to which she could show	No canvas 36

图 4　瓯海关气象观测记录表（4）

瓯海关《医报》（1878.04.01—1879.03.31）

梅威令医生有关温州卫生状况的报告

在上次的报告中[①]，我已经从卫生角度，对该港口主要特点进行了详细描述；但定居在当地的外国居民规模太小，因此我还有很多细节写得不够周全。在进一步报告之前，我需要提一下温州城的纬度，先前报告刊载的当地纬度应修正为北纬 $28°1'30''$，经度则无误。

1878 年 8 月，一场霍乱侵袭温州城。其间有两名欧洲人染疫，其中有一人死亡。第一例病例出现在英国皇家海军"拿索"号上，应朋友皇家海军格雷汉姆医生的邀请，我与其一同前往诊治。

简单而言，我或许可以指出，在尝试过大多数常规治疗手段后，最有成效的还是干热疗法。我们按照"费忽"号船长柯克尔的做法，即将病人放在两个锅炉中间。病人身体被维持在 120 华氏度的温度，并允许他大量饮用冰水。患者很快有了反应，当船第二天早上出航时，他已经迅速康复。

第二个致死病例，起初看起来并不严重，但由于感染者是一位刚刚分娩 9 天的女士，这一不利情况加剧了某些其他不利条件，否则结果也不会如此出人意料。

此次霍乱持续时间并不长，总体上中国民众遭罪也不如去年严重，虽然仍旧得不到任何治疗——当地患者——毫无疑问，在这种情况下，最后的死亡率一定随之高涨。

过去一年里发生的第二起死亡病例，是一名外地患者。病人被带到温州时，已处于瘴气性血毒症晚期，且病情从未出现过好转。据她自己讲，病人之前一直居住在内陆城市一所条件极差的屋子里，四周全是臭水沟和

[①] 《海关医报》第 15 期，第 38 页。

排水道，并且很难获取良好食物。在她病情的最后一个月，呕吐了大量胆汁淤渣。她的身体器官正常，但脾脏除外，病人脾脏出现明显萎缩，仅比一个小鸡蛋略大。

外国居民的健康状况总体上相当好，鉴于这座港口总是拥有卓越的气候条件，因此这一结果非常符合预期。有两个婴儿出生，不过，有一个胎死腹中。此次分娩，虽然极其复杂且持续时间很长，但并没有什么地方值得特别说明。母亲在产后已经迅速恢复。

现在仅容我呈上本次报告的最后一部分——气象表（见图 1、图 2）。

1879.]　　　　　　　　WÊNCHOW.　　　　　　　　61

ABSTRACT of METEOROLOGICAL OBSERVATIONS taken at WÊNCHOW from 19th April 1878 to 31st March 1879.

DATE.	BAROMETER.		THERMOMETERS. Dry Bulb.		Wet Bulb.		HYGROMETER. Temperature of Dew-Point computed.		Elastic Force of Vapour.		Humidity. 0—1.		SELF-REGISTERING THERMOMETERS. Maximum in Air.	Minimum in Air.	RAIN IN 24 HOURS.
	9.30 A.M.	3.30 P.M.	9.30 A.M.	3.30 P.M.	9.30 A.M.	3.30 P.M.	9.30 A.M.	3.30 P.M.	9.30 A.M.	3.30 P.M.	9.30 A.M.	3.30 P.M.			
	Inches.	Inches.	°F.	°F.	°F.	°F.	°F.	°F.					°F.	°F.	Inches.
1878.															
APRIL:— Max.	No barometer.	No barometer.	69.	70.	68.	68.5	67.2	67.30	.666	.716	.969	.976	75.	70.5	1.
Mean			64.4	63.6	60.8	62.6	61.37	60.72	.551	.542	.899	.908	65.3	56.1	.3
Min.			58.	58.	57.	55.	55.1	55.4	.446	.439	.683	.766	58.	53.	.000
MAY:— Max.			87.	86.	80.5	79.	76.6	84.8	.862	1.195	.969	.976	88.5	80.	.8
Mean			76.5	75.8	72.6	71.8	70.61	71.24	.754	.825	.832	.856	79.1	69.8	.2
Min.			66.	68.	64.	62.	62.8	60.8	.572	.533	.710	.716	63.	70.7	.000
JUNE:— Max.			89.	88.	82.	83.	80.0	80.8	1.044	1.044	.945	.946	89.1	82.2	1.4
Mean			79.9	79.4	76.5	75.	76.86	73.17	.820	.809	.797	.816	81.5	75.1	.4
Min.			72.	72.	64.8	62.2	.013		.592	.360	.630	.577	74.7	67.5	.000
JULY:— Max.	30.01	29.98	91.	94.5	84.	88.	81.9	86.2	1.089	1.250	.778	.847	84.	85.5	.4
Mean	29.88	29.78	87.2	88.1	82.1	85.1	76.4	74.0	.981	1.000	.763	.734	84.6	76.7	.4
Min.	29.56	29.62	82.5	79.	78.5	77.	74.4	74.0	.850	.837	.766	.771	84.6	76.7	.000
AUGUST:— Max.	30.04	30.05	93.	93.	84.5	86.5	83.8	85.7	1.158	1.230	.962	.990	97.		2.8
Mean	29.89	29.86	87.7	84.4	81.1	80.1	76.2	76.7	.919	.928	.757	.771	88.5	79.9	.7
Min.	29.76	29.75	70.	70.5	69.	69.5	71.5	74.	.689	.707	.541	.593	77.	70.	.000
SEPTEMBER:— Max.	30.57	30.50	89.	85.	84.	81.	78.9	78.4	.987	.971	.847	.964	82.	82.1	.8
Mean	29.95	29.88	81.9	78.5	76.3	74.9	75.	72.4	.868	.795	.797	.816	85.1	76.2	.4
Min.	29.44	29.30	73.	72.	68.	65.	63.8	63.0	.592	.360	.710	.710	68.	68.	.000
OCTOBER:— Max.	30.38	30.34	84.	84.	79.5	77.	76.35	74.6	.906	.842	.803	.878	92.	81.5	.6
Mean	30.18	30.22	72.4	71.57	67.69	67.69	66.84	60.21	.524	.521	.447	.397	75.77	65.9	.4
Min.	29.99	29.98	59.	59.	49.	52.	40.	45.7	.246	.307	.364	.405	60.5	51.5	.2
NOVEMBER:— Max.	30.46	30.45	77.	70.	71.	65.	66.8	61.0	.536	.536	.696	.731	69.	66.3	1.4
Mean	30.30	30.30	62.8	62.0	57.26	56.	55.50	50.6	.441	.368	.670	.657	66.3	55.	.567
Min.	30.15	30.15	55.	56.	49.	49.	45.0	48.0	.299	.335	.690	.716	61.	45.	.000
DECEMBER:— Max.	30.52	30.52	74.	72.	67.	67.	62.1	63.0	.557	.576	.663	.734	62.	62.	1.6
Mean	30.31	30.29	57.4	53.4	48.7	48.4	44.0	45.2	.288	.301	.608	.635	57.9	45.6	.63
Min.	30.05	30.04	38.	38.	35.	31.	28.5	21.2	.153	.109	.616	.616	42.	28.	.000
1879.															
JANUARY:— Max.	30.54	30.53	67.	67.	62.	62.	53.0	53.2	.482	.406	.740	.871	68.	52.5	1.7
Mean	30.20	30.18	49.9	50.5	46.	43.4	38.2	29.2	.231	.159	.641	.843	54.3	41.	.284
Min.	30.14	30.04	36.	34.	34.	32.	29.8	31.0	.173	.173	.728	.816	30.	42.	.000
FEBRUARY:— Max.	30.46	30.46	70.	64.	63.	63.	57.4	62.1	.472	.558	.630	.919	73.	57.5	—
Mean	30.24	30.22	56.8	52.1	51.7	49.8	46.6	47.5	.329	.318	.643	.843	55.7	44.6	—
Min.	29.88	29.83	38.5	42.	37.	38.	27.0	33.2	.143	.200	.611	.749	45.	33.	—
MARCH:— Max.	30.50	30.44	70.	68.	66.	62.	62.8	55.4	.572	.439	.780	.715	74.	61.	2.5
Mean	30.19	30.17	55.3	54.	51.3	47.8	47.3	44.0	.288	.246	.744	.680	58.47	44.	.6
Min.	29.80	29.84	42.	41.	38.5	41.	37.8	36.2	.149	.214	.553	.640	45.	38.	.000

图 1　瓯海关气象观测记录表（1）

MEAN ABSTRACT of READINGS taken during period from April 1877 to February 1878, and that from April 1878 to February 1879 inclusive.

	BAROMETER		THERMOMETERS				HYGROMETER						SELF-REGISTERING THERMOMETERS			
			Dry Bulb.		Wet Bulb.		Temperature of Dew-point computed.		Elastic Force of Vapour.		Humidity, 0—1.		Maximum in Air.		Minimum in Air.	
	9.30 A.M.	3.30 P.M.	9.30 A.M.	3.30 P.M.	9.30 A.M.	3.30 P.M.	9.30 A.M.	3.30 P.M.	9.30 A.M.	3.30 P.M.	9.30 A.M.	3.30 P.M.	9.30 A.M.	3.30 P.M.	9.30 A.M.	3.30 P.M.
Highest point attained by any instrument in each period, viz.:—	*Inch.*	*Inch.*	°F.	°F.	°F.	°F.	°F.	°F.					°F.	°F.	°F.	°F.
9 months of 1877 and 2 of 1878...	Nov. 30.57	Dec. 30.50	July 88.	July 91.	July 82.	Aug. 85.	Aug. 82.	Aug. ...	Aug. 1.222	Aug. 1.092	June .992	July .942	July 94.5	...	July 88.	...
9 " " 1878 and 2 of 1879..	Jan. 30.62	Jan. 30.53	Aug. 93.	July 94.	Aug. 84.5	Aug. 88.	Aug. 83.8	July 86.2	Aug. 1.158	July 1.250	Jan. .987	Aug. .990	Aug. 97.	...	July 85.	...
From April 1877 to February 1878 (inclusive):— The mean max.	30.28	30.23	74.2	78.	70.2	73.3	68.1	70.1	.720	.762	.917	.852	81.8	...	70.6	...
" " mean	30.09	30.06	65.5	68.1	62.9	64.8	60.2	61.9	.609	.601	.832	.798	69.6	...	61.8	...
" " min.	29.87	29.79	57.	58.9	54.5	55.2	51.8	53.5	.456	.474	.764	.695	60.9	...	53.4	...
" " range	.41	.44	17.2	19.1	15.7	18.1	10.3	16.6	.264	.288	.153	.157	20.9	...	17.2	...
From April 1878 to February 1879 (inclusive):— The mean max.	30.37	30.35	80.	78.5	77.	67.5	71.7	72.4	.807	.848	.818	.893	83.	...	73.4	...
" " mean	30.15	30.08	70.2	69.	65.6	65.	61.8	60.6	.565	.598	.707	.757	72.7	...	62.7	...
" " min.	29.87	29.84	59.	59.	55.	54.7	51.2	55.9	.436	.434	.636	.662	62.7	...	53.8	...
" " range	.50	.49	20.8	19.5	22.	12.8	20.5	16.5	.371	.414	.182	.231	20.3	...	19.6	...

* 1 day.

N.B.—As during the greater part of 1877 there was no gauge available at the port, the rainfall has been omitted from the above table. It must also be recollected that during the first three months of the second period the barometer was not kept, hence the averages given for this period, and relating to that instrument, are only for eight months, and must therefore be taken for what they are worth, as indicating the mean atmospheric pressure of the second epoch when contrasted with the preceding one.

图 2　瓯海关气象观测记录表（2）

　　注意：该港 1877 年的大部分时间未能实现有效测量，降雨量数据已被省略，如表 1、表 2 所示。另外还需要指出，1878 年头三个月的气压也没有记录，因此这一年设备实际上记录的仅仅是 8 个月的平均值。所以在将此数据当作 1878 年平均气压与之前数据做比较时，必须清楚其价值。

　　去年我把气象设备借给海关使用，但海关在 1878 年 2 月已经停止气象观测，并把设备还给了我。因此，我便开始自己记录，但并不包括风速和云层状况；关于这些内容的数据，海关也没有相应记录，所以今年这方面的记录与去年相比不那么完整。

　　为了避免误解，我或许应该做点说明，当代理税务司说我的这些设备"很普通"时，他一定是误听人言［详情参见 1877 年《贸易报告》］。我只能说，这些设备来自国内最好的生产商，我不时会将这些设备的数据与标准进行比较，结果发现相当精准。我有理由相信，因为提供的温度计存在"误差指数修正"，所以导致了海关对设备缺陷的主观臆测。我无须提醒那些对气象观测非常熟悉的人，所有设备得出的数据都需要必要的修正，不能因此而降低对设备优越性的信心。

这是我在温州的这个职位上所写的最后一份报告，我曾想过在总表之前写一份摘要，将 1877 年 4 月至 1878 年 2 月、1878 年 4 月至 1879 年 2 月这两个时期进行比较，可能会发现一些有用或有趣的东西。如前文所述，我遗漏了两年当中 3 月份的记录；这原本应是我的职责，但由于当时设备已经转手，且形势所限，导致气象观测被临时性中断。我只增加了有关露点、蒸气压以及湿度的相关数据，并按 1857 年出版的格林尼治系数进行计算。测量仪器被朝南安放在城市户外的阴凉处，雨量器则在离地 4 英尺处放置。

瓯海关《医报》（1881.04.01—1881.09.30）

玛高温医生有关温州健康的报告

在外国人居住在温州的 70 年间，由于人数一直很少，且不重视气候对健康状况的影响，造成当地气候记录相当匮乏，本报告当中出现一些推断的内容，也就在所难免。

从医学地理学的层面来看，温州无疑是一个地方性城市，它拥有 8 万 ~ 9 万人口，算上其所辖各县，其人口数量约为 50 万。温州离大海约 15 英里，位于永嘉江①，或瓯②江的右岸，这条河流发源于将浙江省西南部和福建省分开的山脉地区，靠近钱塘江和闽江源头；上述山岭和海岸构成了温州"李希霍芬南山"的一部分。这些海岸边的山岭或山丘，形成的时间并不久远，山海交汇处，形成一系列深水湾，深水湾又逐渐被冲击层填满，形成平原，从前被海水冲刷的地方，目前陆基线已相当稳固。山谷里会突兀地冒出一些山丘，形如孤屿。浙江省大片土地，从前大部分是沼泽地。除了面向大海的方向，温州实际上是被长满松林的群山所包围，但经过长时间开垦，这里已成为富饶的水稻之乡。

由于其海洋性环境，温州多雨，降雨之多，帝国诸港无出其右。温州如同美国一样，也会进行森林采伐，但看上去并不能改变当地潮湿的环境。温州有明显的雨季，时间从 5 月中旬持续到 9 月，并且在其他月份中，也经常会下雨。然而，对于这里的外国人来说，温州可能是中国最为健康的地方。由于降雨和海风的缘故，温州夏天的炎热能够有所缓解，温度很

---

① 原文为"Pungcha"，怀疑是"Yungcha"误写。根据弘治朝《温州府志》，瓯江别名为永嘉江、永宁江、慎江、蜃江、温江，并没有玛高温医生记载的"Pungcha"。——译者注

② 瓯（ou），这个名词原本指代整个地区。现在则成为温州的古雅名称；从词源学上讲，与法国杜伊勒里（Tuileries）的用法相同。

少超过 90 华氏度，而冬天温度也很少低至冰点。一个北方病人，可能会因为北方空气中的臭氧、正电、氢过氧化物或任何导致长江以北气候特殊性的原因而受到过度刺激，而在温州，他可以吸入一种极好的能够使体质得到改善的不一样的空气。南方病人在高纬度地区，就如同被刺穿的薄纱，他们同样可以在温州躲避严寒。总而言之，温州拥有极为舒适的气候，这里没有干燥寒冷的北风。在夏天，那些来到此地的旅行者可以在各小岛畅游、垂钓，这种体验可以使身心得到放松与满足。而在冬天，他不需要长途跋涉，就可以如同站在阿尔卑斯山那般高度的"世界屋脊"上俯瞰平原。如果力量超群，体魄健壮，那么他还可以成为人们心中的捕猎能手，因为在当地，人们深受那些残忍的老虎和其他猛兽之困扰。不幸的是，尽管这个港口对于病人来说是具有吸引力的，但同时也是没有吸引力的，因为这里没有合适的住所。但对于那些能够自己应付困难的人，温州是一个很好的度假胜地。

通过温州植被可以更好地了解当地的气候。温州是混种榕树生长的北部边界，但是仍然具有热带的一些基本特征。此地还是棕榈树能够生长的最高纬度，就像北方的栗树和低矮的橡树一样。这种树木也可以用于工业生产；温州还是一种独特柑橘的高产区，作为一种开胃良品，著名的温州苦柑橘（瓯柑），也被称为口味温和的金鸡纳柑。瓯柑的果膜味苦，果肉则不然；其果肉本身极为甜美。

以上粗略呈现了温州的一般概况；但温州也有山洪、海上台风与暴雨，这些灾害会摧毁良田，其破坏性影响偶尔也会造成饥荒和瘟疫。有关自然灾害的记录可以在本土地方志中找到，这些信息对研究气象学很有价值。我附了一张表格，涵盖了过去 15 个世纪以来有关的记载，范围包括浙江与福建部分沿海地区。但首先我要对资料来源进行说明（见图1 至图 3）。①

帝国的每个省、府，甚至每个县都有一大堆被称作方志的资料，这些地理志记录了与地理、公共工程、建筑与庙宇、祥异现象、自然名胜历史、

---

① 泉州、福州、温州和宁波等地区的暴风雨、洪水、干旱与饥荒记录，纬度范围在北纬 24°40′ 至北纬 30°02′ 之间，经度范围在东经 118°50′ 至东经 121°22′ 之间。

Record of Storms, Floods, Droughts and Famines in the Departments of Chüanchow, Foochow, Wênchow, and Ningpo, situated approximately between latitude N. 24° 40′ and N. 30° 02′, and longitude E. 118° 50′ and E. 121° 22′.

Abbreviations.—S.W., storm wave; Ty., typhoon; St., storm; Fl., flood; Fa., famine; Dr., drought; Sp., spring; Su., summer; A., autumn.

A.D.	Moon.	Chüanchow	Foochow	Wênchow	Ningpo	A.D.	Moon.	Chüanchow	Foochow	Wênchow	Ningpo
291	4	...	...	S.W.	...	1216	...	...	Dr.	...	Dr.
293	6	...	...	St., S.W.	...	1217	...	...	Fl.	...	...
304	...	...	...	Fa.	...	1217	...	...	Ty.	...	...
480	4	...	...	...	...	1220	...	...	...	...	Dr.
648	8	St., S.W.	...	...	...	1221	...	...	Fa.	...	...
663	7	...	...	S.W.	...	1222	...	...	Dr.	Dr.	...
674	Sp.	...	...	Fa.	...	1224	A.	Fl.	...	...	...
684	6	...	...	St., S.W.	...	1233	3	...	...	Fl.	...
689	7	...	...	Fl.	...	1233	8	...	...	Fl.	...
768	A.	...	Fl.	...	...	1240	6	...	Dr.	...	...
783	6	...	...	Dr.	...	1241	...	...	Dr.	...	...
784	8	S.W.	...	...	...	1240	6	...	...	...	...
791	...	...	...	...	Dr.	1246	...	...	Fl.	...	...
797	4	...	Fl.	...	...	1248	...	...	Fl.	...	...
840	...	...	...	...	Fa.	1352	...	...	Dr.	...	...
841	...	...	...	...	...	1295	...	...	Dr.	...	...
984	8	S.W.	...	...	...	1297	...	...	...	Fa.	...
1004	...	...	Ty.	...	...	1278	6	...	...	Fl.	...
1001	8	...	...	Ty.	...	1279	...	...	Fa.	...	...
1005	8	...	Ty.	...	...	1291	6	...	...	...	...
1029	...	...	Fl.	...	...	1293	6	Dr.	...	...	...
1066	8	St., Fl.	...	...	...	1297	7	Fl.	...	S.W.	...
1067	6	St., S.W.	...	...	...	1308	...	St.	...	S.W.	Fa.
1093	A.	...	...	...	Dr., Fa.	1324	...	St.	...	...	Fl.
1094	...	...	...	...	Fa.	1330	...	...	...	...	Fa.
1101	...	...	Dr.	...	...	1332	...	...	...	...	...
1110	...	...	Dr.	...	...	1333	A.	Fl.	...	Fl.	...
1126	...	...	...	St.	...	1343	A.	...	...	St.	...
1130	A.	...	...	...	...	1344	...	...	...	...	Fa.
1133	1	...	Fa., Fl.	...	...	1345	S.	...	...	Fa.	...
1134	9-10	...	Fl.	...	...	1346	S.	...	...	...	Dr.
1135	5	St., Fl.	Fl.	...	...	1347	...	...	...	St., S.W.	...
1149	...	...	...	...	...	1349	...	...	...	...	...
1150	...	...	...	Fa.	Fa.	1350	7	...	...	Fa.	Dr.
1152	...	...	...	S.	...	1354	...	3 Tides	...	...	...
1159	...	...	...	S.	...	1356	6	...	St.	...	...
1160	7	...	Fl.	...	...	1357	...	...	...	S.W.	...
1163	...	...	...	Fa.	...	1363	8	...	...	S.W.	...
1165	...	...	...	Fa.	Fa.	1367	...	St.	...	...	...
1166	8-17	...	...	S.W.	...	1376	7	...	...	S.W.	...
1171	5	...	Dr.	Fl.	...	1377	...	Fl.	...	...	...
1171	6	...	...	Dr.	...	1381	6	Fl.	...	...	...
1174	...	...	...	...	Fa.	1389	...	...	...	Fa., Dr.	...
1178	5	...	Fl.	...	S.	1399	...	Fl.	...	...	...
1179	6	...	S.	...	Dr.	1417	...	Fa.	...	...	...
1180	Su.	...	...	Fl.	...	1426	...	...	...	...	Ty.
1183	...	...	...	...	Dr.	1432	6	...	...	...	Ty.
1185	...	...	...	...	Dr.	1446	5	Fl.	...	...	Dr., Fa.
1188	...	...	Dr.	...	Dr.	1449	...	...	...	...	Fa.
1189	...	...	Fl.	...	...	1456	...	Dr.	...	...	...
1192	4	...	Fl.	...	...	1457	S.	...	...	...	Dr.
1195	A.	...	...	...	Ty.	1459	...	Dr.	...	...	...
1195	A.	...	...	...	Fa.	1467	1	...	...	Fl.	...
1203	6-7	...	...	...	...	1478	...	...	...	...	Fl.
1205	...	...	Dr.	...	...	1479	...	Fa.	...	...	...
1210	1	...	Fl.	...	...	1480	...	...	...	...	S.W.

图 1 历年自然灾害情况（1）

RECORD of STORMS, FLOODS, DROUGHTS and FAMINES—continued.

A.D.	Moon.	Chüan-chow.	Foochow.	Wênchow.	Ningpo.	A.D.	Moon.	Chüan-chow.	Foochow.	Wênchow.	Ningpo.
1481	8	...	...	...	...	1624	A.	...	...	...	Dr.
1483	8	...	St.	...	...	1627	7	...	...	...	Fl., Dr.
1486	Sp. to Su.	Fl.	...	...	...	1628	8.	...	...	...	Fl., Fa.
1487	9	...	...	...	Dr.	1628	7	...	...	...	St.
1489	Sp.	Dr.	...	...	...	1633	...	...	...	...	Dr., Fa.
1490	6	...	...	St.	...	1635	...	...	...	...	Fa.
1491	...	...	...	Fa.	...	1637	6	...	...	...	St., Dr.
1493	...	St.	...	...	S.W.	1638	...	...	...	...	St., Fl.
1494	7	St.	...	...	...	1639	...	...	...	...	Dr., Fa.
1499	4	Fl.	...	...	...	1640	S.	...	...	...	St.
1500	12	Dr.	...	...	...	1640	8	St.	...	...	...
1502	...	Dr.	...	...	...	1641	...	...	...	...	Fa.
1504	9	Fl.	...	...	...	1642	...	...	...	...	Dr., Fa.
1505	...	...	...	...	Fa.	1647	...	...	...	...	Dr.
1509	...	...	...	...	Dr., Fa.	1649	8	Fa.	...	...	...
1514	...	...	...	...	Dr., Fl.	1650	9	St.	...	...	Dr.
1512	...	...	...	...	Dr.	1651	...	...	...	Ty.	...
1513	...	...	...	Fa.	Fa.	1653	A.	...	...	...	Dr.
1514	...	Dr., Fa.	...	...	...	1654	A.	...	...	...	Dr.
1529	8	St.	...	...	...	1656	6	...	...	...	St.
1524	...	...	...	...	St., S.W.	1655	...	...	...	...	Fa.
1525	...	...	...	...	Ty., Fa.	1658	5	...	...	...	St.
1527	...	...	...	Dr., Fa.	Fa.	1660	7	Ty.	Ty.	...	...
1535	8	...	...	...	St.	1662	A.	Ty.	Fl.	...	...
1536	...	...	Dr., St.	...	...	1664	A.	Fl.	...	...	...
1538	...	...	...	...	S.W.	1665	6	Fl.	...	...	...
1540	...	...	...	...	S.W.	1666	...	Dr.	...	...	St.
1542	Sp.	...	...	St.	...	1668	...	...	...	...	Dr., Fa.
1542	A.	...	...	Dr.	...	1669	7	...	...	Fl.	...
1546	...	Dr., Fa.	...	Fa.	Fa., Dr.	1670	...	Dr.	...	...	...
1548	...	...	...	St.	...	1671	...	Dr.	...	Fa.	...
1555	9	...	...	St.	...	1672	...	...	...	...	Dr.
1558	7-8	...	...	St.	Dr.	1674	8	...	...	Fl.	...
1562	...	...	...	St.	...	1675	6	...	...	...	Fl.
1569	7	...	...	St.	...	1676	A.	...	...	...	Dr.
1570	...	...	...	...	Fl.	1677	4	Fa.	...	...	Fl.
1575	6	St.	...	St.	...	1679	8	...	...	...	St.
1576	...	...	...	St., Dr.	S.W.	1680	...	Fa.	...	...	...
1579	5	...	Fl.	...	Fl.	1681	A.	Dr.	...	Fl.	...
1585	7	...	...	...	Fl.	1682	...	...	...	Dr.	Fl., Dr., Fa.
1586	6	...	...	...	Fa., Dr.	1683	...	...	...	Fl.	...
1587	...	...	...	...	S.W.	1684	4	...	...	Dr.	...
1589	7	...	...	...	St., Fa.	1686	...	...	...	...	Dr.
1592	8	...	Fl.	...	...	1688	5	Fl.	...	...	...
1595	5	St.	...	...	...	1690	...	...	...	S.W.	Dr., Fa.
1597	8	Ty.	Ty.	...	...	1692	...	S.W.	...	...	Dr., Fa.
1599	...	...	...	...	Fl.	1694	...	...	...	...	Fa.
1601	...	Fl. Ty.	...	Ty.	...	1698	...	...	...	...	Fl.
1602	6	Fl.	...	...	...	1699	4	St.	...	...	...
1603	9	Fl.	...	...	...	1700	9	...	...	Fl.	...
1604	8	Ty.	...	...	...	1702	8	...	...	...	Dr., Fa.
1607	8	Fa.	...	...	...	1704	...	Dr.	...	...	...
1608	5-6	Ty.	...	Dr., St.	Fa.	1707	S.	...	...	Dr.	...
1609	5	...	...	Fa.	Fa.	1711	...	...	...	...	...
1610	5	...	...	Fl.	Fl.	1713	...	...	...	Fl	...
1612	...	St.	...	...	Fl.	1714	S.	Fl.	...	...	...
1614	A.	Dr.	...	Ty., Fa.	...	1718	6	...	...	...	Dr., Fa.
1615	A.S.	3 Tides.	...	...	...	1719	8	Fl.	...	...	Dr., F.
1615	A.	...	...	Fl.	...	1721	5	...	Dr.	...	Dr.
1616	8	Fl.	...	...	...	1722	...	...	...	...	Dr., Fa.
1617	...	Fa.	...	...	...	1723	6	Ty.	...	...	Dr., F.
1618	...	Fa.	...	...	Dr.	1724	7	...	...	...	Dr.
1620	S.	S.W.	...	...	...	1725	6-7	Fl.	Fl.	...	...
1621	6	...	...	...	Dr.	1729	7-8	...	St.	...	Fl.

图 2　历年自然灾害情况（2）

3

RECORD of STORMS, FLOODS, DROUGHTS and FAMINES—*continued.*

A.D.	Moon.	Chüan-chow.	Foochow.	Wênchow.	Ningpo.	A.D.	Moon.	Chüan-chow.	Foochow.	Wênchow.	Ningpo.
1729	A.	Dr.	...	...	Dr.	1809	...	...	...	...	Fa.
1731	7	Fl.	...	...	...	1810	...	...	...	Ty.	...
1734	7	...	...	St.	...	1814	...	...	...	Fl., Dr.	...
1738	9	...	...	Fl.	...	1818	...	...	...	...	S.W.
1739	...	...	...	Dr.	...	1819	3	...	...	St.	...
1741	...	...	...	Dr.	...	1819	6	...	...	St.	...
1745	7	...	...	...	S.W.	1820	6	...	...	St.	Dr.
1747	A.	...	...	...	Dr.	1821	A.	...	...	Ty.	...
1749	...	St.	...	...	...	1823	Sp.	...	...	St.	...
1752	...	...	...	...	Fa.	1832	...	...	...	Dr.	...
1753	...	St.	...	...	Dr.	1834	...	...	...	...	Fa.
1756	8	...	...	...	Fl.	1835	Su.	...	...	Fa., Ty., Dr.	...
1758	...	Fl., Dr., Fa.	...	...	...	1836	6	...	...	Dr., S.W.	...
1759	...	Fl.	...	...	Fl.	1839	7	...	...	Fl.	...
1760	A.	...	...	...	Fl.	1844	8	...	...	St.	St., Fl.
1762	...	Fl.	...	...	...	1847	7	...	...	Ty.	...
1769	6	...	...	...	St.	1848	...	...	...	...	Dr.
1772	A.	...	...	...	Fl.	1849	4	...	...	St.	...
1796	5-6	...	...	Dr.	...	1853	8	...	...	...	St.
1796	8	...	...	Fa.	...	1854	6	...	...	St.	...
1799	...	...	...	...	Dr., Fa.	1856	7	...	...	Ty.	...
1801	6	...	...	Ty.	...	1858	8	...	...	Ty.	...
1805	5	...	...	Ty.	...						

图 3　历年自然灾害情况（3）

人物传记、风土、贡赋与武备等相关内容，这些资料的编撰类似于年鉴，"地方志"看上去是更为合适的术语，对于某些资料，用"杂记"描述可能更为贴切。地方志上的早期记录，通常是照抄通史，或来自地方传统文献。较为晚近的记录资料，会被保存在衙门里，这些内容大多是由某些学者和家族提供的。但这些公共档案通常没有得到很好的保管，当需要重修方志时，士绅们又不得不利用他们的私谱进行补充。大约一个世纪或者更久，才会重修一次方志，通常情况下，旧的版本会被淘汰，并且不会永久保存。如下面附表中的内容，在外国通常会被像统计员这样的人格外珍视。另外一个需要说明的是，要正确理解方志的附录。对于地方志而言，县的资料，往往要比省、府资料更为详尽。举例来说，县志的瘟疫记载的详尽程度，比省、府方志的记载更令人担忧。这些方志的问题在于，记录不够严谨和准确。有些记录过于浅表，甚至存在错解，但这些记录毕竟是将信息保存了下来。

在图1~图3所提到的港口中，只有泉州真正靠海，而其他港口离海潮都还有一段距离。

有关温州和宁波的记录更为系统和全面，这是由于参考了这两个地方的县志，而其余则仅参考府志。县志都是最近新修的，而府志的最后一次编修距今已有 150 年。

有关饥荒的记录，常见的是地方上因为饥荒而造成死亡人数多少，没有关于食人现象的记载，但是对于穷人而言，卖儿卖女这种无奈之举并不鲜见。①

只有当洪水强度和破坏程度很高时，才会被记录，洪水摧垮堤坝，淹没城镇，改变地貌，使百姓的生命受到伤害，庄稼受到损失。洪水急流的突然性，尤其是飓风或地下水暴涨引发洪水的情况，使人们认为这是超自然的结果。人们认为飓风是一条龙，是一个盘旋上天的怪物。江河暴涨，则被归因于"蛟"（它是龙和蛇杂交后的生物），当"蛟"将要化龙时，就会引发洪水。

有关飓风引起风浪的灾害，一般被记载为"海潮"。

根据文献记载，有两次出现"一日三潮"的记载，这样的情况并不是周期性潮汐，仅属于个别现象。根据《申报》记载，该现象在上海发生过，时间是 1880 年 10 月 28 日。这次属于小潮，水位较低，仅有 0.15 英尺②，时间也比较短。同时，也有报道称，前一天从海上刮来一股来自东北方向的大风。也许就是这股海风导致了这次奇异的海潮，这样的海风在上海是时有发生的，但一日三潮实属罕见。最后一点需要说明的是，根据同样的报纸报道，1851 年也曾经发生过类似事情。最早有关该事情的记录是上海的地方文献，发生时间是 1347 年 6 月 23 日③，"上海浦中午潮退，未几复至，人皆异之"。通过记录可以得知，这样的水位异常并不是通常的潮汐。在平江和嘉兴附近的运河和湖泊，水位也曾突然上升了 4 ~ 5

---

① 根据王凤洲《纲鉴全编》记录，在 153 年至 1640 年期间，在有关饥荒的 35 次记录中出现 6 次食人事件，其中两次是父母吃他们的孩子和孩子吃他们的父母。有关 620 年至 1643 年的干旱与饥荒情况，可以参阅何斯德（A. Hosie）发表在《皇家亚洲学会华北分会杂志》（*Journal of the North China Branch of the Royal Asiatic Society*）上的文章。

② 原文当中没有标单位，根据当时的习惯以及后文内容，怀疑应是 0.15 英尺。——译者注

③ 根据《山居新话》的记载，此事发生在至正七年 8 月 12 日，即 1347 年，玛高温对历史年份的换算常有误差。参见杨瑀《山居新话》，清知不足斋丛书本。——译者注

英尺，① 此后再有类似事件的发生是在 1634 年 8 月、1642 年 8 月、1648 年 7 月 21 日、1661 年 7 月 26 日、1662 年 7 月、1719 年 7 月 19 日、1754 年 8 月和 1778 年 8 月。文献中仅记其事，少有备注。这些个案发生的时间大都是在台风肆虐的季节，也可能是暴风雨加剧了这些现象，文献并没有相关探讨的记载。出现这一自然现象的原因，就如同先前提到的那样，也必将从其他方面寻找。尽管缺少数据来证明同时还有地震或海水泛滥等灾害的发生，但是通过推断可以肯定这些灾害一定同时发生过，因为引起这些灾害的源头是东亚沿海火山板块的剧烈运动。②

关于海底火山运动的猜想可以通过温州沿海附近发生的一些现象得到验证，时间是 1166 年的夏天。海面异响三日，海上出现大量泡沫，泡沫如铜钱一般。这种现象被解释为"有蛟出水"，据说这条蛟有 10 英尺那么长。③

对于那些想比较同一纬度沿海和内陆地区气候差异的气候学家来说，处州（即丽水）的地方志资料相当丰富。该府位于温州西部，并与温州接壤，境内皆山地，海拔不高。据该府的灾害记录记载，1511 年以来的 352

---

① 玛高温博士：《对上海临近地区过去十三个世纪宇宙现象的观察注解》，《皇家亚洲学会华北分会杂志》1858 年 12 月 23 日。"Note on Cosmical Phenomena observed in the Neighbourhood of Shanghai during the past 13 Centuries," *Journal of the N. - C.B, Royal Asiatic Society*. Read 23rd December 1858, by D. J. Macgowan, M. D.

② † Analogous to the abnormal waves that flood the China coast are those which impinge on Tungking:—"Un phénomène surprenant est que quelquefois la marée, après avoir descendu pendant environ trois quarts d'heure, remonte subitement et les canaux qui les autres jours ne sont pas navigables à marée basse, le sont pendant tout le cours de la journée.

"Il y a quelques années sur une des côtes du Tunkin est survenu un événement très extraordinaire. On a entendu un bruit effrayant plus fort que celui que peut produire la plus fort canonnade ; et ce bruit a été suivi d'une violente irruption de la mer, qui s'est avancée jusqu'à plus de deux lieues dans l'intérieur des terres, y a porté des arbres déracinés et des débris de bâtiments, et au bout de douze ou quinze heures s'est retirée dans son lit, ayant noyé nombre d'hommes et d'animaux et détruit plusieurs villages. Ce même phénomène avait eu lieu environ cinquante ans auparavant."—*Exposé statistique du Tunkin, de la Cochinchine, du Camboge, du Triampa, du Laos, du Lac Tho, sur la relation de M. de la* BISSACHERE, *Missionaire dans le Tunkin* : Londres, MDCCCXL.

③ 根据《永嘉县志》卷三十六记载："乾道二年，是年夏，海门有蛟出水，长丈余。既而塔头陡门水吼三日，海上浮钱，有父老识之曰，海将以钱鬻人，风潮必作矣。至八月十七日，飓风挟雨拔木飘屋，夜潮入城，四望如海。四鼓风回潮退，浮尸蔽川，存者十一"。——译者注

年间，飓风有 5 次，洪灾有 49 次，饥荒 19 次，旱灾 44 次。①

在上述记录中，中国人所说的"飓风"通常包括我们所说的台风或气旋在其中心区域所引起的灾害。

灾难性的飓风与台风（造成灾害才统计在内）在 18 世纪里共发生过 16 次。

中国的沿海居民和水手非常善于预测飓风。"当日光出现晕圈时，其光如虹，并且肉眼可见，那么这种现象就预示飓风的来临，这种征兆被称为'飓母'，若鸡犬都默不出声，此时也必有飓风出现。"这是一种出现在夏、秋间奇特的风，风从八面而来。据《温州府志》的注释记载，有一种草②可以预示台风的来临，被当地人称为"知风草"。③

从大禹治水到现在，中国人民为了保护自己免受洪灾之苦，同洪水做英勇的斗争，大禹所治理的黄河被称为 ——"中国之殇"，黄河不断考验着中国工程师们的技艺，并证明中国已经无计可施。当中国还没有获得有关治理河道的水文学和气象学的知识时，她又如何能够治理这个长期性的水患问题呢？对密西西比河洪灾的调查工作，④ 已经成为高登先生在治理伊洛瓦底江时的参考对象，测量工具也正不断丰富与进步。在不同时间段对水流和排洪量进行系统的测量，在不同水位时，对河流沉积物的数量进行测量，这些关于所有河流及其支流的数据，对于外国商务而言至关重要。在中国的某些水域，使用雨量测量仪和温度计进行测量，对于将来进

---

① 1650 年一名 3 岁的幼儿夭折，被埋在临近其父母在遂昌（Suichang）的花园里。"一场雷震（不是闪电，在中国，这是一种有害的现象）击中了坟墓，幼童因而复活。"这名幼童的埋葬时间以及坟墓构造，在原文中都没有提及。如果我们能知道所有相关信息，那么就有可能证明理查森医生（Dr. Richardson）的观点，即当血液不是变成胶状而是维持液体状态时，生命就可以进入半生半死的状态。但结局令人感到痛苦，这名不可思议复活的幼童，随后被他的父亲献祭。因为一名恶邻指认这个小孩事实上是"雷震子"，这对父母没有将这起事件上报官府；于是父亲残忍地将这个可怜的幼童杀死了。

② 参见乾隆朝《温州府志》卷十五下"风痴草"条。——译者注

③ 关于温州 11 个月的气象观察记录，可以参见 1878 年 5 月《海关医报》中梅威令医生的报告。

④ Humphrey and Abbot, *Reports on the Mississippi*, Washington, 1861 - 1879; *Reports on the Irrawaddy*, Robert Gordon, Rangoonm, 1879, 1880.

一步的水文调查至关重要。同时还可以将这些数据，与印度和缅甸所做的观测做出对比，研究整个大陆共同存在的洪水特征，发现这些地方出现的干旱、饥荒之间的相互关系。同时这里也存在一个可供讨论的问题，即这些地方出现的自然灾害是否存在着周期性。另外，这些气象状况与太阳耀斑有什么联系，是否存在着周期。对于海关部门来说，对水文进行测量并不是什么难事，通过这些测量可以呈现自然状况，并解决同中国渔业相关的一些问题。

在总税务司的指示下，大清海关已经从事气象观测好几年了，研究者已经掌握了一些珍贵的数据，并适时地运用于实践中。现在相比欧洲和美国，只有一件事情还有欠缺，即缺少统一的观测标准，这也是日后测量工作能够进一步展开所必需的。这项欠缺也是目前观测出现一些问题的原因。1879 年 9 月在维也纳举行的国际大会已经要求国际气象委员会制定统一标准，这对于相互间的交流是一个重要机遇，至少可以形成一个统一的、标准的观测方法，也有利于制定标准化表格，用以日常记录，同时也便于世界各地观测点的实际操作。该要求已经得到普遍遵从，现在地球已经被影像化，同时其大气状况也被影像化，这两种过程是同时进行的。只有观测同时进行，实际发生的海潮、飓风和洋流运动才能被精准记录下来。徐家汇天文台负责人能恩斯告诉我，在去年 1 月前，他把他所记录的数据送给了华盛顿美国陆军通讯长，他的观测时间是当地时间 8 点 49 分，美国华盛顿时间 7 点 35 分，但是为了同时观测，他需要对时间进行调整，因为 1 月 1 日的气象观测需要提早 35 分钟，或者说，徐家汇需要在晚上 8 点 14 分观测才能与美国同时。按照维也纳大会任命国家气象委员会给出的解释，即在华盛顿的下午，中国同时需要提前 0.8 小时做观测，这也是海关需要遵守的规定。海关观测者在该地区的测量范围很广，同时也是按照国际测量的标准进行的。如果这样的观测能够维持在 1 天 3 次，那么这样的测量结果就符合科学标准，并且最终被运用于商务，只要通过这些数据做出的天气预测足够简明，水手们就会接受我们权威的风暴预测。他们并没有发现，在风暴中心会产生八重的风向，气压表也不会在风暴中心地带下降或者上升。风暴在中国海的路径演变需要进一步的调查，到目前为止并没有足够的数据。最新版的气象数据并不是一个满意的结果。另外，现在仍然需要去解释，飓风整体是如何从中心上升的。总之，在这片海域有关飓风的研究课题需要投入更多的精力，包括水手和科学家都应为之努力。我其实对自己所做的研究成果并不满意，即根据雷德菲尔德、雷德和皮丁顿的研究成果，在 1853 年我曾就此问题用中文出版过一本大纲性的书籍，① 这本书后来在日本由萨摩藩的藩主再版。我很想销毁这本书，再出修订本。在每一个中国海关都建立气象观测站，这种主张可能看起来很怪异，但我以为是可行且适当的，所用的仪器既不是很贵重，也不是很复杂，根据纽约气象天文台的主管德雷珀医生的说法，不需要购买图像式气压计，普通气压计的主要构件不过是块表盘。② 美国通讯监测站每年的花费是 300 银圆，这并不包括支付士兵薪水和发电报的费用，但他们的观测结果既全面又细致，比海关监测站所用的花费又少很多。③ 另外，为了促进农业发展而做的天气预报，为磁力研究、大气电流研究、辐射测量等做的相关检测，这些都不是海关和商业所关注的项目。但关于太阳辐射和大气吸收利用太阳热量的研究将会对预防干旱和缺水起到极大的促进作用，并且对商业产生的价值并不比农业产生的价值少，同海关收入也有直接的关系。总之，我恳请海关气象观测者能够采取这套公制系统，并将这种方法应用于中国。④

中国是一个美丽、富饶、人口稠密的国家，想要对中华人种进行简单归类是很难的，与周边国家相比，中国人在身体与智力方面并不占优势。他们外表纤弱，身材矮小，并且脑袋较小。很少有人能活到 70 岁，在浙南地区，很少有学者考过省试。当地民风淳朴，友好热情，遵纪守法。

---

① 《航海金针》，宁波出版，由布朗先生（J. C. Bowring）资助。
② 德雷珀医生曾在 1880 年 1 月 3 日《科学美国》增刊中，对气象设备做过这样的描述。
③ 参见哈森将军（General Hazen）的《1881 年美国陆军通信兵团报告》（*Report of the Signal Corps for 1881*）。
④ 在台湾，相较于温度与气压测量，更为重要的是地震数据记录——这个岛的地震密度，与日本或吕宋相当——其地震区域包含沿海地带。这里有一条关于候鸟的有价值信息，最近苏格兰东海岸的灯塔不断捕获候鸟。布朗（Brown）先生与科尔达（Cordaux）先生遵照规定，将情况发了出去。美国海岸也发现了与欧洲类似的情况，即鸟类不断冲撞灯塔；由此来看，也许海岸灯塔在这片沿海地带不堪使用。

但当地乡绅将百姓作为奴隶看待，中国人严重依附于宫庙，因此被认为是一个虔诚的民族，宗教团体通常被认为易于感染和传播疾疫，这主要是因为他们身体素质差。而如今，中国人又沾染上鸦片，身体素质更是每况愈下。

温州到处都是水渠和湿地，海拔与水平面大致相同，这样的地形因素，就决定了它成为间歇热的多发地。每年春季，很多时候一直持续到秋季，间歇热会在当地肆虐，有的村子甚至有一半的人染病。总体来看，此病形式多样，但绝大多数患者的症状较轻，而对于那些初来温州的外地人来讲，他们的症状与当地人则不一样，当他们适应这里的水土和气候后，病情就不会再加重。当那些苦力和穷人染上该病以后，他们因为太穷而没有能力接受治疗。病人只能在大街上随地而卧，随着病情的发展，病毒就会扩散，只要他们能撑完整个病理期，就会慢慢自行恢复。但如果再染上败血症的话，身体就会逐渐变得憔悴，这时候最容易感染其他疾病，甚至丧命。每日或隔日发作的病例较少，并且也容易得到治疗，症状随着天气转凉会自行消失。隔日疟如果持续的时间很久，就会病情反复，最终变得不可治愈，在持续一年或两年以后，最终丧命。

给人的第一印象是，该病发生在夏末秋初时节，推测可能与稻田有关。每年5月，会同时种植早稻和晚稻，在轮耕的田地里一片一片地种植。早稻在8月份成熟并收割，而晚稻也已经长得半熟。已经被收割的早稻田因此裸露在太阳的炙烤下，然后疟疾就会出现。但是，我们不能断定疟疾的出现与田地一定有关，或产生疟疾的病毒就是来自稻田。当地居民也不认为疟疾与他们的田地有任何关系，这种说法被认为是没有合理依据的。远在古代，中医已经认识到砒霜在治疗疟疾方面的功效，虽然中医在给病人开药内服时相当克制，但因为缺乏药剂学知识，无法通过更改剂量有效减弱其毒性。

在世界范围内，也许没有任何国家像中国那样遭受那么多的传染病，同时也没有任何国家像中国那样保留了大量关于这方面知识的连续性记载，这主要包括有关肠热病的报告与治疗情况等，这些理论从元典时代一直流传至今。在希波克拉底撰写《危险期天数》的几个世纪之前，黄帝就被记载曾提到过此事，即身体有自我修复的功能，这是他在与他的医生和官员的谈话中提到的，其内容涉及医学和病理学。此时医生的权威逐渐开始形成，等级制度在当时还不存在，希腊的阿斯克列皮阿德斯曾对希波克拉底的治疗方法和药物进行改进，但中国没有出现这样的人；中国保存下来的医书，充分展示了中国人的聪明与观察能力，详尽地阅读中国医书将会很有价值，但实事求是地说，很多内容在今天已经不再实用。同时，中国医学史存在着一定的断裂性。有一本书叫《温疫论》，这本书几乎每个医生都人手一本，该书作者认为 1400 年来，中国治疗温疫①的方法都是错的，在这期间造成无数人枉死。该书出自一位苏州医生吴有性之手，写于 1641 年，但该书一直是以抄本形式流传，直到 1805 年一批具有公益精神的学者才将其正式出版，我现在看的是 1852 年的版本。②

根据吴医生的记载，从晋朝（265 年）到其所处时代期间，有关温疫理论的错误观点一直相当盛行。医生常常误认为普通的发烧，是季节性症状，也是季节更替出现的正常现象，但吴有性认为温疫是由一种"疬气"所致。在他撰写该书时期，当时中国的浙江、江苏、山东、直隶正遭受着严重的瘟疫③，吴有性认为，造成这种大规模死亡现象的原因并不是瘟疫本身，而是错误的治疗方法。中国人一般将热病称作"伤寒"④，也许更确切地名称应该是"稽留热"。此病系冬天常气自肌表而入，没有传染性，且每年都有。⑤ 温疫疬气与此不同，疬气从口鼻入，且口鼻通乎天气。前者能够汗解⑥，后者无法汗解。除了这位伟大的医学革新者的著作，我看

---

① 玛高温用"epidemic fever"来翻译吴有性的"温疫"，但按照现代温病学，更准确的对应概念应该是"外感热病"。——译者注

② 根据书籍日期。

③ 吴有性认为温疫（epidemic fever）就等同于瘟疫（epidemic），玛高温在这里接受了吴有性的这种主张，读者需要知道，吴有性的这种主张是比较激进的。——译者注

④ 玛高温在这里指的"伤寒"，是中医里的"大伤寒"概念，是指张仲景六经辨证范围的"伤寒"。——译者注

⑤ 关于热病最早的医学著述，是汉代张机（张仲景）的《伤寒论》，他的成就在公元前 200 年至公元 200 年之间，无人能出其右。无数后辈医家继承了张机的学说。

⑥ 指中医"汗法"，治疗八法之一，是通过开泄腠理，调和营卫，发汗祛邪，以解除表邪的治法，又称解表法。——译者注

了许多医书，再也找不到关于瘟疫的专著。

凡是从事中国医学史的研究者，都不能绕过吴医生的《温疫论》。以下是我翻译吴医生论述中的一段文字，居住在中国的外国人，可能没人会意识到空腹进行户外锻炼的危害性——吴医生记载的这件事，直到进入现代之前，可能都没有引起过医生们的注意。这位与著名的哈维①同时代的人物记述称，三人冒雾早行，空腹者死，饮酒者病，饱食者不病。②

以下是该省瘟疫肆虐情况的附表（见图4），时间从这些瘟疫在当地被记录时开始。该表参考了省志、大部分府志和一些县志；就目前来讲，这份表已经非常精准，但如我前面已经说明的缘故，所参考的地方志还存在许多漏洞。

图4虽然缺乏细节，但绝非不实记录。除了一些特别情况之外，表格记录的传染病可能多为肠道疾病，但根据中国文献的术语，记录常指的是"疾病在同一时间影响到所有人"，这张表广泛地包含了许多疾病。此表展现的仅是一省的传染病情况。总体而言，方志编撰者总是会在干旱、洪水、饥荒、内战的后面记录瘟疫。

从浙江省的情况可以看出，爆发战争的地方与那些山区地方相比，瘟疫要更为频繁和严重，战争波及小的地方受到的瘟疫影响相对有限。

根据记载，致病物质引发瘟疫的情况只有一例。1638年，一场瘟疫由杭州波及东阳，该病是由一名女童携带而来的，她被卖到这个邻近的城市，无亲无故。这场瘟疫的传染源并不是空气，而是她所穿的衣服。根据

---

① 哈维以颠覆前代血液循环理论著称，作者这里是在用吴有性类比哈维的革命性成就。——译者注

② 吴医生引用了《伤寒论》（Shanghan，汉代）某些有趣的词源学现象，以展示"温病"这两个字的文本起源，温病是一种不正常的热疾。人们首先省掉了"温"字的"氵"，然后加上了"疒"，从而构造出了今天使用的"瘟"字。类似的还有"疫"字，这个字最早写作"徭役"，指百姓如同仆人般，临时性地为政府服务（类似西方的劳役租佃制度），瘟疫与徭役一样，任何地方、任何家庭都无法避免；随后"役"字加上了"疒"变成了"疫"字。因此词典编纂者，解释"疫"字时，认为它是由"疒"（代表疾病）和"殳"（代表标枪）组合而成的观点是错误的；正确的解释是，"疫"是由"疒"（代表疾病）和"役"（代表劳役租佃）的缩写组合而成。

RECORD of EPIDEMICS in the PROVINCE of CHÊHKIANG.

A.D.	Moon.		A.D.	Moon.	
95	4	Hsianhsing districts.	1333	3	Preceded by a flood.
758	...	Preceded by drought and flood.	1334	...	Western part; preceded by drought and famine.
783	...	Preceded by drought and flood.			
791	Autumn	Western part of the province; preceded by drought.	1361	Summer	Shaohsing, two districts.
			1363	...	Shaohsing, two districts.
806	Summer	Eastern part of the province.	1385	...	
829	Spring	Western part of the province.	1403	7	Shaohsing, two districts.
833	Summer	Hangchow and west.	1414	7	Throughout Hangchow, Hsianhsing and Ningpo.
870	...	The entire province.			
1001	...	Entire province.	1417	5	Kinhua; epidemic, leprosy.
1195	...	Hsianhsing; preceded by famine.	1435	Winter	Hsianhsing, Ningpo and Taichow.
1131	6	Hsianhsing and western part of province; preceded by famine.	1443	...	
			1446	3	Ningpo and Taichow; preceded by drought.
1144	...	Hangchow.	1463	...	Hsianhsing.
1147	Autumn	Hangchow.	1480-1	...	Hsianhsing; for 2 years.
1165	...	Linan and Yuyow; preceded by famine.	1493	...	Kiahsing; preceded by floods.
1173	Sum., Aut.	Hangchow.	1510	...	Huchow; preceded by floods.
1182	4	Hangchow and Linan.	1511	...	Huchow; preceded by floods.
1188	Spring	Hangchow.	1512	Spr., Sum.	Pingwu. Reappeared next year.
1194	6	Western part.	1513	...	
1195	3	Linan, Hsianhsing; preceded by famine.	1516	5	Wênchow.
1196	5	Hangchow.	1526	Summer	Yuyow and Hsianhsing; preceded by drought.
1197	3	Hangchow.	1546	"	Wênchow; preceded by drought.
1199	Summer	Linan.	1547	...	Kiahsing; preceded by drought.
1204	5	Hangchow.	1589	...	Epidemic leprosy over several districts, preceded by unprecedented rains.
1208	...	Yuyow; preceded by drought.			
1210	Summer	Linan.	1589	...	Chichau; preceded by floods and famine.
1211	"	Hangchow.	1590	...	Hsiaoshan, a district of Hsianhsing; epidemic leprosy, its reappearance.
1212	2	Hangchow.			
1275	4	Hangchow.	1591	...	Epidemic leprosy in Changhua district, Hangchow.
1284	7	Hsianhsing.			
1304	Spring	Hsianhsing, Ningpo and Taichow.	1622	...	Ningpo.
1305	7	Hsianhsing; preceded by famine.	1624	Summer	Ningpo; preceded by drought and famine.
1308	7	Hangchow, Yuyow and Ningpo; preceded by drought and famine.	1628	...	Ningpo.
			1634	...	Chichow.

A.D.	Moon.		A.D.	Moon.	
1643	6	Hangchow, and year succeeding.	1718	6	Siangshan.
1652	Autumn	Ningpo.	1757	...	Pinghu.
1660	Sum. & Aut.	Wênchow.	1806	...	Wênchow; small-pox.
1673	Sum. & Aut.	Siangshan.	1811	...	Ningpo; small-pox.
1678	...	Lishui.	1820	Autumn	Wênchow and Ningpo; Asiatic cholera.
1680	...	Pinghu.	1821	...	Wênchow and Ningpo.
1681	...	Ningpo.	1834	Autumn	Ningpo.
1710	...	Siangshan.	1835	Spr., Aut.	" with dearth.
1715	...	Taichow, preceded by famine.	1864	8, 9	Ningpo.

图 4 浙江省传染病记录表

《本草》毒物学一章的记述，旧衣服会含毒。

晚近的地方志修撰者，在涉及瘟疫时，会使用更详尽的专有名称描述瘟疫，比如天花和亚洲霍乱。令人高兴的是，他们的前辈修撰者，在针对某些特殊传染病时，也会进行专门描写，许多有价值的信息得以传承下来——例如我们由此得以知道"疠风"[①] 的存在。据记载，1417 年金华曾暴发一场

---

① 疠风即麻风。——译者注

疠风病；1589 年绍兴也曾经暴发严重的疠风病，该地很大一部分地区都受到影响；而邻近杭州城的昌化县在 1590 年也出现过疠风患者。

14 世纪早期有关瘟疫暴发情况的记载并无多少，1558 年以后的一段时期，浙江降雨增多，降雨有时从秋季一直延续到冬季，时间长达三个月以上。在 1558 年，浙江北部疠风流行，如图 4 所示，处州府也出现了疠风，但只知道疠风是在降雨后出现，并不清楚疾病的其他详细情况。该瘟疫暴发得非常突然，并且没有任何征兆，而关于疠风病的记载，在长江沿岸的各省以前并没有出现过，福建沿岸或者更多的是在广州（或更南的地方）曾经有过疠风病的暴发，也是其起源地。绍兴是疠风病暴发的代表性地区，患者症状通常为双腿肿胀，世界上还没有任何一个地方如绍兴一样，受到这么大规模的影响，或许是出于其他原因，比如其低洼的地形（绍兴海拔只比水面高出一码）。该地区疠风所呈现的症状，与沈朗仲《病机汇论》中所记载的一样，患者皮肤溃疡，身体出现可怕的肿块和溃疡，痛如虫咬。鼻梁发炎塌陷，手指也会出现类似症状。然后头发和眼睫毛会脱落，视力下降，声音沙哑并且最后失声。除非病情较轻，否则无法医治。我非常希望能够很快在中国从事这方面的研究，以考证疠风与西方黑死病之间的关系。有人认为西方中世纪的黑死病起源于中国，该病从东亚一直传播到欧洲直至大西洋沿岸地区。

关于瘟疫的信息，只能在地方志（而非通史著作）中才能找到，搜集工作的辛苦程度可想而知。[①] 在王凤洲《纲鉴全编》的简史记录中可以很快找到相关记载，而其中记录的瘟疫则依次发生于 1052 年、1054 年、1275 年、1279 年、1308 年、1313 年、1564 年、1583 年、1589 年、1642 年和 1644 年。

温州有许多关于霍乱肆虐的记载，这些信息对于今日的病理学研究者来说可能无用，却是中国瘟疫史研究者感兴趣的内容。对于下面我将要呈现的内容，首先我要提醒读者，虽然印度的病理学家有不同意见，但权威学界普遍认为，印度是霍乱的起源地，霍乱起始于 1813 年的新德里。也有

---

① 我在县志与府志中发现了关于“祥异”的章节，但这些资料越来越难以获取，为此我需求帮助——将相关章节抄出来；在此我要为此或以其他形式给予帮助的人表示感谢。

很多不会被广泛引用的学者，比如某些梵语、希腊语和阿拉伯语地区的研究者，主张霍乱起源于东方的其他地区，他们认为今天的霍乱是百年沉寂后的再次暴发。更为重要的是，霍乱不仅在印度流行，也在欧洲与美洲流行，这些相反的霍乱病因学理论，表明霍乱治疗和预防手段具有复杂性，必须把它限制在一定区域范围之内。与非传染性疾病相比，即便没有好的传染病治疗办法，也必须建立有效的卫生行政制度。有人认为，霍乱通过人与人之间传播，传播的媒介就是水；其他人则更强调霍乱起因的风土性，他们认为人并不是疾病传播的媒介，微生物是通过空气传播，空气与土地中的霍乱病菌，在满足一定自然条件后，会发酵到空气中，从而引发传染病流行，水里并不存在所谓的肠道毒物或某种特殊疾病的毒物。然而持后一种主张的人，大体上仍旧要求洁净饮用水，并推行卫生章程。

中国浩如烟海的文献与地方志，也许能为解决有关霍乱的争论提供资料，尤其是关于前面提到的第一个问题，即霍乱历史起源的问题，但根据我的调查，实际所得有限——几乎不可能找到决定性的证据——另外我也要承认，在面对这样宏大的研究时，区域性的研究无疑具有局限性。马六甲的中国人是最早一批感染印度霍乱的人，1819 年该霍乱从水路经由暹罗传到马六甲，同时也传到宁波。根据一位 70 岁的老者回忆，霍乱出现以后，这座城市遭受巨大的灾难，这名老者是一位当地人，这是宁波有关霍乱的最早记录。在当地，霍乱被称为"蟹爪病"，此病往往发病突然，致命性强，很多患者来不及医治就死在大街上，一位法国的病理学家称这种现象为"发病即死"。我所看到的唯一关于霍乱的专著来自嘉兴的一位医生①，据作者记载，霍乱首先爆发于浙江和江苏的交界处——嘉兴。此次霍乱发生于 1821 年，因为疾病的特殊性，作者以"脚筋吊"或"吊脚痧"② 对其进行命名，根据作者的记载，当时医生按照中医普通霍乱的方

---

① 指清代徐子默的《吊脚痧方论》。——译者注

② 玛高温在这里提到了三个概念，即中医里的"吊脚痧"和"霍乱"概念，以及西医里的"霍乱"（cholrea）概念。在本文中，按照徐子默的主张，能够对应西医"cholera"概念的应该是"吊脚痧"。玛高温为了区别中医霍乱与西医霍乱概念，将中医霍乱称为"ordinary cholera"，但有时为了行文方便，也不加区别地直接称为"cholera"。本文在翻译时，将中医里的"cholera"翻译成"中医霍乱"，以方便读者阅读。——译者注

法医治这种突然呕吐的疾病，造成严重后果，百无一存。作者认为中医霍乱"因热而成"，这就需要用凉泻法进行医治。中医霍乱发于阳，吊脚痧发于阴；中医霍乱为热，吊脚痧为寒，对于吊脚痧就该用温经通阳之法治疗。两年之后，霍乱卷土重来，这是因为不存在有效的治疗方法，霍乱在帝国境内迅速蔓延开来，1860 年浙江省染疫的情况特别严重。[1] 几乎每一个夏季都会发生这种大规模的传染病，从一个地方蔓延到另一个地方，直到现在才被认为是瘟疫。在中国的这一地区，这种类型的"干霍乱"（指发生在干旱的夏季）也被称为"痧"，[2] 该术语包括疝气、中暑、中风等其他病症，这些症状会突然出现。在广州，该问题比其他地方都严重。该地居民认为，这种被称为"痧"的疾病从他们的先人开始就已经存在，他们认为祖祖辈辈都受过这种亚洲霍乱的影响。在广州，痧症被认为是地方性疾病，甚至会在冬季出现。在去年冬天，上海浦东许多村庄也出现严重的印度霍乱。冬天与夏天的最大区别在于，冬天，这种传染病的致命性会有所降低，会有三天的发病期，即病人不会马上死去，而是会支撑三天时间。[3] 至于为什么会有这样的区别，根据中国人普遍的说法，这主要是由

---

① 根据克利耶（Cleyer）的《1873 年美国霍乱》（*Cholera Epidemic of 1873 in the United States*）记录，"霍乱于 1669 年在中国出现，可能来自马六甲（Malacca）"。而蒂尔（Gentil）在他的《东方之旅》（*Voyage aux Indes Orientales*）中指出，霍乱于 1769 年在科罗曼德尔（Coromandel）出现后不久，它就在中国盛行。西蒙斯（D. B. Simmon）医生在他的关于《日本霍乱》（*Cholera Epidemics in Japan*，参见 1879 年 9 月《海关医学报告》）的详细文章中引用了这些权威论述。这些作者所拥有的信息来源并没有出现。我不知道他们的论述应该有多大程度的重要性。除了西蒙斯医生之外，德贞（John Dudgeon）医生在 1872 年 9 月的《海关医学报告》中已经讨论过这个问题。不幸的是，我现在无法查阅那篇论文，这篇论文无疑包含了我可能做出更好解释的信息。在 1877 年 9 月的《海关医疗报告》中，万巴德（Patrick Manson）医生花了几页篇幅介绍了在中国流行的亚洲霍乱（Asiatic cholera）。1843 年 9 月的《中国丛报》（*Chinese Repository*）中有一篇关于宁波霍乱的论文，而该刊 1851 年 8 月也有我本人关于同一主题的几段论述。

② 在这个港口，最新霍乱爆发是记录在税务司麦克基（Mackey）先生 1878 年的温州贸易报告（Wenchow Trade Report）中。在 1878 年 8 月和 9 月间，霍乱盛行，而且是非常致命的。

③ 《申报》1881 年 2 月 19 日。

于夏季干旱，水渠会遭受严重污染（但根据温州当地人的观点，出现霍乱原因在于长时间的雨季和过量的雨水，因为长时间的雨季过后往往会伴随着瘟疫的出现。关于热病、疟疾和天气的关系，他们坚信疾病都是四时不正之气所致）。毫无疑问，这种被称为印度霍乱的瘟疫在中国北方被认为是一种新的疾病，但也有很大的可能，这种疾病以前就曾存在，只不过是长时间消失后，在今天再次出现而已，许多方志附录中记载的"疫"可能就是"霍乱"。我们知道，在最近的文献中，"疫"确实就包含有"霍乱"。李中梓的《医宗必读》远较其他医书更为提纲挈领，该书认为转筋只是普通地方性霍乱的一种特殊形式。① 但吴有性认为，转筋和霍乱虽然很相似，但两者是截然不同的疾病。吴有性医生同时引证，人们不会认为"突然性的吐泻"是通过人与人进行传播，但这确实是一种新型传染病，其传染机制与热病、疟疾相同。我目前所有能收集到的资料显示，印度霍乱，或者说流行性霍乱，对于中国来讲是一种全新的疾病，这种疾病并非通过肠道病毒在人与人之间传播，而是通过空气里的微生物传播；这种疾病受到大气与土壤的影响，因此总的来说，对霍乱采取隔离检疫是无效的。这个结论，直接反对西蒙斯医生和万巴德（Manson）医生的观点，他们的观点来自对最近日本和中国霍乱情况的细致考察。我从未听说过中国政府通过检疫措施，挡住过传染病的流入。② 西门医生还顺带用了一段引文，指出在麻疹流行期间突然出现了霍乱病例，病人在麻疹尚未康复时，又染上了霍乱，这让我想起了1851年我所写的一篇类似文章。"1848年秋季（霍乱初流行），宁波暴发了麻疹瘟疫；虽然当时并不认为是恶性麻疹，但因此丧命的人还是不少。麻疹在中国东部沿海发生战争的地区极为普遍，流行范围包括整个太平洋沿岸，直至萨摩耶德人的居住地，在那里麻疹尤其致命。根据一名俄国官员的报告，俄国在西伯利亚所有的殖民地都出现了麻疹，大量居民死亡。他们在阿留申群岛的人口损失了一大部分，而在阿拉斯加东南部的锡特卡，原有人口600人，一个月之内就损失了80人。除了一些欧洲人外，几乎所有的人都感染了麻疹，城里充满了恐惧与死亡的气氛，太平洋上的密克罗尼西亚群岛几乎也出现了麻疹流行，桑威奇群岛更

---

① 《医宗必读》（1637年）。

② 德贞医生曾在《海关医报》上写过关于霍乱的文章。

是遭受毁灭性打击。在中国，当地人和外国人都会受到感染。值得注意的是，麻疹在这片区域从热带一直传播到寒带时，霍乱也从伏尔加河流域传播到了美国的密西西比河流域"① 西蒙斯医生可能是根据美国赖辛森群岛的相关资料得出上述麻疹流行潮的结论。

去年冬季和春季，除了上海出现霍乱外，还爆发了麻疹和天花，前一种在苏州府邻近地区暴发，后一种则出现在南昌，南昌地属相邻的江西省。在苏州的大部分地方，很多孩子染上麻疹，症状并不是轻型的，而是恶性的——十例中有九例存在生命危险，麻疹病主要被归因于气候的反常，当时冬天出现严重干旱，随后又出现雨季。在南昌暴发的天花往往起初极危险，而最终能化险为夷。② 可怜的患者家人不得不去天花宫求神，祈祷他们孩子能够康复。天花、霍乱、麻疹在该地区同时性、连续性的出现，具有重要的传染病学价值。作为对中国传染病学研究的贡献，我罗列出了该省的瘟疫流行情况，大多数瘟疫我都只能以编年的形式简单列出来——正如我前面所做的，这种简单罗列可能占到总数的一半，这是因为该省的 11 部方志中，我只能吃透其中的 5 部。

除文献之外，在五灵庙一块凿刻的碑文上，也有关于瘟疫的记载，可以补充文献的不足。③ 根据这上面的资料可以得知，在几十年前，温州每年春天和夏天都会遭受瘟疫的侵袭，感染瘟疫的人会被自己的近亲送到废弃的庙宇里隔离，只给他们提供一些简单的残羹冷炙。在夜间，没有人敢私自外出，他们害怕在夜间碰上瘟神。1579 年④当地知县决定解决这件事，他将年纪大和有阅历的人召集起来，并向他们询问情况。一些人建议免费施药，一些人建议要将被抛尸荒野的人尽快埋葬，还有人建议举行大规模的祈福活动，以平抚导致疾病的疫鬼，并在江边举行"傩逐"的仪式。林知县则提出了更加综合性的看法，以适应时局的需要。知县主张用

---

① 《中国丛报》（*Chinese Repository*）1851 年 8 月。
② 《申报》1881 年 2 月 12 日。
③ 据《永嘉县志》，五灵庙最早修建于万历二十四年，咸丰元年重修。《永嘉县志》仅收了明代碑文，并没有清代碑文，玛高温在这里看的应该是咸丰年间的原碑。——译者注
④ 这篇碑文记录的时间是万历二十六年（1598 年），此处应是玛高温医生换算公历时出现了错误。——译者注

节俭和精神力量去战胜疫鬼，为此他当众宣读了一段训诫——第一，人有五伦（君臣、父子、夫妇、兄弟、朋友）；第二，天有五行（水、火、木、金、土）；第三，味有五辛（甜、苦、酸、辛、甘）；第四，体有五脏（心、肝、脾、肺、肾）；第五，心有五（?）情（喜、怒、哀、惧、爱、恶、欲）。① 林知县这段五点论的要旨在于具体应用，即要对饮食、全部的生活方式进行革新，只有这样才能改善卫生状况。对于百姓的建议措施，至少老者的建议受到了采纳，另外兴建了一座供奉五位瘟神的特殊庙宇（迄今为止，这些瘟神在许多庙宇中都还在受到供奉）。当地人热情高涨，计划很快付诸行动，五灵庙在一个月内就拔地而起，庙宇结构坚固无比。为了修建庙宇，知县拿出了衙门里的罚款，富人拿出积财，普通百姓则义务出劳力，并拨出田地作为庙宇的香火祀田，以供应平时开支。当读到这位杰出的知县庆贺瘟疫消失时，我感到非常喜悦。

也许会显得太过冗长，但我在这里还是要加上一段关于五瘟神②的记载，当瘟疫发生时，无论官府还是民间，五瘟神都受到普遍信仰。根据记载，开皇六年③（591），突然有鬼怪凌空接近皇帝；这些鬼怪由"五力士"组成。皇帝询问他的大臣，力士出现是凶兆还是吉兆，大臣回复到，"力士们"是上天派下来的五鬼，分别代表五种瘟疫，即春瘟、夏瘟、秋瘟、冬瘟和总管的中瘟；大臣还说出了五瘟使者的姓名和绰号，这五位都是历史上的名人。五瘟神身披不同颜色的袍子，分别为：青、白、红、黑、黄；各自手持器具，如铁锤、长杓、宝剑等。"等等，"皇帝接着问道，"有办法避开灾难吗？"大臣回复道："没有办法，这是上天所降，无法治之。"这一年，全国都出现了瘟疫。6月27日，皇帝下令兴建庙宇，并敕封五瘟神将军名号。隋、唐两代，庙宇都会举行仪式，以避免激怒这些可以引发瘟疫的"力士"，现在这件事看起来相当"不可思议"。

---

① 原文如此，玛高温医生在这里打了一个问号，后面记述的实际不是五情，而是七情。——译者注

② 可以参考《三教源流搜神大全·卷四》中的《五瘟使者》。五瘟使者分别为：春瘟张元伯、夏瘟刘元达、秋瘟赵公明、冬瘟钟仕贵、中瘟史文业。——译者注

③ 应是开皇十一年6月。——译者注

在一些富裕的城市——如宁波——瘟神往往具有崇高的形象，每个行会和街道辖区都会修建壮丽的瘟神像，其中一个形象是一位乘坐马车的女孩，看起来就如同盛开的莲花，铁条巧妙地穿过裤腿，支撑神像凌空而立，在祈禳游行中给人以仙女般的感受。祈禳节日总会在天热时举行，但这种仪式本身恰恰会造成突发性疾病。

在温州城，当地百姓为了除疫，甘愿忍受巨大痛苦，以证明他们的赤诚。他们会手持高温的花瓶，走上很长的路，并用钩子挂在自己手臂的肉上，枝条从臀部一直斜插到手上，手臂借此被固定在平举的姿势。根据最近编撰的当地府志，对庙宇瘟神的崇拜不足以驱逐疾病，温州尤其容易遭受瘟疫的侵袭，这都是大气变化的缘故，即便温州已经堪称帝国最干净的城市。

根据儒学的观点，主张其门徒应该劝阻民众进行盲目崇拜，尤其是事关卫生事务时。最近遵行这条教训的政治人物是江苏巡抚①；他关闭了寺院，勒令僧人还俗，并索还寺庙占据的不义之财。南宋的大臣张子智②也曾这样做过，他原本是江苏省常州知府。1295 年③常州府瘟疫大作，患病者，十有九室。他努力减轻和抑制瘟疫的影响，建立施药局并免费派药，但全然无效。没人来求药；所有需要消除瘟疫、寻求帮助的人，或为自己，或为朋友，都会前往瘟神庙，据说庙里的僧侣能够驱魔，并售卖咒语和护身符，这些僧侣还主张符咒是避免或治疗瘟疫的唯一手段，并反对使用药物；听说此事之后，知府亲自前往瘟神庙查看，他看到中间的怪兽神像容貌冷酷，两旁的神像则是丑陋无比，无数的信众正在受到蒙骗，于是知府下令关押所有相关人等；随后让他的士兵吃饱饭并大量饮酒，再让喝醉的士兵去毁灭神像，并将寺庙夷为平地。在士兵们清醒过来并意识到他们的渎神行为之前，这项军事任务早已完成。同时知府命令鞭打妖僧，并强迫他们还俗。当地城镇的居民，全都非常好奇，知府如此大胆破坏神

---

① 这里的江苏巡抚指的应是谭钧培。谭钧培上任后发布"苏藩禁条"，下令禁毁淫祀，时间应在 1880 年左右。——译者注

② 可以参考宋代《夷坚志》中的《张子智毁庙》。——译者注

③ 1295 年南宋已经灭亡，此处年份明显错误。根据《夷坚志》的记载，时间应是庆元乙卯春夏间，即 1195 年。——译者注

像，会遭到何种天谴，但不久，皇帝便召张子智入京，担任吏部郎中。不幸的是，后世的统治者并没有模仿或继承张子智的做法。自然而然的，医生们会组织起来反对僧侣的欺诈行为，但僧侣们站在广大民众的立场，也承认其超自然助力的成功，需要有过往时代医生医术的帮助，其中一些医生还被僧侣们封为圣职；比如在中国到处都能找到的药王庙，药王类似国外的医神埃斯科拉庇俄斯，虽然在中国历史中，还找不到具有阿波罗之子这样声名的人物。"药王"是对一系列显耀医家的尊称，但这些药王没有一个是正规医生，或写过医学典籍，这些人都是相当成功的江湖骗子，其中一些甚至是外国冒险家。最早有资格建起药王庙的人是扁鹊①，此人活跃于周威烈王时代（公元前 468 ~ 前 440 年②），祖籍是郑国人③（今开封府），但住在卢国，因此扁鹊也被称为"卢医"。扁鹊起先是开旅馆的，自从碰到长桑君之后，长桑君在 1 个月之内，每天都传授给扁鹊某些医术，并向扁鹊保证能够成仙，扁鹊学会用肉眼看穿石墙，并洞察人的身体系统和五脏六腑。此后扁鹊擅长诊断疾病，大多数隐疾得给他的医术让路。晋定公有一个大臣，财富无与伦比，晋定公十一年，这名大臣病倒，宫廷医师全都束手无策，于是找来卢医进行医治。扁鹊诊治时病人已经昏迷 5 天，但吃了扁鹊开的药方后，不到 3 天就恢复了意识。病人康复后，赠给扁鹊 2 万亩土地。但扁鹊没能活着享受这份荣誉，一名宫廷医师刺杀了扁鹊。通过解剖，扁鹊建立起了解剖学知识和脉象理论，他的著作如《扁鹊神应针灸玉龙经》对针灸和艾灸贡献良多，但这本书可能是假托扁鹊的伪书。根据《四库全书总目》记载，这本书可能出自元代。④

738 年，京师出现了一个奇怪的外国人；他身穿天鹅绒的袍子，头戴纱帽；脚穿怪鞋，手持拐杖；腰上围着几十个葫芦，葫芦里装的都是药，

① 关于扁鹊的这段材料，可以参考《史记》中的《赵世家》与《扁鹊仓公列传》。——译者注
② 应为公元前 425 年至公元前 402 年，另外关于扁鹊的生卒年份还存在争议。——译者注
③ 玛高温医生在这里错会了"秦越人"的意思，误以为"秦越人"是扁鹊的籍贯，但关于扁鹊的真实籍贯，一直还存在争议。——译者注
④ 如果《凤洲纲鉴》的记载是正确的话，那么在迈耶斯（Mayyes）的手册（*Manual*）中，关于扁鹊籍贯和出生日期的引用，则存在很大错误。

并免费发给那些患病的人。这个怪人的名声传入皇宫，并得到了皇帝的召见，此人自称"得道人"，来自印度①。皇帝非常欣赏此人，命人给他画像，并册封为药王。他的真实姓名叫韦古。根据《闽杂记》的记载，药王庙或扁鹊庙也被称作卢医庙。另有一种说法认为，药王菩萨即韦古，是苏门答腊人。也许他在离开印度后，先去了苏门答腊并成名，之后才来到中国。韦古并不是佛教徒，却具有极高的宗教地位，他也不是婆罗门或回教徒。7世纪末，武则天篡取皇位，并统治了华人这一黑发种族。一名叫韦善俊②的道教医家，由于如和尚一样苦修，再加上医术精湛，深受武则天赏识。韦善俊总爱带着一条名叫"乌龙"的黑犬，并受到百姓的爱戴，被尊为药王。在今天能够看到的药王画像中，还能看到韦善俊所亲近的黑犬，值得注意的是，西方古典时代和中世纪，也存在类似亲近犬科动物的情况。传统上，西门·马古斯③与其他擅长黑魔法与骗术的古代医生们，都偏好随身带一条黑犬。16世纪著名的医生和哲学家科尼利厄斯·阿格里帕，同样圈养一条黑犬，胡迪布拉斯称其为"地狱犬"，"这不仅是条杂种狗，还是这位神秘主义哲学家兼医生的导师"。但民众对韦善俊的信仰并不牢固。在唐代④，韦善俊可能很快就被人遗忘，但在宋代，一位重要大臣的遭遇使人们又唤起了对他的记忆。这名大臣声称幼时在病中见到了韦善俊，他牵着黑犬，一如其生前。神灵指引生病的幼童服下药片，幼童照着服下药片，紧接着出了一身大汗，病情立刻痊愈。幼童长大后执掌国政，命人绘制了药王像，并加以供奉，韦善俊的大名再次得以流传。苏州因其医学领域的万神殿而自豪。从前这座庙仅供奉三皇，即伏羲、神农和黄帝——这三位都是近乎半神的先代君王，后来又增加了大禹，四神都因其医术而受到尊崇。1692年⑤又以岐伯、雷公、伯高、鬼臾区、少俞、少师配享，现在这座神庙被称为"药王庙"。⑥很显然，不能将药王庙里供奉

---

① 根据《闽杂记》原文，韦古是疏勒人，即今天的南疆人，并非印度人。——译者注

② 可以参考《太平广记》中的《韦善俊》。——译者注

③ 《圣经》中的人物，与使徒同时代人，一切异端之父。——译者注

④ 可以参考明代《琅琊代醉编》，材料中的大臣指韩亿。——译者注

⑤ 根据乾隆朝《苏州府志》，此事当在康熙三十年，即1691年。——译者注

⑥ 以上大部分内容，都出自《集说诠真续编》的引文，作者黄伯禄（字斐默），上海，1860年。

的这些神，错误地类比为中国的科拉庇俄斯。

根据中国的炼丹术，石黄①，即二硫化坤，可以用来预防疾病，并且具有辟邪的作用。中国人会在五月初五端午节这天，将少量雄黄和朱砂一起放在酒中饮用；此外还将其涂抹在幼儿前额以辟邪。

传染病的疯狂，已经引起了生理学家们的注意，并且理应将其作为国家医疗的分支，纳入关注的视野。虽然还无法完全掌握，但关于传染病的这些信息，对于公共事务的管理者来讲非常有价值。下面几段关于传染病的内容，对于一些专业读者而言，也许没有太大价值，但对于一般读者而言，多少会有一些意义。1876 年曾经出现过一本专著《治蛊摘要》，是一名大方的无名氏所写，这位具有公共精神的绅士，是江苏②常州人。这本书还提到了一起事件，外国居民们对此事一定还记忆犹新——这就是曾经引发过恐慌的神秘剪辫子③事件——鉴于此事在帝国大范围内造成心理和身体痛苦，这本书的目的在于，一方面要在巫蛊来临后传播有用的知识，同时为患者提供治疗手段，并抑制巫术的影响，另一方面这本书还向读者们展示了关于这起奇异事件的神秘上古传说。下面我所叙述的内容，主要来自这本书和我自己的观察，在这起事件中，举世瞩目的妄想持续了数月之久，整个帝国陷入奇怪的迷乱状态。关于之前的巫蛊情况，我知之甚少；但在作者国家的地方志中，记录了之前发生过的类似妖术事件。中国发生妖术事件的时间，依次为 1464 年、1529 年、1596 年、1657 年和 1753 年。中国第一次发生妖术狂热事件的时间，几乎与欧洲英诺森八世发布敕令、掀起女巫狂热事件同时。庆幸的是，这些谬误在中国没有因为宗教狂热而加剧，虽然"妖"这个字在词源学上和女人有关，但中国人很少会沉

① 即雄黄。——译者注
② 原文作"Kiangsi"，即江西，但清代江西并没有叫"Changchau"的府、县，再加上《治蛊摘要》这本书目前可能已经失传，无法查证。且太湖流域自明代以来就是妖术流行的地区，因此怀疑应是江苏常州，而不是作者所写的江西常州。——译者注
③ "纸人"和剪辫子狂潮使得朝廷最后颁布了诏令［见《京报》（Peking Gazette，1876 年 10 月 15 日）］，另外浙江巡抚也有相关报告［见《京报》（Peking Gazette，1876 年 11 月 9 日）］，这些文件显示出，中国政府认为狂热事件是针对基督教传教士。玛高温医生在温州这样的小城，未必有途径能够看到《京报》原文，他看的可能只是《万国公报》上的《京报全录》。——译者注

迷于将女人当作妖人。妖术、魔法、恶毒、媚惑，这些词语构成了"女人"和"巫师"结合后的形象。根据 17 世纪中期一名作家的叙述，1657 年的瘟疫，是由一名扬子江北部地区的妖人所引发，这些妖人曾在清江和常州出没。他们拥有能使人神魂颠倒的力量，通过"催眠术"，在户外他们只需呼唤路人的名字，就能引诱路人，并将其拐卖到别的城市，这种妖术与"邪眼"（evil eye）① 类似，虽然蛇妖诱人的传说在东亚乃至世界范围内并不流行。这些被催眠的人，会被施法者卖到苏州和常州的中间商手上，且备受压迫；中间商因此受到严惩，有些妖人被迫退出常州，并转往杭州继续作恶。大约一星期后，常州有鬼魂出没，整个社会都深受其扰。由于各种灵异现象，没人敢在晚上睡觉；房梁和屋瓦会发出可怕的声响，人们能够看到模糊的幻影，且恶臭难闻，幻影有时有一配克②大小，有时又会突然暴长到房屋那么大，事实上，这个黑暗魔鬼变化多端，举例来讲，有时它能变成巨嘴、星眼的狐狸，有时又能变成马或狗的形象。这些鬼影巨魔进入房屋后，会将人生生闷死，或将人抓伤，直至血尽人亡。虽然一些剑客试图捕杀妖人，但最后死的都是他们自己。这些妖人只害怕一样东西——那就是喧闹声。通过不断敲打金锣和木盆，同时不断大声喊叫，时间从日出一直持续到日落，就能将幽灵从房子里赶出去，连续七天，就可以让异象彻底消失。此事发生及之前的相当长一段时间，纸人妖法也让百姓深受其害，妖人可以通过纸人进行施法，尤其是加上受害人的断辫后，这种妖法成为当地人苦恼的来源；妖人会将断辫覆盖在纸人上，由此获得剥夺生命的权力。周医生家里曾住过一名临时房客，这名房客对周医生讲，他售卖的护身符可以破除一切符咒。此人售卖护身符的价格非常低，购买者络绎不绝，但一些不怀好意的人声称，这名房客就是妖人；一个暴徒将这名房客扣住，并将其扭送至知府处，衙门为了逼供，最后将其拷打而死。我们的作者指出，他一直对妖人诡计这一传统说法的真实性感到怀疑，但巫蛊的流行，又使他相信恶魔的说法并不夸张，在恐慌的气氛日渐上升时，他曾亲眼见过妖，这是一种能够摄人魂魄的恶魔。它们的

---

① 古罗马和古希腊都有关于邪眼伤人的传说，最出名的当属希腊神话中的蛇形女妖美杜莎。——译者注

② 容积单位，1 配克 = 2 加仑。——译者注

眼睛如同闪亮的镜子；能够像幽灵一样消失，作者立刻背诵了一段咒语自救，这段知名的咒语能够破邪，且相当押韵。后来，作者开始从事这一主题的研究工作，并搜寻前代解决巫蛊之患的有效方法；另外他也在书中补充了自己和其他当代研究者的相关成果。他所采用的标题是《治蛊叙言》（意译），即关于蛊虫的治疗方法，蛊虫这种说法最早源自古代炼丹医家的著作，这些古代医家认为世上存在七种寄生虫，或者说"毒蛊"，蛊虫会折磨病人的身体系统，普通治疗手段对其完全无效，只能使用驱邪的方法，再结合诸如解毒剂这样的药物，才能祛除蛊虫。那些妖人所使用的妖法就是同这些蛊虫有关，因此除妖也被称为驱虫。论蛊毒之术，两广地方，最为知名。

纸人代表着被妖人捕获的受害者，妖人将纸人作为工具，以驱使灵魂。妖人会通过一切手段进入民居，然后通常是通过受害者的断发，伤害居民；妖人拥有断发后，就可以随时召唤受害者的魂魄，使其成为妖人的鬼奴，按照中世纪的说法，就是"世仆"——自然，受害者会因为失去魂魄而死。有时妖人会将鬼怪附在纸人上，将针插入受害者的身体，或是在受害者皮肤褪色斑点处印标记。有时这些恶魔会伪装成小贩，通过商品进行哄骗，受害者往往因为商品极低的价格而上当。常州就有人曾因此而遭害。此人买了一把剪刀，当晚他就用这把被施了法术的工具，切断了自己的喉咙；一名可怜的九江外地人，买一个甜瓜，当夜他就听见有人叫自己的名字；起来以后，并没有见到任何人；天亮以后，却发现自己的所有头发都被剃光了。

另外一种妖人或擅使妖术的医生摄人魂魄的方法，是通过动物做中介——比如老鼠、蝙蝠、麻雀、甲壳虫等，事实上，任何动物都可以成为他们犯罪计划的工具。

受到这种神秘疾病侵害后，病人首先会感到胃痛；然后病毒就会在人身体里四处扩散。如果受害者是儿童，那么数天之内就会丧命；成年人通常可以活 100 天左右，但有时也能活 2～3 年，然后突然暴死。

治疗这些疾病必须使用医学药物和辟邪咒语。因为磁铁丸具有吸力，所以被当作治疗的主要药物使用，根据不同情况，也会使用其他药物作为辅助。泻药和催吐剂也扮演着重要角色；如果病人能够将人发、猪鬃、竹屑排出体外，那么就能够获得康复。如果有人发现自己的辫子短了一截，那么他必须再剪掉 1~2 英寸，然后将其在阴沟里泡 80 天。只有通过这种方法，才能切断断发、病人与巫师的联系。最保险的办法是放置咒语，符咒由当局颁发。当疯狂的传染病开始流行时，恐惧的民众会请求官府为了公众和世俗利益介入。1876 年时疫发生时，江苏巡抚发布告示，并进行驱鬼逐疫。总督请道士设置代表疫病的恶魔纸像后，首先会与恶魔进行搏斗，他会散发一些他发明的写有汉字的符咒，这些符咒会被放置在居民的门上，或佩戴在身上作为护身符——符咒的神秘含义只有恶魔才能理解；之后他会开始念道教创始人老子（生活在公元前 6 世纪、公元 666 年被神化为太上老君）的咒语，然后他会在黄纸上用朱砂写下来，随后烧掉，灰烬则被吞下。这些符咒的词句三字一读，读作："祈上君，以天力，以地力，斩恶鬼，灭其魄；勿使留，勿使生。往兮哉，汝鬼物。我灭汝，表与血，尽成灰！我（祈求者）谦信，请上君，如律令。"道士会花几分钟写符咒，然后把烧掉的灰烬吞掉。最后，总督向民众保证，官府完全有能力处理疫鬼，并挫败所有企图搅乱人民魂魄和国家稳定的阴谋。

为进一步加强干涉力度，人们寻求道教最高领袖的帮助。最高领袖是世袭都，有时被称作"天师"，他被认为能够战胜恶魔（中国恶魔的概念并不是产生于中世纪，而是产生于古典时期），这是官方才有的能力；遇到紧急情况时，他会发放符咒或护身符，这些东西在 1862 年被用来抵抗霍乱。很少有房屋的门上不挂符咒，也很少有人不在帽子或袖口上带护身符。在疾病流行的最高峰，每栋房屋的门上都能看到符咒，外国人可以由此了解到当地民众身体与精神上的不安。这些符咒很容易识别，认得这些符咒，有时也会有些用处（见图 5）。

图 5①是太上老君符，这种护身符几乎到处都在用（另有一些则在特殊场合用）。符咒抬头有神秘的三点，另有一个非常规的汉字。中央写着"太上驱邪潜形遁迹普照吉祥太上律令敕！"两边则画有北斗七星。另外还写了受命令的六种鬼的名字。图 5②是天师符，它被用来驱魔和进行占卜，也被当作护身符佩戴。图 5③具有与上述两道符相同的功能，一般被放置在门上；这道符只有开头能够识别，作者并不能了解其深刻内涵。散布者将此符称为"长"，学名叫"天师"。这道符都是简单的字母，发符者还向我请教了一些他所患的小病。我得知他来自龙虎山。在其宫殿内有无数被封印的罐子，这些罐子里都被封着恶魔。他被任命为整个帝国

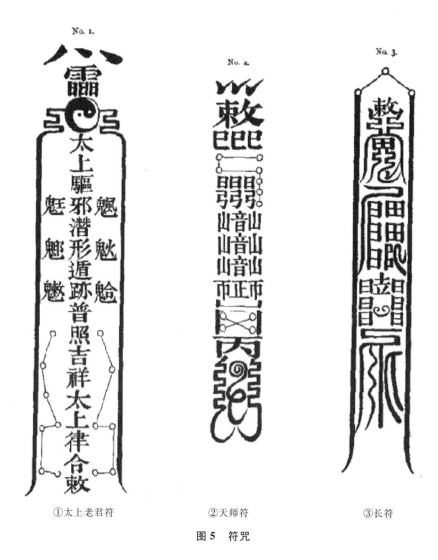

①太上老君符　　　　②天师符　　　　③长符

图 5　符咒

道观的监理。其魔法的强大能够凌驾于宇宙精神之上，保护国家和家庭免于灾祸。

我们的作者列举了无数使人受折磨的妖术，他指出人们可以用两种方法对付妖术；一种是用破布、狗血或其他一些脏东西；另外一种则是使用正统的书写符咒，以及朗读符咒以达到辟邪驱邪的目的。《大学》或《中庸》的第一章，或是《易经》64 卦，又或是爱国殉道者田凤洲（音译）的诗句，它们都是些不明其意的乱语。儒家经典有时也被认为具有辟邪的作用，新建的房子里会在木盒里盛放四书五经。通过以上手段，再辅助以其他措施，如在腰带里佩戴药物、在房里悬挂桃树枝、拉弓驱邪、击鼓、点火等，鬼怪就会被驱逐。

前文所讲的传染病大概流行了 8 个月，流行病遍布广东至长江北部，乃至西部的两湖地区。据估计在这段时间，有些秘密暴力团体正在借机煽动恐慌。有一些信徒在大城市里通过剪人辫子制造恐慌，随后又在公共场所宣布他们自己也是被剪掉辫子的受害者。一旦出现某些病例，人们就会让巫师制作纸人，如果有人做噩梦，或在皮肤上发现污点，或是患疝气，那么这都是妖术的缘故。总而言之，城市里一切错乱事情的发生，中风、自杀、物品遗失、非同寻常的噪声、梦境以及幻影都被认为是隐形的敌人妖术的缘故；更广泛的迷信认为，妖术会导致体弱的人得脑病。

在其有关治疗的叙述里，作者提出了一些预防措施。妖术常常寄身于鸦片馆、茶叶铺、庙宇或隐藏在深山、林间、洞穴里。士绅和老人应找出一切可疑的人，逮捕这些可疑的人并将其送官。这里提出了值得注意的警告，有些黑帮结成巫师搜捕队，并以此为借口劫掠旅行者，他们会把外国制造的针藏在受惊吓的人的行李里，然后借此勒索，受害者常常被迫屈服。如果碰到有的旅客身无分文，这些暴徒会扒掉其衣服甚至取人性命。这些事情并非夸大其词，在《治虫撮要》里有相关的记述。不仅是无赖会做这种事，恐慌的村民有时也会对行商做同样的事情。普通百姓在暴怒之下，总是会把陌生人扭送到衙门进行司法审查。我们的作者对被怀疑是妖人进行司法审查的场景做了一些描述。在湖北有一名间谍被送到衙门里进行审判——审判包括用刑——犯人既不招供也不怕痛，但被揭去其腋窝与脚底的药膏后，犯人从喉咙里吐出了恶心的物质，他大叫并说出了真相，承认一名巫师让他去剪头发，每簇头发付 1 美元，用针刺人则给一半钱，在人身上做标记给的钱更少——总之一句话，这名不幸的人承认了所有指控。由此发现了这名巫师的踪迹，他在白天扮作僧侣，到处化缘或传法，晚上就扎纸人，纸人则承载有间谍的魂魄。从上文的观点来看，如果一个人在晚上突然苏醒并出现窒息症状，那么就应该用一块洗碗的抹布盖住病人身上的斑点，并派人出去寻找施法的媒介，此人一般就在附近房中睡觉。这名睡着的媒介被找到后，往往呆若木鸡且魂魄已失；用抹布包住他，再将其送到知县那里去。在无锡，用这种方法共抓到 5 名妖人。

在安徽宁国，敌视教会的人宣称在教堂里有纸像，并领着暴民冲击教堂，指认满篮的纸像作为证据，这些纸像都是这些人栽赃放在教堂里的。民众被彻底激怒，暴力和流血随之而来。暴民领袖企图到首都去继续告状，却被总督投入监狱，暴乱自此被控制住。

如同 1876 年那样广泛的恐慌并不常见，但疯狂行为在有限的地区还是时有发生，《大清律例》对相关情况有所规定，散布谣言为有罪，这对维护公共安全极有必要。我再举两个引起恐慌的例子，一名女士习惯于早上在城墙上散步，她被要求说明自己的意图。她并不是一个失控的疯子，这一点被她的邻居证明，邻居说这位女士唯一的反常就是喜欢外出做好事。最后裁定这名女士企图在城墙上散布纸人，以达到蛊惑驻军和当地居民的目的。为了破除她的法术，所有人都在晚上上街击鼓、燃爆竹、大叫，以此破除阴谋并保证公众的安全。

有时恶棍会通过一些凶兆在城镇里引发动乱。在温州还没有开埠之前，就发生过这样的例子。一名文人挑起了一场争端和诉讼——此人文笔很好，并靠其才智为生，被认为精通洋务，人们不仅尊敬他，更十分惧怕他，他由于卷入了一起无法解决的经济事务——宣称自己发现将有一起大灾难在温州降临。具体是什么灾难他无法确定，但规模肯定很大，他说有一艘船只装满了外国女人，这些外国女人全都面目可憎，长着红色的毛发，很快就会达到瓯江河口。如果有需要的话，民众会把温州唯一的传教士给赶出去，因为人们认为所有事情都与这个无赖有关。造成的结果是，人们像躲避麻风病人一样躲避这名传教士。实际上，外国人有时确实具有一些神秘的气质，一个外国人通常力大无穷，且带有居高临下的傲姿，又常常带着一根手杖。当时人们还不知道可爱的绅士为何物，仅仅知道外国人都是瘸子，只有靠手杖才能支撑身体，并且有能力把城市搅得天翻地覆。正当事件快平息时，这名文士又收到消息，说魔女已经到达河口，他宣布自己已经尽到对公众的责任，接下来他要去照看自己家庭的安全并把他们带到内地，红发魔女只能望其后尘。在他将行李打包好之前，富人们已经带着妻妾、儿女、家什全都挤在了码头上。商业已经暂停，店铺因此关门，人们因为惊骇完全不知所措；他们向官府寻求帮助。道台派人召来传教士，说自己为此事相当生气，并立刻发布安民告示，动乱得到平息。这件事情发生在很久之前——所有动乱都是由那名文人引发的，他只有通过这种办法才能离开温州。事后所有人都开怀大笑，唯有文人的债权人们笑不出来。

最近《申报》上记载了两名医疗巫师的故事，这两人企图在靠近湖区的乡村修炼法术，并对部分地区施法。这两人是美女，却假装未婚，并暗示自己是仙女。她们声称能够用符咒祛病，但如果有人减少供奉的钱物，她们可以通过咒语让人重新患病。当疾病在那个地区发生时，这两人获得了对当地的支配地位。没有一个人不需要向她们缴税——穷人每年都要缴1美元，富人要缴100美元或更多。她们派几十个男人帮自己收费，这些仆从的行为与强盗无异，这些人所展现的破坏性比火灾或洪水更强烈。

对当地人日常生活的一瞥展示出对当地进行教化是多么的有必要。有必要去传播看得见与看不见的关于宇宙的观点，在这一点上，期刊报社是最重要的机构，这就要求报纸尽力驱除迷信与无知的乌云，而迷信与无知正是大清帝国虚弱的根源，人们需要逐渐使其消散；西方清楚地知道，黑暗沉闷的时代已经不再被容许继续存在，虽然不快，但稳步的变化正在急促发生。

这是对中国人无知与迷信生活的一瞥与揭露。但他们并不像我们处在黑暗与沉闷的中世纪时那样对巫师感到狂躁，他们好像并没有因为多灾而受到妄想的影响，据估计，欧洲人在那个时期将900万人送上了火刑架。令人高兴的是，经过逐渐的启蒙与解放，我们的先驱们得以冲出陆地，将正确的观念撒播到全世界，期刊报纸在其中做出了杰出的贡献。

最近巴西的达·西瓦尔·利马在其国家发现了印度脚气病，随后西蒙斯医生在日本也发现了该疾病，这表明这种疾病流传的范围比我们想象得要广的多。根据我所翻译的中国文献，以及口头调查，这种病被描述为"疟疾腿"，也就是脚气，与日本人对该疾病的命名一致（脚气）。我对印度病并不熟悉，我以前并不知道中国与印度的此项疾病相同，直到我阅读了西蒙斯医生关于日本"脚气"的论文。

查询有关疟疾腿的文献，上溯至模糊和定义不清的时代，历史总是与神话交织在一起；有必要对这一时期的中国考古学进行批判性研究，相关主题很难通过医书进行印证。但这些问题都是交错在一起的。《内经》中就有关于脚气的记载，另外《灵枢经》也有记载，无疑这是现存关于脚气的最早论述，公元前2697年，黄帝撰写了《内经》，但《内经》是否如此古老实际上并无根据，否则周代或孔子的编年史不会对其毫无记录。根据沈朗仲的《病机汇论》，"厥"（此字的本意是指一种抛石工具，常常与某

种疾病名连用并作为后缀）就是"疟疾腿"，汉代被称作"慢风病"，到
了宋朝其定义才逐渐明确；但并不指单一疾病，而是指一系列厥病。这方
面最早的专著《脚气治法总要》①，该书原本早已遗失，但在《四库全书
总目》和《永乐大典》中有副本。该书有两卷，最后一卷包含有 46 种药
方。自宋代开始，出现大量对治疗此病的系统论述。该疾病被认为有两种
类型，分别与积水型脚气和萎缩型脚气相符，病如其名，这都是根据西方
研究来进行病原学划分的。"疟疾腿"是由土壤传递的毒素所致。这又有
两种类型，一种是温湿所致，另一种是湿冷所致。在一年当中的任何季
节，站在潮湿的地方、流汗突然受抑制、某人突然因为天气或情绪而燥
热，以及在此情况脱光衣服都会导致此疾病的发生；另外，根据尊敬的皇
帝陛下的说法，饮酒荒淫也会导致得脚气。湿热脚气的脉象会很快；湿冷
脚气的脉象则很慢。当毒气从腿上升到心脏后，人的心智就会受到影响，
病人开始咕咕哝哝，他们毫无食欲且剧烈咳嗽，坐立不安又呼吸困难，且
小便不利。温湿脚气患者的腿会非常疼痛，并会伴有热病；湿冷型脚气患
者的四肢并无痛感，也不会出现发热。两种类型患者嘴都会发黑，皮肤和
肌肉都有痛感，尤其是胸侧痛感更明显，青筋会突出；这些症状会逐渐在
脸部和头部显现。此外，脚气还与湿度有关，错误饮食也被认为会导致脚
气。为什么中国至今还没有发现这一疾病的行踪？这是因为这种疾病并不常
见，且这种疾病一定程度上是一种阶层病，另外在中国的外国医生也很少治
疗这种疾病。现在脚气病既然已经引起注意，相信很快就会有相关报告出
现。一名中国海关官员的母亲患有该病，病情来得很急，一周之内病人即告
不治。当地医生认为是脚气病所致，从报告来看，应该属于温湿类型。

有理由相信，东京流行的就是脚气病，而非阿贝·理查德所谓的
恶风。②

---

① 《脚气治法总要》出版于 11 世纪后期至 13 世纪后期，东京安德森博士再版的著述
可能就参考了这本书。参见他有关这方面的论文，以及盖伊医院（Guy's Hospital）
报告。

② * "Le mauvais vent (Sinicè, morbific vapour!) est une autre espèce qui nous est inconnue. Le mauvais vent ou l'impression subite d'un air froid, chargé d'exhalations locales, glace tout d'un coup le sang et fait mourir sur le champ plusieurs personnes; d'autres ne sont qu'estropiées de quelques membres: le plus souvent, la bouche se déforme et tourne comme dans une attaque de paralysie. Lorsque l'impression est légère on en guérit en se réchauffant. Il y a des remèdes spécifiques contre ce mal s'ils sont administré à temps."—*Histoire naturelle, civile et politique du Tonquin*, par M. l'Abbé RICHARD, Chanoine de l'Église royale de Verelai: à Paris, MDCCLXXVIII.

　　一场破坏性极强的瘟疫在包括水牛在内的牛畜中流行。引人注意的是，1877年秋，几乎每一种家畜都因为瘟疫而出现了大规模死亡（之前的夏季曾出现过霍乱流行）。凡是长角的牛畜，包括奶牛、水牛，以及马、山羊、猪、犬、家禽，几乎全都遭了瘟——牛科动物得的是牛瘟；山羊得的是口蹄疫；至于其他家畜的相关情况，我目前掌握的信息尚不全面。道台是一位仁慈的绅士，他严格强化法律（但南京知府执法更严，一名穆斯林因为违犯禁令，而被斩首），禁止屠宰牛畜，并且会给那些牛畜已经老朽的农民以补偿，出于对老牛的怜悯，道台建起了一座收容站，让老牛能够在收容站中得到照顾并安享余生。棚屋建在西门，里面一共有数百头这样的老牛，但由于不小心引入了一头瘟牛，这些老牛不久全都病死了。温州地区牛瘟盛行的原因还需要进一步查明；此次牛瘟影响到了浙江全省，并且蔓延至临近的江苏、安徽两省。

　　两年以后的1879年，蒙古的小公牛和骆驼也遭受了瘟疫，结果导致卡尔甘和库伦之间的茶叶贸易受到严重影响。按照《牛经》的记载，可以通过牛畜粪便或带有黏液的呕吐物，来判断常规牛瘟的病症，但这本书没有太多其他有价值的信息值得翻译。猪瘟通常并不会与牛瘟同时出现。波特·史密斯医生曾在汉口发现了旋毛虫，[①] 万巴德医生在厦门也发现了旋毛虫（参见上一期的《海关医报》），证明了寄生虫在中国的普遍存在。虽然万巴德医生曾指出，由于中国烹饪猪肉的方式，这种疾病在中国可能极为罕见，但通过进一步的调查，也许就能够找到旋毛虫病的病例。

　　温州不仅是鸦片产区，也是鸦片进口的通道。中国人会在国产鸦片里掺杂印度鸦片——通常会掺巴特那鸦片，而不是马尔瓦鸦片[②]。当地鸦片因为生物碱含量不足，相较而言，会在短时间内对吸食者的身体造成刺激；在吸入这些鸦片两或三个小时以后，吸食者会渴望吸入更多。在此评论使用鸦片所造成的腐化与病态，也许超出了我的工作范围，但从医学的

---

① 《中国药物学与博物学》（*Contributions to the Materia Medica and Natural History of China*）。本书在海关总税务司赫德的资助下，于1871年出版于上海，作者在封面指明，该书供医学传教士和当地学生使用。——译者注

② 巴特那鸦片也叫"公班土"，马尔瓦鸦片也叫"白皮土"。"白皮土"的价格略高于"公班土"，这也是选择掺"公班土"的原因所在。

观点来看，烟瘾会影响到人类繁殖，我们需要用医学手段改变吸烟者。9
个月前，内地会在温州建立一家医院，专门为眼科病人和鸦片吸食者服
务，负责人是杜思韦特先生，在这段时间里，超过 200 名患者得到了救治，
所有瘾君子在接受平均 4 个星期的治疗后，都能戒除烟瘾并离开医院。①
来此医院进行治疗的病人，除了支付伙食费外，并不需要支付其他费用。
北京德贞医生治疗的病人平均每天吸食 4 钱 5 厘鸦片，杜思韦特医生的病
人平均每天只需吸食 3 钱 2 厘的鸦片。当地对戒除烟瘾药物的需求很大，
城墙上贴得到处都是吹嘘能够完美戒除烟瘾的药物广告；许多所谓的秘
方，都宣称曾受到外国人的赞助，这种策略对他们的销售很有好处。鸦片
在某种形式上正是戒烟药的成分，这些戒烟药非常有效，因此无须怀疑其
疗效。说来话长，早在 1844 年我曾采用过一种治疗方法，也许可以称得上
"彻底的"方法，这种方法与我前面讲的渐进疗法不同。这种疗法包括，
要求病人接受治疗后，在第一次习惯性上瘾时就保持克制，并要与因为突
然戒断导致的可怕后果做斗争。戒断鸦片数小时后，会导致患者出现脱水
性腹泻，紧接着出现遗精现象，腰椎部位也会疼痛难当，并最终导致虚
脱。为了支撑痛苦的病人不在这一治疗过程中被压垮，需要让病人服用兴
奋剂、收敛剂和补养药，并提供滋补的饮食，直到新形式的刺激能够勾起
病人的欲望为止，至此病人算是跨过了那道坎，并和过去的生活说再见。
酗酒对于这些病人来说是绝对不允许的，即便是对采取渐进疗法的病人来
讲，在减轻戒烟药剂量的过程中，戒酒也不是难事，最后病人常常能将酒
瘾和烟瘾一起戒掉。接受渐进疗法的病人，当他们再次受到烟瘾的诱惑
时，他们因为感到只要借助药品就会很容易得到治疗，稍微放纵一下自己
的烟瘾并不会有什么危险，但结果常常是毁灭性的，对于接受"彻底"疗
法的病人来讲，他们对生不如死的折磨感到恐惧，对他们来讲没有什么比
接受重复治疗更恐怖的了，因为已经受过这样的痛苦，便很难复吸。无论
是从身体层面还是从道德层面来讲，病人都翻开了人生的新篇章，其身体
的所有官能都开始逐渐恢复男子气概；但这些人从此会更容易患疟疾和黏

---

① 在我写下上述内容时，杜思韦特先生撰写的《第一次温州总医院与戒烟所年度报
告》（*First Annual Report of the Wenchow General Hospital and Opium Refuge*）已经出
版。我将其中与本文主题相关的有用的信息附于其后，见图 6。

膜炎——这似乎是在暗示，麻醉剂能够让人对上述疾病免疫。我曾在很多年前发表过鸦片烟瘾的治疗方法①，后来这种方法被福州的奥斯古德医生所采纳，另外他又找到了一种新药物，即水合氯醛②，这种药物可以用来满足病人的上瘾需要。

ANTI-OPIUM HOSPITAL STATISTICS.

Number of patients admitted	213	Number of patients incurable	2
„ „ cured	209	Expelled for bad conduct	2

NUMBER OF YEARS SINCE SMOKING WAS COMMENCED.

9 had smoked 1 year.	4 had smoked 9 years.	1 had smoked 19 years.
10 „ 2 years	14 „ 10 „	2 „ 20 „
21 „ 3 „	11 „ 12 „	1 „ 21 „
18 „ 4 „	4 „ 14 „	5 „ 23 „
25 „ 5 „	13 „ 15 „	2 „ 24 „
29 „ 6 „	5 „ 16 „	5 „ 25 „
12 „ 7 „	4 „ 17 „	1 „ 29 „
17 „ 8 „	3 „ 18 „	

AGES OF PATIENTS.

Under 20	3	Over 40 and under 50	52
Over 20 and under 30	64	„ 50 „ 60	14
„ 30 „ 40	79	„ 60 „ 70	1

AMOUNT OF OPIUM CONSUMED DAILY BY EACH MAN.

7 consumed 1 mace.	41 consumed 5 mace.	3 consumed 9 mace.
23 „ 2 „	17 „ 6 „	5 „ 10 „
45 „ 3 „	11 „ 7 „	1 „ 12 „
49 „ 4 „	10 „ 8 „	1 „ 15 „

Average, 4½ mace.

4½ mace per day is 1,642 mace, or 10 catties 4 liang=13 lb. 6½ oz. avoirdupois, per annum.

If we consider those who have entered the hospital as fairly representing the opium-smokers of this city, and accept the lowest native estimate of the number of smokers—i.e., half the adult males,—then reckon the population at 80,000, we shall find there are at least 10,000 opium-smokers in the city.

At the above average of 10 catties 4 liang per annum, 10,000 men would require 102,500 catties of prepared opium for their yearly consumption. Crude opium loses in the process of preparation about one-third in weight; accordingly, 102,500 catties of the extract represents 132,950 catties, or about 1,329 chests of the crude drug.

As only 58 chests of foreign opium paid Customs duty here last year, a great quantity must be smuggled, or brought overland from Ningpo, to supply the market.

QUALITY OF OPIUM SMOKED.

69 smoked Malwa.	15 smoked Patna.	119 smoked native.

The Indian opium contains from 8 to 15 per cent. of morphine. The native drug is only about one-third that strength as it is sold in the shops, but in the Suian district, about 30 miles south of Wénchow, a very superior drug is produced, which those who smoke it declare to be equal to Patna. An opium planter from that district told me that a great quantity is annually sent over the borders to Fukien, where it is sold as Indian opium. It does not become soft when exposed to the air as the Wénchow and Taichau drug does.

	FOREIGN.	NATIVE.
Largest quantity smoked daily	8 mace.	15 mace.
Smallest „ „	1 „	2 „
Largest quantity eaten	1 „	5 „

TIME SPENT IN HOSPITAL.

Longest	40 days.
Shortest	8 „ „

Average, 21 days.

On leaving the hospital each man takes a supply of tonic medicines, so the average period of treatment is about 30 days.

---

① 《中国丛报》1851 年 8 月。

② 水合氯醛是安眠药的主要成分。——译者注

The following statistics will show the work done during the past 12 months:—

GENERAL HOSPITAL STATISTICS.

Number of out-patients treated during the year 4,030
    ,,   in-patients ,,   ,, ... 45

NATURE OF DISEASES TREATED.

Eye Diseases:—		Eye Diseases—cont.	
Purulent ophthalmia	47	Amblyopia	40
Gonorrhœal ,,	9	Abscess of orbit	2
Granular ,,	86	General Diseases:—	
Conjunctivitis	46	Syphilis	32
Entropion with ulceration of cornea	1,626	Rheumatism	68
Granular lids	205	Ulcers and abscesses	146
,, ,, with ulceration of cornea	1,030	Ague	57
Superficial ulcers of cornea	190	Bronchitis and asthma	90
Deep ulcers of cornea	27	Pulmonary consumption	8
Pterygium	98	Dyspepsia	107
Iritis	9	Anemia	103
Cyclitis	3	Hepatitis	5
Cataract	2	Nasal polypi	3
Night blindness	15	Harelip	1
Asthenopia	20		
		TOTAL	4,075

OPERATIONS PERFORMED.

For cataract	2	For abscess of orbit	2
,, pterygium	98	,, harelip	1
,, entropion	160	,, nasal polypus	3
		TOTAL	266

图 6　杜思韦特医生所提供的温州普通医院与鸦片吸食者治疗医院
首份年度报告统计

　　值得注意的是，在戒断鸦片后，病人会迅速出现遗精现象，这应与病人之前在妓院中，为了延长性高潮，将鸦片作为壮阳药服用有关，因此不断吸食鸦片所导致的阳痿现象，也就不足为奇。如果鸦片能够导致阳痿，那么对于经常有人认为吸鸦片是中国的全国性恶习的说法，就可以通过评估中国的人口增长，来进行检验。

　　据《鸦片海关报告》①显示——第一，如果每个人平均消费 3 钱鸦片，那么外国供应的鸦片数量仅能满足 100 万人的需求；第二，中国总人口约为 3 亿；第三，中国本土鸦片产量至少与进口鸦片数量相当，因此吸烟者仅占到总人口的 1/200。② 一般情况下，除了较少例外，只有部分男性吸鸦片，这些受害者没有人会在 20 岁以下，根据我们所能掌握的更为精确的数

① 《中国帝国海关·特辑·第 4 册·鸦片》，据海关总税务司命令出版，上海：总税务
　　司署造册处，1881 年。
② 原文作 1/300，根据作者提供的数据，那么吸烟人口起码应该在 200 万人以上，即
　　吸烟人口要占到总人口的 1/200 以上，而不是 1/300。——译者注

字，中国 20 岁以上吸食鸦片的人数大约超过 600 万①。也许我们可以说，中国有 1/60 的成年男性消费外国鸦片，而同等数量的人消费本土鸦片；换言之，20 岁以上的成年男性中大概有 3.5%② 的人吸鸦片。另外，根据我本人所做的调查，中国本土鸦片增长的数量是外国进口数量的 4 倍以上，这可能表明相当大比例的女性也在消费鸦片。鉴于中国人口的不断增长还能造成生计压力，情况或许不如想象的那么糟糕，但考虑到这些烟瘾者的后代肯定会不断退化，并且也会承续这一趋势，继续沉迷于这种令人阳痿的癖好，那么对于统计估算进行藐视，或对政治经济学家的看法视而不见，就显得罪大恶极了。③

中国药物学的价值理应受到认可，目前也已受到外国人的关注，因此中国的食物学也值得进行研究。中国有关烹饪和饮食的规定相当多。比如，中国人会特别注意一顿饭当中有哪些食物不能同时食用；食物在单独食用时是健康的，但混合食用时可能就会对身体有害，甚至产生毒素。最为典型的例子就是蜂蜜和葱混合在一起。在有些省份，常有人借此法自杀，因此死亡的案例常常能够见诸报端。《本草》曾引用过伟大医生孙思邈的观点（在 7 世纪初被封为医圣），认为生葱和蜂蜜混在一起会导致腹泻，如果是炒过的葱和蜂蜜混在一起则会致人死命。毫无疑问，将这两种食材混在一起相当不明智，长久以来，中国的医学权威都普遍认为这种混合会产生毒素。类似的，蜂蜜和枣也不能同时食用。鳝鱼和甘蔗也不能一起吃。最近上海就有因为同时食用螃蟹和柿子而死人的报道。

为了寻找有关色盲的信息，我已经在帝国内的诸省份搜寻多年，我会找到诸如画家、染工，以及其他同颜色打交道的从业者，然后询问他们是否在视觉上存在缺陷，但我并没有找到色盲存在的证据。最近，通过杜思韦特先生，我获得了他在本地医院的帮助，有超过 1000 人提出申请，希望在这所戒烟所里获得解脱，而我则借此机会对申请人进行了检查。另外我

---

① 原文作 6000 万，但 6000 万这个数据明显不合逻辑，根据后文内容，应是 600 万的笔误。——译者注
② 根据作者原意，吸食鸦片者比例应为 1/30，即约 3.33%。——译者注
③ 一部公正的中国鸦片编年史，定不会忽略一些作者对乡村地区鸦片种植的评论。在去年（1880 年）11 月，半官方的《新报》（*Hsin Pau*）就曾以相当聪明的笔调，为鸦片种植和在经济方面的可利用性进行辩护。

还对炮艇①船员进行了体检，检查的结果是，我没有找到道尔顿症（色盲）存在的证据。② 即便色盲在中国存在，也一定极为罕见，没有证据能够证明，中国人视力或感知器官存在缺陷，相反在华的欧洲人和美国人却存在这样的疾病，这似乎是在暗示色幻觉是种族性疾病。根据对印度铁路工人应征者的体检，发现了色盲患者，这些色盲患者可能并不是纯种的当地人，而是印欧混血人。最近的研究发现，努比亚人也完全没有色盲这种缺陷。

根据调查显示，在美国人和欧洲人当中，有5%~7%③的人是色盲，他们不能正常区分红色和绿色，比如信号灯的颜色。中国沿海有上百名或更多的引水员，其中有些人就因为是色盲而不被允许从事这一职业。最近西方也在立法进行这种常规色盲检测。在巴尔的摩，最近就有一位引水员由于不能区分红色和绿色而被撤销了从业执照，尽管他有25年的从业经历；这样的例子显示，虽然存在这样的缺陷，但是并没有造成严重后果，重要的是海事当局通常不会关心职员识别正确颜色的能力；同时巴尔的摩的案例似乎证明了波尔先生④的观点，他自己就患有"二色视觉症"，对于色盲的机器操作者和领航员而言，他们不会比正常人出现更多错误，不会把红色当成绿色，也没有火车或船只因为这样的问题而出现事故。

种牛痘在许多省份取得进展。大城市的儿科医生，经常会在日常工作中施行种痘，但施行这项新技艺最多的人，却是那些专门以此为职业的种痘师。不幸的是，这项伟大进步的推行，并不是一帆风顺。令人不安的是，种痘师的疏忽或欺诈，会使全社会因为种痘作伪而感到失望。一场不同寻常的天花流行，由于毒性有轻有重，也会使得人们不再相信天花种痘的效果，从而导致灾难性的后果。如果人们看到"种痘"无效，可能会因此失去对天花预防的信心——这种危险正在威胁社会，知府有必要下令只

① 海关巡逻艇"凌风"（Ling Feng）号船长法罗（Captain Farrow），以及一些大清帝国炮艇的船长，非常友好地允许我对他们的船员进行体检。

② 色盲患者会将检查用的彩虹色认作是暗褐色，有些患者则会认作为黑色，顺带一提，黑色在中国相当流行。

③ 威尔逊医生（Dr. Wilson）在1154人中（这些都是接受体检的人），发现有17.7%都是色盲。

④ 《道尔顿症》（*Daltonism*），威廉·波尔撰，皇家学会会员，《当代评论》（*Contemporary Review*）1880年5月。

符合资格并有执照的人，才能施行种痘。杜思韦特先生告诉我，金华的佛教僧侣也在施种牛痘，他们的寺庙最近接纳了无数怀抱啼哭婴儿的母亲。母亲们相信，通过僧侣向佛祖的祈祷，种痘一定会成功；类似于兄弟会，人们会围在现场，举行神秘又壮观的仪式，金华的僧侣看起来已经在当地垄断了这种新式种痘技术。同样的，施行牛痘的世俗医生，在种痘过程中也会强迫病人举行一些超自然的仪式，医生们会指引处在潜伏期的病人，去某些神庙进行朝拜。一名当地的基督教种痘师由于不愿意采用这种欺骗手段，反而失去了所有的病人，迫使他另谋他职。

目前来看，牛痘接种并不会迅速取代人痘接种，人痘接种技术是由西藏（1023~1055年）传入，这种方法可以缓和天花的毒性，而正如我前文所述，天花是一种输入性疾病，它是由名将马援从当时湖北的化外之地带回中国的。

在《自然》杂志上，有两位作者发表了有关"手部皮沟"的研究，他们向我咨询了中国的相关情况。① 正如标题所示，这是一个同时关系到法医学和人种学的问题，本报告的以下内容，正好回应他们的问题。

根据福尔茨医生在日本对指纹的观察，发现指纹具有种族性和某种遗传性。赫谢尔先生则从政府机构的角度来研究这个问题，他在印度主管20年的文书登记工作，在印度用手盖印与亲笔签名具有同等效力，以此为手段防止冒名和抵赖。杜利特尔在他的作品《中国人的社会生活》中曾描述过类似风俗。我现在还没能查到当地将手印视作亲笔签名的文献。对于这种做法是否在古代法庭适用，我感到怀疑。当地见多识广的人告诉我，他们认为手印流行于汉代之后；果真如此的话，那么就可以证明，埃及发现的手印是世界上最早的手印。目前，中国的衙门会要求犯人在签署认罪状时，按下拇指指纹——男右女左——根据记载，这与古代埃及的情况类似，古埃及会要求犯人在认罪时用拇指指甲盖印——这与中国用手指头盖印的做法非常像。这种手印被称作"指模"，在中国的法庭具有重要意义。没有犯人的供状，任何犯人都不能被合法处决，而供状必须要有犯人的手印才能生效。虽然没有直接的强制力要求罪囚按手印，但顽固的罪犯

---

① 两位作者是东京筑地医院的福尔茨（Henry Faulds）与英国牛津的赫谢尔（W. J. Herschel），在《自然》上发表的日期分别为：1880年10月28日和1880年11月25日。

也许会遭到拷打，直到他愿意在判处死刑的供状上按手印为止。在军队里，为了防止冒名顶替，也会采取手指画押的方式；温处镇总兵就在他的军队中推行了这项制度。对于文书而言，如果采用这样的形式，就不会被轻易伪造，而且相较于照片，也更难抵赖——指纹还不止这么简单，在人的一生中，虽然外形可能发生巨大改变，但指纹会陪伴一个人从摇篮走进坟墓；时光不会在指纹上留下一丝褶皱。军队造册，除了要描述一个人的外貌，还要备注上此人手指螺旋形指纹与松树状指纹的数目。这叫记"螺纹"，中国人将梭形螺纹称作"箕"，螺旋纹则被称作"斗"。① 在某些民事契约中，尤其是卖儿卖女的契约，由于当事人不会写字，就会被要求按手印，以防止冒名或抵赖。当有人卖子女时，他的父母需要在卖身契上按下指纹；当一名男子想要休妻时，也需要在休书上用整个手掌盖印；当有人想要卖掉自己的妻子时，买家需要卖家的双手、双脚全部在契约上蘸墨盖印。中国的专业算命师傅几乎可以通过任何身体器官，去预知未来，这里面当然也包括手相，但指纹并不会受到特别关注。业余的算命师，就如吹嘘头部"隆起"的颅相学家一样——实在是很浅薄。这些业余算命师认为，幼童手指"斗"与"箕"的数量，就能决定他们未来的命运，俗话说得好："如有九斗，一世不愁。"

从种族学的角度来开，我发现中国人的指纹与欧洲人的指纹，没有什么相异之处。依据我的观察，极少会有构造一致的指纹，从法医学的角度看，指纹可能具有重大价值，但我并不认为指纹存在遗传性。

奎宁因其具有抗疟疾的价值，深受中国人青睐，但令人遗憾的是，由于价格高昂，大多数百姓并不能获取这种药物；这是国家之恶，在温州地方政府理应关注这个问题，我有理由相信，温州府应该做出更多努力，以减轻疟疾所造成的痛苦。

从荷兰人和英国人在爪哇与印度试种金鸡纳树的结果看，上述地区都适合移植金鸡纳树，因此我认为非常有必要，把这种做法推广到云南和帝国其他南方诸省。另外一个值得种植的诱因是，金鸡纳种植园已经成为印度当地税收的重要来源，其生产的金鸡纳富含生物碱，每英亩的产量大约

---

① 晚清军队中，除了"花名册"外，常常还会有一本"箕斗册"。——译者注

价值8000美元①。虽然金鸡纳树已经在各国成功移植，但随着南美的金鸡纳树林遭到迅速破坏，世界范围内一定会出现奎宁荒。借此之时，我非常希望看到帝国中央政府，或是南方的各总督，能够采取行动，大规模地引进这种桉属树木，以预防对帝国最大利益造成损害的疟疾热。在无数被热病折磨的村庄里，潜伏着村民们狡猾的敌人，一些私商已经开始引进和种植这种桉属树木，在这些无价树木的树荫足以为村民们提供庇护之前，商人们必须寻求并得到政府的帮助。我曾在中国做过最为成功的尝试，是由霍巴特镇植物园的阿伯特博士向我慷慨提供的种子和指导，我选择了能够在南部最高纬度和最高海拔生长的种子，希望它们能够经受住上海或宁波的寒冬。但我在上述港口试种的金鸡纳树大多死掉了，很少有树能够挺过三年，也许在更靠南的区域种植会得到较好的结果。

根据最新的观察，还不能充分确定这些抗瘴气的异域树木是否可以在阿尔及利亚和加利福尼亚存活，即便金鸡纳木的预防药性被夸大，由于其木材的独特价值，② 大规模栽种也还是有利可图。像最近左宗棠大臣在甘肃的种树行为，与历史上任何壮举相较，都可以说是无与伦比，他在甘肃引进了有用的植物，这样的伟业不需要大肆宣传就能获取人们的支持。

现在帝国政府支持外国年轻科学家的研究，但以科学研究名义进行的人体解剖请求，通常仍会遭到拒绝。无论是在陆军还是海军，一名正式合格的外科医生，如果没有尸体进行解剖，就不能有效地展示人体构造，解剖学知识是军事艺术最重要的分支，③ 而这方面的知识必须通过实体解剖

---

① 根据1880年上海出版的《画图新报》第一期的记载，当时上海一瓶上等奎宁价值3美元，劣等价值0.5美元。又根据1888年《申报》上济和堂的医药广告，奎宁每瓶1美元，而乌鸡白凤丸仅要100钱。——译者注

② 我曾专门叙述过金鸡纳树，相关内容已经在傅兰雅先生（Mr. Fryer）编的《格致汇编》中出版。1879年，郭姓前任大臣（ex - Minister Kuo）为此向我索要种子，希望能够在南方的湖南成功种植（这里的郭姓大臣极有可能是湖南湘阴人郭嵩焘，据《郭嵩焘先生年谱》，郭氏于1879年3月26日迫于国内舆论压力，辞去公使职务，自英国回到上海）。

③ 玛高温医生在这里是想利用清政府重视军医的态度，迂回的为人体解剖开禁。晚清政府偏重军医发展的纲领性文件，可以参考1901年张之洞和刘坤一的《江楚变法会奏三折》，其中提到"至医学一门，以卫生为义，本为养民强国之一大端，然西医不习风土，中医又鲜有真传，止可从缓，惟军医必不可缓。"——译者注

才能获得。目前在人体解剖这一问题上，还是谨慎为好，但我相信流行的偏见一定会迅速被克服。即便保守如中国，也能在古代找到解剖的先例，我们应该提醒中国人关于孝武帝①用犯人进行活体解剖的典故，援引此先例，也许可以说服中国人用死刑犯尸体进行解剖。459 年②，悦般国使团抵达北魏皇宫，悦般国起先属于匈奴部落，其南部边境是天山山脉的火山地带。使团中有一名幻人，自称能够割人喉脉，击人头令骨陷，虽血出盈斗，但只要用了他的药，伤口就会止血并愈合，且不会留下疤痕！如果不是渴望推动医学知识的进步，那么必定是在好奇心的驱动下，皇帝下令用一名囚犯进行试验。试验的结果相当成功，一个月内，囚犯的伤口完全得到了愈合。皇帝厚赏了这名幻人，并开始推动这项研究。值得注意的是，这种具有神奇疗效的草药，在中国的各大名山中都能找到。③

在之后的朝代里，我们发现有一名总督，他为了探究解剖学，下令取出了 40 名罪犯、孕妇和儿童的内脏，并且让有经验的医生对内脏进行检验。④ 这里可能有相当大的争议，即一个有好名声的皇帝，是否应该让囚犯遭受解剖，但如果一名总督如此残忍地进行活体解剖都无罪的话，那么知府当然可以将被斩首的尸体用于解剖，想想看温州城的百姓是多么热切地希望目睹刽子手，从罪犯身上活生生地掏出心脏来，所以只要小心行事，就不会引发众怒：温州常有上千人亲眼见证残忍的行刑，而被挡在外面看不到的人，还会对前者艳羡不已。

中国人公开进行处决，是希望多少能够遏制犯罪，但现在尸体切割所带来的刺激，却逐渐变为一种所有阶层都能享受的娱乐。代表中国医学领

---

① 据《太平寰宇记·一百八十六卷》和《北史·西域传（第九十七卷)》，这里应该是北魏"太武帝"，而不是"孝武帝"。——译者注

② 据《太平寰宇记》和《北史》，此事发生在太武帝真君九年，应为公元 448 年，玛高温医生的推算有误。——译者注

③ 《太平寰宇记》(976—983)，第 186 卷。据《四库全书总目》介绍，这部著名的地理学著作，目前全书尚存 193 卷，但原书不止此数。根据我的阅读，我找到了对悦般国的如下描述："日三澡漱，然后饮食。"值得注意的是，这并不是蒙古部落的生活习惯。

④ 《中华帝国自然历史录丛》(法文)，第 8 册，第 261 页。此论丛由耶稣会士韩伯禄创办。——译者注

域最高权威的《本草》①，也能找到支持解剖的证据。该书记载，曾有一名贵人，与家奴同时出现腹痛的病症。家奴不久因病死去，此人于是将其尸体剖开，发现了一只赤眼白鳖，他用尽各种药物，都无法杀死这只白鳖；一次偶然的机会，他得知马溺可以溶化白鳖，他推测马溺虽然迄今仍是一种未知的药物，但一定能解决他的腹痛问题；于是他试着喝下马溺并得到了治愈。自此之后，药典在记载治疗内脏肿痛和其他许多疾病时，马溺都会享有崇高的地位。如果此人不是对家奴进行过解剖的话，也许我们永远都没法知道马溺的医药价值。通过援引上述事实，也许能够逐渐让中国人，接受我们提出的革新。

气象信息补充，1882 年 1 月——中国海出现了相当多且颇具毁灭性的台风，给今年画上了句号，根据记录，今年至少发生 20 次以上的台风，最后一次台风大概在 12 月末。必须承认，某些气旋被重复统计过两次，但这样的异常气象，确实是空前的。值得注意的是，4 月末频繁出现大雾天气，与平时相比，大雾持续的时间更长，范围更广。哥伦布对在好望角所遭遇的雾有如下描述："可能只有刀才能把它们切开"，这段话非常适合形容 4 月末的温州海岸和扬子江。此外，在 12 月份，大气压力指数非常高，许多地方的指数都大过以往。温州虽然地处 30.02 等压线，但无液气压计显示温州的气压达到了 31.20。这与江海关的标准气压计并不相符。根据《申报》记载，今年气候极端反常，江苏和浙江北部都出现了多次瘟疫流行——秋疫流行，幼儿受害最深，12 月开始苏州出现了产褥热病情。有许多患者不治身亡，最近在十天之内，有几十位妇女被这种流行病夺走了生命。

① 这段材料可以参考《本草纲目·五十卷·马》。据《本草纲目》，李时珍这段材料引自东晋祖台之的《志怪》，另外东晋干宝的《搜神记》也有相同记载。——译者注

瓯海关《医报》(1881.10.01—1882.09.30)

玛高温医生有关温州健康的报告

温州外国居民人数有限，过去一年多能免于疾病，但由于雨季格外漫长，热病与霍乱性疾病流行多于以往，温州良好的总体卫生状况至此中止。穷人是主要受害者，除了要忍受恶劣的居住条件之外，他们还要因为稻谷为淫雨所毁，而遭受粮食价格上涨的痛苦。从卫生角度看，下半年情况恐怕也不容乐观。令人遗憾的是，由于杜思韦特先生将内地会医院迁往烟台，在此港口进行有关疾病调查的机会已不复存在。

本次雨季不仅妨碍当地一般卫生状况，而且起始早、持续长、雨量大过往年——由此造成一场灾难性洪水，洪水横扫南山北部流域，导致本省西南尽数糜烂，赣、皖两省南部、鄱阳湖与扬子江下游同样泛滥成灾。初经劫难，骤然之间，我们也难以搞清楚，上述天灾到底在多大程度上能够被证明引发了诸种疾病。

中国流行病备录

《海关医报》卷首的总税务司通令强调要重点关注各地流行病问题，并进行所谓的普查式研究；因此我认为，当发现相关疾病在帝国境内流行时，无论身在何处港口，都应详尽地将其记述在医报内。

我掌握到的内陆流行病相关信息主要来自华文报纸记者，这是我接下来所述内容的主要资料来源；本文资料虽略显单薄，但对气候学与流行病科学也不无贡献。

通过观察这些华文报纸上的医类信息，我认识到气象与地气影响是造成疾病的原因。1881年夏季气候格外反常，再加上紧接着秋、冬两季的情况，能够很好阐述我的上述理论。反常天气包括一系列台风，共计有二十场，其中一些持续影响到秋季。接着温州出现"暖冬"现象，与今年欧亚大陆北部地区所流行的天气状况很类似；起码就欧洲东北部来讲，确实出现了前所未有的暖冬。随后，华北地区河港开始出现封冻，而解冻则早于往年。同时，中国冬季气压指数往往很高，而温州本年尤其高于往年。只有通过统计数字，才能确定气象环境对公共卫生的影响；但由于缺乏生命统计资料，我们也许可以利用某些具有内在一致性的"民俗学"知识作为替代。通过各地零星报道，能够清楚地发现，当大气状况能够影响到大面积区域时，如果出现低压气旋就不会出现传染病扩散，如果出现高压反气旋则会发生疾疫流行。

我将附上一年内我所找到的全部华文报纸上的公共卫生信息，并依据季节将其分为四个部分——这个方案较为符合中国习惯，他们通常认为某种类型疾病，差不多总会在一年中的特定时期流行；举例来讲，春季有"疫"，如斑疹伤寒和天花；夏季有"痧"，如痉挛性霍乱；秋季有"痢"，如腹泻和疟疾；冬季有"瘟"，如良性热病。

1881 年 10 月、11 月和 12 月

南京（古都，位于扬子江右岸）——记者注意到，在早秋时节，由于反常高温，造成许多人中暑。9 月 20 日阵雨，略有降温，但随后气温又迅速回升，即便静处也汗如雨下，夜晚简直难以入眠——不久出现了恶性霍乱流行，幼儿受害最多。

秋季，南京城里田鼠出现异常死亡。死鼠最早在江对岸出现，不久，古都西郊也发生类似情形。老鼠最初从邻近住宅的洞里涌出来，随后不断跳跃、翻滚，最后扑地而死。人们将死鼠装在箱篓里，直接丢进水渠。与平常所见相比，这些死鼠毛色暗淡且尾巴更短。这表明底层土壤明显有毒，与瘴气引发云南鼠疫（然后再由老鼠传染给高级动物与人）的情况类似。庆幸的是，南京地下的瘴气没有对地表生物造成影响，地下动物之间也没有出现交叉传染。

苏州（地处湖区，坐落在扬子江之南、大运河之上——该城是丝绸文化的中枢，也是天下户口繁盛的膏腴之地）——去年夏季，由于寒暑交错，疟疾与肠道疾病肆虐流行，幼儿害病最多。有关瘟神降临的消息广为流传，民众放弃寻医求药，寺庙内反而人山人海，常规治疗被完全忽视。

恶劣的健康状况，从夏季一直延续到秋季；疾疫蔓延超出了医生的能

力，他们无法对病人进行适当照料——造成疾病的原因，在于不合时宜的寒风，再加上间歇性的炎热天气所致。疟疾（ague）和腹泻（diarrhea）极为流行，且非常致命，尤其是 10 岁以上幼儿，往往患病当日即夭折。有些情况下，甚至会出现全家同时死亡的惨事。

扬州（坐落在扬子江之北、大运河之上，地形特点与后文所述的汉口类似）——夏季过后，气候更为炎热，无数致命的霍乱病例开始出现，而治愈率尚不及 20%。与此同时，兽瘟开始在牛、马、猪、狗等家畜中流行。除兽瘟外，宁波与汉口也传来类似消息，上海亦遭其害，本次时疫异常盛行。极有可能是沿着浙江与江苏北部海岸进行传播。

汉口，据 11 月 22 日报道——11 月以来，气候异常温暖，民众仍需穿夏衣，且飞蚊成群；由于异常炎热的天气，汉口患病人数很多，但并不致命。当地母鸡死亡率极高；这些家禽患病往往相当突然，并很快奄奄一息。

1882 年 1 月、2 月和 3 月

杭州（位于钱塘江、杭州湾河口，为大运河起点）——据报道，2 月初时，冬季气候寒热无常，导致幼童中出现大量炎症病例，一些患上喉症的儿童由于没有得到及时治疗，数小时内即遭丧命（可能指的是"白喉"）；至该报道撰稿为止，天花流行依旧存在，虽然采取了一切预防措施，保证孩子们待在家里，饮食也被严格管控，但仍有幼童患上天花。此外，那些 40～50 岁、接受过种痘的人被限制不能离床，他们脸上往往长满脓包；这些人虽然看起来病情严重，但不致命，7 天后即可自动康复。当地医生认为疫症是由风气不畅、四时不正所致——再加上寒热无常——同时他们认为疫症属于假性天花——水痘（可能指的是"水痘"）。水痘往往被认为是春季健康状况良好的吉兆。

苏州——当地夏、秋两季健康状况恶劣，人们认为冬季可能会有所好转，但棘手的疫症依旧流行，目前出现了产褥热病例，其治愈率尚不及 1/10；人们发现对此疾病束手无策。数日之内，几十名妇女相继病逝。另外一篇报道指出，由于伤寒热流行如此之广，妇女患病人数如此之多，甚至导致织物价格看涨。

扬州——去年冬季气候温和，继之以雨雪，来年必是丰年。但当地阴

（寒）阳（热）不调，致使疾疫流行，尤其是幼童，多患喉症，数小时内即遭丧命——目前人们对于其病理还一无所知。

1882 年 4 月、5 月和 6 月

南京——冬季温和少雨，导致春季健康状况恶劣；春季一般性疾病多为慢性病，极难治愈。

南昌（位于鄱阳湖南岸），据 5 月报道——前一季节，气候极为多变——晴雨无常，寒热交错，继之以狂风暴雨，暴雨带来的降温导致疾病高发，虽不致命，但极难治愈。症状看起来与疟疾类似，但绝非疟疾；病人状况时好时坏——这有点像是某种特殊病，应谨慎防治。另外，当地还出现了猪瘟，有人因为食用瘟猪肉而生疮。

广州，据 5 月 10 日报道——粤省出现旱情，导致在有些地区，近一半粮食歉收。且疾疫流行，幼童患病最多。一场雨后，严峻形势方得缓解。

1882 年 7 月、8 月和 9 月

扬州——7 月，该城及邻近地区，再次出现霍乱流行。一年之前，有近 4 万人染疫，而本次霍乱肆虐更甚以往。上次霍乱，是自北向南传播。今年路径则相反，疫病是自南向北传播；霍乱疫潮甚至北及京津，两地都出现了轻度病例。不幸的是，一个月后，这一地区又出现了三种类型的热病。第一种类型患者主要是男性，由于寒风胜于暑热，因此引发热病，其病情复杂多变，有些病人在患病第 7 天至第 10 天，病情会发生变化，开始退烧并且康复；另有一些病人，在患病第 3 天至第 5 天，病情发生变化，其全身会出现瘀斑并最终死亡。第二种类型患者主要是女性，患者首先会浑身发冷，然后发热，症状持续不退；还会伴随出现嘴巴干涩的症状，而降温疗法则完全无效；此病生还率不及 20% ~ 30%。第三种热病患者主要是幼童，患者首先感到发冷，同时满脸出现斑疹，与麻疹类似；如果出疹明显，表明病情正在好转，如若不然，病情可能发展为锁喉症，最终致人死命。

广州，据 8 月 1 日报道——该城突然出现疫情，患者首先会极度口渴并大量出汗，随后嘴部流涎，舌缩入喉，并窒息而死。医生指出，对于这种病症，用热猪油滴在舌头上，即可帮助舌头复原。

汉口（位于长江左岸，地处汉水河口）——据当地医生报告，秋季出现了腹泻病例，患者在初期如果不接受治疗的话，则会变得相当棘手。同时，疟疾（agues）异常频发，春季往山东运粮的船夫，常因此丧命。这些船夫在回程途中开始出现腹泻，这是在山东水土不服的缘故，因此船夫患疟疾的人数格外多。

苏州——该城同样遭受霍乱肆虐。之前出现过疟疾与腹泻流行；从这些疾病的持续时间看，可能属于慢性型。

宁波——夏末，由于天气炎热，宁波当地发生了一场牛瘟；随后瘟疫扩散至马、狗及山羊。通常家畜很容易染上瘟疫，但像本次这样的规模，并不常见。奶牛和水牛，两三次拉稀之后必死无疑，病情通常仅持续数小时。1778 年也发生过类似牛瘟，其烈性之强，超过以往人类所知的任何一次——造成 80% 的牛死亡。这并不是一种新瘟疫，虽然众所周知，但却唯独 1778 年这一次来得格外猛烈。此后，每年秋季都会发生牛瘟。

宁波南部山区的奉化和台州，出现了病菌栖息地（指的可能是炭疽杆菌），这种微生物常使得牛患上脾病，当地极少有牛能够幸免。同时，当地还出现了马瘟，可能是马鼻疽；上海的矮种马几乎在同时也染上了这种疾病。有关犬类流行病的消息，相对较少。患病犬会突然出现痉挛，并迅速死亡。为人所熟知的是，中国犬类会因为丝虫（filaria）堵塞心脏而死。宁波的狂犬病病例似乎相当多，每年总会发生几起致死病例。

台湾北部——一支布防在台湾北部的湘军分遣队，全都染上了热病；报道中没有提到热病类型，目前仅能知道这种热病能够致人死亡。目前人们发现，相比于沿海地区，内陆地区的人更难适应台湾的水土。其间多雨天气，士兵又被派往筑路，这使得他们更易染病；再加上缺医少药，使得情况雪上加霜。

瓯海关《医报》（1883.04.01—1883.09.30）

玛高温医生有关温州健康的报告

　　自温州第一次遭到印度霍乱侵袭之后，总是会反复出现流行。值得注意的是，截止到目前①，温州今年夏季没有出现霍乱流行。但中国其他地区，从广州到牛庄，从海滨一直延伸到宜昌甚至更西的广大区域，都出现了霍乱流行。最近，有一人因为食用河豚中毒。另外我最近有机会观察麝香作为一种药物的价值，中国人普遍将麝香当作药材使用，除此之外没有什么值得报告。

　　有一名海关职员长期遭受风湿病的折磨，在台湾时几乎被泡在碘化钾里接受治疗，又因为患上疟疾要依靠金鸡纳进行治疗，最近又患上腰椎痛，忍了 10 天后，病人才开始寻求医治。他在看病之前，已经自行使用过药物，他在整个腰椎部位都涂抹了松脂油。有 4 晚的时间，疼痛让他无法入睡。我使用了一些常见的中国麝香药膏（仅仅一小撮），并在其中加入了大概 4 格令的麻醉药。两小时后病人安然入睡；第二天早上病人痛感明显消退，三天后症状完全消失。

　　与此同时，我以同样的方案治疗了一名脚踝扭伤的外国居民。

　　这名病人大约在扭伤 11 小时后开始接受治疗。与常见的意外事故类似，病人受伤部位出现肿胀，且疼痛难忍。在接受治疗 10 小时后，病人疼痛减轻，并且能够入睡，第二天早上关节部只有按压时才会出现痛感。15天后病人部分恢复了行走能力。数天之后，除了关节部有略微僵硬并持续一段时间外，病已经完全恢复。血管破裂造成局部青紫，大概持续了 5个星期，可见损伤的严重性。

　　中国人告诉过我一些在短时间内恢复的严重病例。在上述病例中，对

---

① 两周之后，霍乱开始肆虐，并且流行了数星期之久，但范围并不广。

病人使用水蛭吸血疗法并无效用，而擦剂疗法或其他疗法的治疗周期往往是使用麝香的四倍。

通过中国作家们的翻译，麝香在西方早已闻名遐迩。麝香有两个来源，一为西部省份的麝香鹿，一为常见于华中地区的灵猫。

麝香鹿遍布于云南、四川、西藏的山地。这种动物非常胆小，常常因为受到惊吓而致死。它们以杜松叶、爬行类动物为食；在它们的胃里曾找到过蛇骨。春天时，这种动物的腺囊开始肿胀。作为分泌物的麝香就会随尿液被排出体外。麝香鹿常会在同一个地方撒尿，并用泥土掩盖尿液。这种地方往往能够得到优质麝香，分量有时能达到 15 斤之多。

当地一名旅行者曾这样描述麝香鹿：

> 麝香鹿习惯在自己的尿液上打滚，以此让自己凉快，并止腺囊的痒。尿液的气味会引来无数蚂蚁，它们会爬上去尽情享用这顿大餐。麝香鹿借由蚂蚁的叮咬止痒，再通过括约肌的闭合，达到赶走蚂蚁的目的。这样的行为反复出现，在蚂蚁的帮助下，雄鹿（母鹿身体里没有麝香）的腺囊得以生产出硬质、类似橡胶的块状麝香。

这篇文章认为，最有价值的东西正是麝香鹿在地上的遗留物，这些颗粒如珍珠般宝贵。麝香的刺激性非常强烈，如果把它们放在花园或树林里，会导致植物无法结出果实。另外麝香鹿小便的地方植物会出现枯死现象，也能反映出新鲜麝香的毒性。麝香能够导致一定范围内的植物绝迹，更远一些则会导致叶子枯黄。有一些植物会对麝香更为敏感，比如荔枝树就很忌讳麝香。如果麝香靠鼻子太近，则会导致炎症，鼻孔里会生出白色的蠕虫。

据记载，742～755 年，一位渔人捕捉的一种珍贵物种被饲养于宫中。用针刺激腺囊，产出的强效麝香单颗重量超过一加仑，混合一半水后的水麝，哪怕在衣服上涂上一点也会芳香扑鼻。取香之后再用雄黄帮助麝恢复伤口。另有一种心结香，是麝因惊吓死后形成的干血块；这种心结香并不在体内形成。对于猎人来讲，麝肉能够解多种蛇毒。在果树林里捕蛇的猎人，往往会在大拇指的指甲上涂上一点麝香，以此防患于未然。

这种有价值的物质从猎人的手上一脱手，马上会被大量掺假出售，往往真香只有 10% 左右。能够实实在在享用这种药物的效力实在是很幸运的事。另外，可以通过麝香内部的毛发来判断其真伪。假的麝香往往用麝腹皮包裹，并混杂灵猫香，极难分辨。

麝香不能与葱属食物共服；长时间随身携带麝香会导致不同寻常的疾病。麝香能够驱毒包括凶邪鬼气；能够驱虫，且能够治疗蛇毒；可以杀死某些植物。若风在骨中，麝香能够祛除风湿，但若是风在皮肉之间，麝香反而会引风入骨，疼痛更甚。昏厥的人在使用麝香后，一经恢复就要停止用药。麝香还能够治疗瓜果食积。麝香只能当作刺激性药物使用，不能作为补药使用。能够治疗各种热病，并有助于难产。一种非常流行的说法是麝香具有巨大的效力，能够用来堕胎，犯罪者往往将其放入酒中一并服下。作为一种安神药物，麝香被广泛使用将麝香放在枕头上能够助好梦并防止梦魇。在治疗虚脱时，麝香能够发挥类似氨气的效力。麝香作为外敷药使用时，能够治疗痔疮，麝香为此目的被广泛地制成药膏，这种药膏会加入蜡和松脂混合而成。这种药膏往往非常浓稠。药剂师在药物中放入充足的麝香，往往会使药物极受欢迎。由于这个原因，上海的药膏需求广泛。

与麝类似的是灵猫，灵猫分布于华中和华南各省，遍及南海山谷区域。其外貌类似猫和狸，属于灵猫科，因此中文将其称作"灵猫"、"香狸"和"神狸"，中国人描述此种动物为雌雄同体。灵猫的阴囊和麝的很像，因此其分泌物常常被拿来假冒麝香。1683 年 M. 博米特在其药史著作里提到了中国的这些动物，他记述道：

> 我在蓄养这种动物几天之后，发现在墙上和栅栏上出现了油腻物，浓稠呈褐色，味道强烈且难闻，于是我每天都会把灵猫的这种分泌物收集并清除出去，过程中并无麻烦出现，灵猫也不喜欢这些分泌物；数月之后，我收集了大概 1.5 盎司。但这些畜生会自己抹去一些分泌物，如果不是这样，我可能会得到更多。

中国人并不会去养灵猫取香，他们会直接杀死灵猫，并割下腺囊，再泡酒并晒干。

麝香除了入药之外，还被用来制成香水。《帝国海关申报表》里记载了此种货物的数额，1872 年至 1882 年 10 年间，中国共出口了 329.38$^1/_2$ 担麝香，价值 2520364 两关平银。汉口是主要的贸易地点，汉口（除了宜昌之外）是离产地最近的港口。天津麝香产自直隶（河北）与山西，山西的产量更多（见图 1、图 2）。

EXPORT of each PORT for TEN YEARS.

Shanghai	*Piculs*	$43.61\frac{3}{15}$ = *Hk.Tls.*	375,527
Canton	,,	$5.87\frac{7}{8}$,,	26,638
Hankow	,,	$218.30\frac{1}{15}$,,	1,731,581
Tientsin	,,	$27.46\frac{10}{16}$,,	191,047
Ichang	,,	$34.13\frac{1}{2}$,,	195,571
TOTAL	*Piculs*	$329.38\frac{1}{2}$ = *Hk.Tls.*	2,520,364

图 1　各地麝香产量

TOTALS for each YEAR.

	QUANTITY. *Piculs.*	VALUE. *Hk.Tls.*	
Total 1873	$21.23\frac{1}{2}$	118,218, averaging about *Hk.Tls.* 56 per catty.
,, 1874 . . .	$24.64\frac{1}{2}$	148,239 ,, ,, 60 ,,
,, 1875 . . .	$25.23\frac{3}{4}$	164,288 ,, ,, 65 ,,
,, 1876 . . .	$25.03\frac{1}{4}$	209,469 ,, ,, 84 ,,
,, 1877 . . .	$57.53\frac{13}{16}$	479,095 ,, ,, 83 ,,
,, 1878 . . .	$42.85\frac{15}{16}$	374,246 ,, ,, 87 ,,
,, 1879 . . .	$37.84\frac{1}{2}$	267,056 ,, ,, 73 ,,
,, 1880 . . .	41.28	283,016 ,, ,, 69 ,,
,, 1881 . . .	23.61	202,802 ,, ,, 86 ,,
,, 1882 . . .	30.11	273,935 ,, ,, 91 ,,
Total for 10 years, 1873–82 . .	$329.38\frac{1}{2}$	2,520,364 { average value for 10 years about } *Hk.Tls.* 76 per catty.

图 2　历年麝香产量

　　没有数据能够用来估计中国国内的麝香消费情况，也没办法知道前面这些数据所列的麝香被掺入了多少假货（见图 3）。

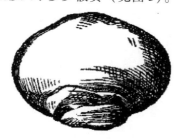

图 3　干燥后的麝香香囊（云南：商店中能够找到的平均尺寸）

食用动物中毒

河豚——病人因为食用河豚而中毒（前文已经提到），情况虽不严重，但常常有人因此丧命，因此我感到有必要将中国人对河豚的研究记录在报告里。

在中国的鱼类著作里，与其他鱼类相比，河豚占据着更重要的地位。陈氏的百科全书①曾引述30位作者，他们在其著作中都提到河豚。很少有鱼类受到如此钟爱，也很少有鱼类会因为含毒而受谴责。如同英国、德国、法国等海洋民族一样，中国人以外形给这种鱼类命名，他们称其为河豚，即"江河中的猪"。河豚在春季时从海洋进入河口，并在扬子江中产卵，为此它们会在江中不顾湍急，逆游将近1000公里。河豚初生时，外貌会显得很胖，此时食用毒性较小。其腹部的肉极为丰腴，被人称作"西施乳"，西施是中国有名的美人。一位作家记述道，河豚之所以肥滑，是因为它食用柳树芽的缘故；但另一位作家反驳这种意见，他认为河豚在柳树发芽之前就已经很肥。如前所述，在长江上游地区，河豚总是与柳树芽同时出现。另一位作家记述，柳树芽对鱼类是有毒的。另外，因河豚有毒，其他鱼类都不敢吃河豚；河豚鼓起来后体积会增大很多。一名超过百岁的作者在12世纪时写了一首有关为吃河豚冒风险的诗作。他首先评价了伟大的诗人苏东坡，并称河豚味美，值得冒死，而像这样的好诗遂成绝响。作者前往在潘阳做学官的朋友处，这位朋友认为南方所产之味美无过于河豚，于是他决定烹饪一些河豚举办宴会。两人落座后宴请宾客入席，就在此时，一只猫扑向餐碟，一直狗也跟着吃起美味；但不久，猫和狗全都中毒而死，宾主全都大吃一惊。他还提到在河南的饭馆里有假河豚菜卖，以他的观点看来，真河豚肉会致命，而假河豚肉只会让食客半死。相比于动物，人似乎不那么怕毒。一位作家提到，猫狗吃河豚总是会死；渔民则说食腐鸟不会吃河豚的内脏，如果这些鸟吃了的话，则会立刻毙命。河豚肝被认为有毒；河豚的眼和血，尤其是接近背部的部分，毒性更强。所有吃河豚丧命的案例，都是因为疏忽而没有采取有效的预防措施，这就需要对江中河豚进行更详细的观察。处理河豚首先要将其彻底洗干净，烹饪的时

---

① 这里的百科全书应是指陈梦雷编纂的《古今图书集成》。——译者注

候一定要煮熟；宁波人十分小心，他们通常会煮 8 个小时。为了进一步确保安全，人们会用中国橄榄或者甘蔗与河豚一起煮。如果有人同时吃河豚和鼠尾草的话，则必死无疑。根据食用河豚不同的部位，中毒情况也会发生变化。河豚的血和肝通常都有毒，食河豚的脂肪会导致舌头肿胀和麻木，食河豚眼则会导致视力下降。在扬子江下游地区，人们吃河豚时会用酒糟将其焖一会儿。有一句谚语是这样讲的，"拼死吃河豚"。女人们用来化妆的胭脂可以解河豚毒，或者用中国橄榄与樟脑一起用水浸泡也能解毒。

虽然地方官员一再发告示，提醒人们不要食用河豚肉，但几乎没有哪个春季不会发生几起河豚中毒事件。最近《申报》上报道，在扬州发生了11 起河豚中毒事故。

有毒的鱼——《宁波地方志》称这种鱼叫"虎鱼"（tiger fish），它的尾巴像针，有毒，可以伤人或杀死其他鱼类；人被蜇伤后会十分痛苦，据说如果将其尾刺扎进树，树会枯死。"虎鱼"和刺猬很像，同时被它咬到也会中毒，肉也有毒。浙江和福建沿海有一种鱼叫"燕红鱼"，这种鱼与"牛尾鱼"很像。"燕红鱼"游速很快，会给潜水采蚌人造成极为疼痛的伤口。更严重的是，"燕红鱼"的尾部有三根刺，也会使人中毒；疼痛会使人日夜呻吟。

人们在嵩阳发现了一种鲟鱼和猪很像，色黄。这种鱼气味难闻，让人不敢靠近，且有毒；尽管如此，这却是进贡给皇帝的食物。

有一种鲶鱼也有毒，尤其是红眼无鳃的鲇鱼。鲇鱼非常忌讳和牛肝、野猪肉或鹿肉一起食用。有一种小心鲨鱼被称为"白鲨"，皮肤坚硬，肉质粗糙，轻微含毒。一些鳗鱼也被认为含毒。有的宁波人在没有人先尝之前，不会吃鳝鱼。人们把鳝鱼养在深水罐里，用强光照时，鳝鱼会跳出来，人们通过这种方法将有害的鳗鱼剔除出去。有些鳝鱼能够把头直立起来，这种鳝鱼不能吃。尾鳍能够直立的鳝鱼也该被丢弃；背部有白斑、无鳃、有"四眼"、肚子上有黑色条纹、重达 4～5 斤的鳝鱼都不能吃。《本草纲目》关于鳝鱼来自死人头发的说法是错的，它们有可能是鳝鱼卵而已。

"石斑鱼"被认为会导致呕吐。这种鱼和蟑螂很像，鱼鳍很长，表面有虎纹。这种鱼没有雄性。据当地记载，雌鱼通过和蛇交配繁衍，其鱼卵有毒。在南方，人们会把这种鱼挂在有黄蜂巢的树上，以吸引鸟类来消灭黄蜂。石斑鱼通常在水面游动，但一碰到人立刻会潜到水底。

还有一种娃娃鱼十分奇特。这种两栖动物生活在山涧地区。其前足像猴，后部像狗；尾巴很长，达到 7~8 英寸；叫声如婴儿，正如其名。娃娃鱼能爬树，因为长时间干燥，因此嘴里总是会含水，它们会在树林里通过树叶和草地来隐藏自己，会把嘴巴张得很大；鸟类因为口渴而喝水时，就会中娃娃鱼的圈套。可以将其吊在树上，让白色流质的毒素全部流出为止。

有一种奇怪的乌龟，书中并无记载，江苏人称其为"灰土龟"或"地公蛇"，因为这种龟的尾巴很长。它会从嘴里喷出类似蜘蛛网的物质和草茎连在一起，被缠住的动物或昆虫就会被吃掉，被捕动物会因为中毒而死；有时人也会因此送命。这种龟被认为眼盲，所以它才会用分泌网来增加触觉。它们通常会在 5 月至 7 月出现。虽然有一定夸大成分，但这却是一种非常有趣的动物。

有的鱼在正常时间被食用很安全，在某些时间段食用就会有害，这些具有周期性的鱼最突出的是鲥鱼。鲥鱼常被制成鱼肝油药物使用。当鲥鱼在扬子江逆流游到四川时，它们在此阶段就会带毒，被称为"有害的鱼"，发生这种变化的原因可能是鲥鱼在长途跋涉过程中过分消耗体力所致。根据监利（湖北一地名）地方志记载，在再也无法向上游动时，它们的速度会像"白色蜗牛"，此时鲥鱼会被大量捕捞；这种捕捞地离海洋大概有 1100 英里。迷信的说法是，女神在它们的头部留下了印记，以将它们留在四川，此时它们变成"有害的鱼"——它们离大海已有将近 1300 英里。鲤鱼有时也会有毒。小溪里会有一种鲤鱼，头部有毒，其背部有两条筋，且血为黑色；这种鲤鱼不能吃。在烹饪鲤鱼时，要避免被烟熏到，否则视力会受到影响。在时疫发生时，或肠不适，或出现便秘，或使用水银时，都不能食用鲤鱼；另外鲤鱼不能和狗肉同时食用。鲈鱼有时也会含有轻微的毒素，即便是著名的松江鲈鱼；如果鲈鱼有"四鳃"，食用就会相当危险；当食鲈鱼中毒时，芦根能够解毒。有一种与鲇鱼类似的鱼会含有轻微毒素。一名作家这样写道，这种鱼"最好与芭蕉叶一同烹饪"。

有些龟也含有毒素，它们的特征为：三足，赤足，独眼，头部或足部不能伸缩，眼部凹陷，腹部有"卜"字纹路，腹部有"王"字纹路，腹部有蛇形图案，这些都不能食用；有一种山地龟被称为"旱龟"，全都不能吃。龟不能和菠菜或是鸡蛋、鸭肉、兔肉一起吃；怀孕妇女如果吃龟肉会导致幼儿短脖；有肺病的人吃了龟后会导致腹部肿胀。这些并非夸大其词，但也可能是误载。不能缩头缩脚的龟被认为是没有"衬"（甲壳边缘的皮质），食用这种龟会导致窒息。有一首金陵谚语，说水龟三足、四足尚可食，五足龟化蛇，六足龟化蝎，含有致命毒素。扬州（江苏）宜城的一座山叫春山，曾在其池塘里找到过三足的龟，被认为是神话人物大禹的化身。这种龟性寒，有毒，食用则死。一个太仓人命他的妻子烹饪三足龟，他吃后躺在床上化为血水，只留下他的头发。他的邻居向知县黄廷深告发寡妇杀夫，知县让一名死刑犯吃下了这种龟肉，死囚立刻化为血水，于是寡妇被当庭释放。博学的《本草纲目》作者，他并不愿轻信其所处时代的上述说法，不相信龟毒足以使人溶解；另一位作者则说吃了之后并不会发生任何事情。另外他还开出了一些含有三足龟的药方。看起来作者没有法医学的观念，知县并没有根据法医学对寡妇进行不利的判决。有时在市场里能够买到三足龟，这可能是在争斗中被咬掉一只足的残疾龟。①

甲壳类动物有时也会有毒；大概有 15 种螃蟹不能食用。螃蟹中毒后，可以服用紫罗勒、芦根汁、南瓜汁或大蒜等。如果妇女在怀孕期间吃了螃蟹，可能会导致胎位不正。螃蟹不能和柿子一起吃。有些含有毒素的螃蟹肉，可以作为打虫药使用。田地和沟渠里的虾也被认为有毒。许多人听过不要吃生蚝的警告，生蚝与其他许多类似的水生贝壳类动物都含有毒素。

毒 鱼

使用毒素毒鱼的方法被称为毒鱼。在远古时代，人类发现了火，并掌握了捕鱼的方法。他们发现死鱼会浮在溪流的表面，于是将有毒的种子抛在水里，鱼吃了后就会浮起来。直到今天，人们还在用这种毒法捕鱼。《古今图书集成》里曾引用过一名作者的话，在中国西部地区，水十分

---

① 这位作者认为三足龟是存在的，但他也引用了另外一位作者对骗子伪造三足蟾蜍的记载，骗子们通过敲碎一足的办法作伪。三足蟾蜍被认为是存在的，在神话时代，它是一种鬼物的坐骑；小孩的帽子上有时会佩戴三足蟾蜍作为护身符。

清澈，人们不用渔网捕鱼，而是在冬季造一艘竹排，在沿河洒下小麦与捣碎的蓼属植物的混合物；鱼吃了后就会浮上，但不久之后鱼会苏醒过来。他们称这种方法叫"醉鱼"。在中国的这些地区，巴豆也常常被用于同样的目的。人们把巴豆磨成粉末抛洒在水里，如同蓼属植物一样，巴豆药性非常强，能够迅速杀死吃了粉末的鱼类和甲壳动物；这些种子会使鱼类的颜色和口感变样，但不会对人体有害。买鱼的人并不会上当，因为从鱼的颜色很明显能够看出差别；但穷人会因为价格便宜买这种鱼。大运河至扬子江流域也有类似的捕鱼方法，知县为了公共健康有时会禁止用这种方法捕鱼。外国人经常会到这些地区旅行，毕竟百闻不如一见。苏州府最近颁布告示，禁止销售"雷公藤"，这种植物能够用来捕杀鱼、龟、贝，且对人体有伤害。在那四个月的时间，这种因为食用毒鱼的病例很常见。

气　象

我要感谢德·阿诺克斯，他向我提供了下列的半年气象观测记录摘要（见图4）。

图 4　瓯海关气象观测记录表

瓯海关《医报》（1883.10.01—1884.03.31）

玛高温医生有关温州健康的报告

在上一次的半年报中，我曾指出，霍乱的传播遍布帝国的许多地区，这座港口却免受其害。但10月中旬我察觉到霍乱开始出现，因此补充了一条脚注进行说明，与此同时，福州、宁波和其他地方的霍乱已经渐渐平息。

在前几个月中，降雨比往常要少，从9月开始疾病多发，与此同时滴雨未下。平时水量充沛的稻田如今已干涸，水渠水量（不再流动，出现停滞）急剧下降，结果造成水渠充斥更多排泄物。值此时节，在江浙两省的海岸冲积平原，某种地气与气象环境很容易诱发发酵病（zymotic disease）。然而，在中国其他地区，类似疾病也会在不同环境中发生，降雨异常通常伴随霍乱的暴发，同时饮用水也会变得非常稀缺且遭受污染。

上一期报告已经提到过1883年暴发的霍乱流行，我补充说明的内容来自当地报刊的摘要。此次霍乱流行范围从广州一直扩展到牛庄的整个沿海地带，甚至从上海扩展到徐州，徐州在扬子江中部的上游区域，距离出海口超过1500英里①；虽然霍乱侵袭了大江中下游所有城镇，但位于支流的城镇未受其害。

成都（四川省会）内地会的爱德华兹医生告诉我，成都没有受到霍乱影响。

广州、汕头、福州、宁波、上海、牛庄、杭州、苏州、扬州、南京、武昌和宜昌的报纸都提到当地出现了霍乱病情，但这些报纸上的信息并没有太大价值。武昌霍乱流行发生在7月和8月（两个月后宜昌也出现了疫情），紧接着是漫长的雨季，直到天气骤然转凉。

---

① 徐州距离上海实际不超过400英里。——译者注

在苏州，药物被证明对霍乱完全无效，最后不得不使用蜗牛进行治疗（病人会出现手指萎缩弯曲的病状），当一些人康复后，人们因而将这种疾病称为"蜗牛头病"。

霍乱在扬州一直徘徊到9月末。据称，在这场传染病中，凡是那些鸦片吸食者都比其他一般人更容易受到传染。

苏州疫情一直延续到10月份，10例病人中有9位丧生。在宁波，霍乱被命名为"午夜月病"，因为这个时间段是该病的发作期和死亡期。"不到1/10的感染者能够幸存下来。"

关于印度霍乱在中国的流行史还有待进一步梳理。以下我所提交的报告所涵盖的信息来自嘉兴徐子墨于1860年出版的《吊脚痧方论》，他认为该种疾病最早出现于1821年。① 徐子墨在书中并未明言疾病来源，但根据宁波医学的传统说法，传染病起源于英国海峡殖民地，然后通过舢板传入福建。疾疫自福建扩展至广东，又进入江西，次及江、浙两省，呈现输入性传染病的特征。

温州的传统说法认为1820年霍乱第一次出现在浙南，如果这种说法是正确的话，那么霍乱从福建传入的可能性极大。我们由此可以接受1820年是印度霍乱第一次出现在中国的起始年份。

这波霍乱慢慢推进至扬子江流域，1825年重庆霍乱暴发的恐怖，至今让人难忘。而向北方向，其传播看起来也是非常迅速，但帝国那一地区的准确信息仍然非常缺乏，从韩国和日本的情况来看，这场霍乱极其致命。

由此在超过40年的时间里，霍乱被认为在流行病学特征的层面上，是遍布帝国各地的地方病，有时霍乱流行会扩展至整个东亚，其他时候则仅在一省或部分省份流行。

在第一次印度霍乱流行中，出现了一个显著和悲剧的谬误。即理论和普遍实践都禁止在温暖气候条件下使用"温药"，同时也禁止在寒冷天气下使用寒药。当这种类型的霍乱第一次流行时，人们仅仅使用寒药，显而

---

① 仅仅一年前，雷夫·W. C. 米尔恩（Rev. W. C. Milne）已经记述过霍乱第一次出现在浙江［见《中国丛报》，《中国出现亚洲霍乱》（ *Chinese Repository* ，"Asiatic Cholera in China"）］，按照规定，1820年应是道光元年。但皇帝下令隔年登基才为元年。

易见的是，一代人的时间过去了，其疗效可谓"百不救一"。我们的作者徐子墨则主张使用相反的温药疗法。在徐子墨的文章中，开篇即提到这种类型的"吊脚痧"古无其名，道光辛巳年（1821）间，才忽起此病。

其症或吐或泻，或吐泻并作，伴有腹痛者，亦有不痛者。肠胃吐泻数次，即两腿抽搐，或手足痉挛，痛愈甚（抽愈甚），顷刻肌肉尽削，渐觉气短声嘶，眼窠落陷，渴欲饮冷，周身冷汗如冰，六脉（每只手腕能够识别出三脉）渐无，半日即死。人患此病，或夕发旦死，或旦发夕死。甚至行路之人，忽然跌倒。或侍候问疾之人，染病先死。

医以寻常霍乱之法治之，百不救一。后知其病起三阴（肺、心、肾），改用温经通阳（积极属性或男性属性，与阴相反，因代表着消极属性和女性属性）之药，如参、姜、附（一种斑叶亮丝草）、桂。病人总是不愿意使用温药，或用药太过保守，导致不能痊愈。富贵人家，尤其不愿意换药。

所可悯者，穷乡僻壤之间，延医不及，城市夜深之际，救治亦难，终至不治。

大抵此症，逢暑热愈炽；值天寒则稍衰。一交冬令，鲜有一日半日便死者；用药虽轻，病人亦能渐趋康复。若在夏秋之间，情况则相反，其症虽轻，而其势骤，倘不急治，或致人死亡。"值此之际"，作者说道，"余乃详载于篇，俾病家可照症选方，惟顾士君子平时识之，以备疾疫。"①

当看到中医药系统描述霍乱作为一种传染病所有症状的非凡恐怖，包括其传染方式，对印度霍乱的命名，以及旧式医生对温补疗法的记述后，中医在接触到此种新传染病的适当疗法的情况下，还会如此长久的存在相当误解，实在令人惊异。中医还会提到睾丸收缩的症状，但在中医著作中，包括徐子墨的著作，都没有提到排尿不畅的症状，在中国有关印度霍乱的报告中，此种症状却常常被提及。

总体而言，印度霍乱不同于中国人所经常提到的霍乱，这种区别仅仅在于其流行特性，前者流动性更强，而后者则固定某一区域。印度霍乱在

---

① 以上内容出自清代徐子墨《吊脚痧方论》，但玛高温医生翻译时在个别字句上已经做了改动，因此译者在回译时仍以玛高温医生英文原文为准，在尊重徐子墨原文的基础上，做适当增减。——译者注

从一个区域传染到另一个区域的过程中，与其发源地恒河流域一样，毫无规律可循，传染往往会跳过某一地区，有时会返回某地造成再次流行，有时又不会。印度霍乱并不是依靠空气或人员进行传播，其遍地暴发似乎在等待合适的土地、大气条件——某地可能有适合的条件，但其相邻地区则可能不具备这样的条件，也可能连续好几年也不会具备适合印度霍乱爆发的条件。印度霍乱的传播历史表明，要么这种疾病是由国外传入的一种特殊微生物所引起，要么从南至北相继暴发疾疫流行，是由于这些地区具备一系列适合致命地方性霍乱流行的环境。

关于苏州霍乱的描述，让我们了解到中国人与西方类似的迷信行为，即相信猫头鹰是凶兆，猫头鹰刺耳的叫声预示着死亡。城市里猫头鹰（枭）尖叫被认为预示着霍乱的来临。人们听到叫声后，会立刻冲出去用火把杀死或赶走它们。猫头鹰看起来会在那些地区不定时出现或消失，其降临往往意味着某人将要死亡。

关于在某些地方发生的驱瘟鬼游行，一位作家在《申报》上做了明智的评论："疾疫流行出自天道，与神、魔无关。民众仰仗迷信，愚昧如狂。"他随后描述了驱鬼的游行过程，他本应该还加上一条这种方法无用的理由。因为这种禳疫游行通常发生在炎热气候下，大量暴露在酷暑环境，再加上过度疲劳，导致参加者更容易受到病变影响。

牛 瘟

1882 年，浙江省北部地区暴发了家畜流行病，流行病波及马、羊和狗——但主要感染者是牛。在上一年，当地牛畜也因同样原因受到严重影响。台州山区曾经暴发过一场牛瘟，当宁波地区的霍乱瘟疫稍有减弱之时，这场牛瘟便传播到宁波。在中国，我并没有发现对口蹄疫的任何记述。

《申报》一名记者建议屠宰染病牲畜以防止瘟疫扩散，并掩埋它们的尸体，以取代抛尸水渠或河流的做法。黄浦江上牲畜尸体极多，松江与嘉兴当局已收到请愿，要求禁止这种行为。但填埋的做法也遭到反对，因为反对者认为任由尸体在泥土中腐烂很不卫生。同一作者还建议使用苦参——这是一种令人愉悦、苦味的根状补剂，将其掺在动物饲料中使用。他还主张使用燃烧的芳香剂对牲畜窝棚进行熏蒸，香烟还可以用来对死者的房间，或者对身患传染性热病等类似疾病患者的住所进行消毒。但他们的医疗看起来毫无效果，这位记者所记述的针对牛畜疾病的医疗措施也不起作用，从牲畜间流行病极高的死亡率来看，中国人对牛瘟可谓毫无办法。

鱼豚中毒

作为我上次报告相关主题的补充，现增补以下内容。4月末，安庆有5人因为食用鱼豚中毒死亡。其中有一家人，父子双双中毒；这对父子，一人吐了出来，另一人虽然服用了催吐剂，但没有起效；最终父子两人还是全部死亡。另一户人家，父母和女儿三人也因为同样的原因死亡。死者生前遭受了巨大痛苦，腹部肿胀，皮肤发紫又僵硬，且口吐绿沫。这也是该类案件唯一对症状进行过描述的报告。看起来扬子江流域的鱼豚中毒现象，比沿海地区要更为普遍，越往上游走，长江里的鱼豚好像就越不适合作为食物，这一点与西鲱类似。众所周知，水手在海上捕捉鱼豚食用不会受到任何影响，像日本人，就很少因为吃鱼豚而中毒。

中国梅毒学备录

本次报告最后一部分包含一篇名为《梅毒史的贡献》的译作，作者是莱比锡的舒伯特医生。作者通过引用日本文献，指出日本早在806年之前就已经出现了梅毒。在长时间从事关于中国梅毒的历史研究和治疗之后，舒伯特医生的文章立刻深深打动了我，我决定以发表短文的形式，提一些值得注意的问题。

除非梅毒在日本有自己独立起源，否则日本梅毒史必须追溯到中国。梅毒在广东是一种常见疾病，其历史可能应追溯到9世纪，随后传播到帝国的各个部分。

中国关于梅毒最早的著作，是北宋御医窦汉卿的《疮疡经验全书》，大概为11世纪医作①，具体时间不详。参考这些早期皮肤病书籍的一个障

① 此书又名《窦氏全书》，根据本书序文的说法，窦汉卿行医于"庆历、祥符之间"。此书将梅毒称为"霉疮"或"杨梅疮"，详见《疮疡经验全书》第十三卷。玛高温医生在本报告中大量引用了《疮疡经验全书》的原文，但玛高温医生翻译时在个别字句上已经做了改动，有的改动还比较大，因此译者在回译时仍以玛高温医生英文原文为准，在尊重窦汉卿原文的基础上，做适当增减。——译者注

碍在于，由于这些书籍早已散佚，今天看到的成书是由隆庆（1567—1572）时期的后辈作者重新辑录而成，使得我们无法区分哪些是后世增添，哪些才是原著内容。这本书虽出自古代，但价值极高，几乎每所医学图书馆里都能找到这本书。全书共 6 卷，分为 13 章。嵩阳（音译）是当时河南的大都会，也是宫廷医生的驻地。

根据我们皮肤病专家的说法，梅毒是从广东传入中原的，当时广东仅以适合拘役而闻名，罪犯被发配到广东，而行政官员则都是因为失宠才沦落至此，换句话说，遥远的南方和中原之间交流甚少。从广东省开始，该疾病扩散到整个帝国，按照我们的纪年，当时应该是 11 世纪晚期。根据舒伯特医生的文章，日本在 9 世纪就已经开始出现关于梅毒的记载，为什么日本的梅毒会比中国核心地区出现梅毒早这么长时间，此处需要进行推测；可能在日本存在着独立起源地，并从日本传到广东。最有可能的是，该疾病是由中国帆船从广东的港口传播到日本，广东梅毒在向北方传播之前，似乎已经在当地流行数世纪之久。假设欧洲的梅毒是由外部输入，那么这一文献足以证明广州就是欧洲梅毒的输出港。这一过程可能是通过陆上商队，也有可能是通过航运，阿拉伯商人作为中间商，在广东和阿拉伯湾之间贩运货物，这一事件如果不是发生在回教纪元（公元 622 年）之前的话，那么大概应该发生在公元 8 世纪。

中国不仅仅是梅毒的起源地（可能是全球享有此恶名的几大发源地之一），同时也是第一个在治疗过程中使用水银的国家。该方法被我们的作者所否定，他认为水银疗法造成病人中毒的副作用，实际上抵消了其带来的好处。结论仍待观察，但他事实上却在以其他形式使用（无意识的）水银。根据他的病因学理论，广东之所以会成为梅毒的发源地，主要在于当地的风土因素：人们在行房事时，因为受到"天厉时行"（malarial cachexia）① 的影响，而造成毒素传染，甚至拥挤道路上短暂的常规接触，也会造成传染——《疮疡经验全书》的这种观点，如今早已被医生们遗弃。

我认为有必要在此引用窦汉卿的原文。他在关于梅毒的章节，开篇写道：——

---

① "malarial cachexia" 可以直译为"瘴气恶变"，这是作者在用西方的瘴气理论比附中医的"时气"理论。——译者注

霉疮（也叫杨梅疮）一症，古未言及。究其根源，始于午会之末，起自岭南之地，至使蔓延通国，流祸甚广，今当未会之初，人禀浸薄，天厉时行，交媾斗精。气相传染，酷烈非常，人髓沦肌，流经走络，或中于阴，或中于阳，或伏于内，或见于外，或攻脏腑，或巡孔窍（眼、鼻、嘴、耳、肛门、尿道）。有始终只在一经者，有越经而传者；有间经而传者，有毒伏本经者。形症多端，而治法各异。

下面是本书对这种疾病之毒的解释，或者说是对五种内脏中梅毒的分别阐释，即肝、肾、脾、肺、心。

肝中毒——毒中肝经，先发便毒，① 嗣作筋疼，疮标耳、项、胁肋，形如砂仁，俗以砂仁疮名之。甚则筋痿不起。传于脾，四肢发块痛楚；移于心，生疮如痣，痛痒交作。毒伏本经，大筋微疼，久则毒发颈项两膝。

肾中脏——毒中肾经，始生下疳，继而骨痛。疮标耳内、阴囊、头顶、背脊，形如烂柿，名曰阳霉疮。甚则毒伤阴阳二窍。

脾中毒——毒中脾经，疮标发际、口吻，或堆手臂。甚则毒伏脏内传于肾；骨痛髓烈，发块百会、委中、涌泉等穴。移于肺，肌肤生癣如花色，红紫褪过即成白癜。毒伏本经，发斑如丹，久则毒结肠胃。

肺中毒——毒中肺经，疮标腋下、胸膛、面颊，形如花朵，俗以"棉花疮"名之。甚则毒聚咽嗌。传于肝，作筋疼。遇月郭空，或天阴申酉时分作疼。

移于肾，作肾脏风，痛痒交作。毒伏本经，生赤白癜，久则毒结膺臆臂膊。

心中毒——毒中心经，疮标肩胸，头部紫黑，酷似杨梅，俗以"杨梅疮"名之。甚则毒攻眸子，传于肺，发喉癣，渐蚀鼻梁，多作痰唾。移于

① 医学理论的历史总是循环往复，正如政治学、社会学理论会随着环境循环往复一样。黑泽尔［Haeser，《医学和传染病史教科书》（*Lehrbuch der Geschichte der Medicin und der epidemischen Krankheiten*），1882 年版，第 259 页］在总结欧洲早期医家对梅毒的观点时认为：

> * [History repeats itself in medical theories just as in political and social theories and combinations of circumstances. HAESER (*Lehrbuch der Geschichte der Medicin und der epidemischen Krankheiten*. Jena, 1882, Bd. iii. S. 259) thus sums up the views of the earliest European writers on syphilis:—" Man dachte sich das syphilitische Gift . . . . . als eine dem kranken Körper in seiner Totalität beiwohnende verborgene Eigenschaft (*totius substantin qualitas occulta*), welche im Körper des Angesteckten vor Allem auf die Leber, den Heerd der Blutbereitung, wirkt, indem sie daselbst eine Veränderung des Blutes, eine Art der *putredo* erzeugt. Durch die von der Leber entspringenden Adern verbreitet sich die Verderbniss zu allen Körpertheilen, am frühesten zu den Genitalien, welche sich vor allen übrigen Organen durch die Weite ihrer *Poren* auszeichnen."]

牌，手足起"鹅掌风"。毒伏本经，十指流痛。我们的作者还对病毒传播的形式和症状进行了以下描述：

是症也，不独交媾相传，禀薄之人，不拘老幼，或入市如厕，即染其症——或即病，或不即病。患者周身剧痛。或不作痛，而传于妻妾；或妻妾无恙，而传于子女。

梅毒是一种经络病，毒有浅深，药有缓急，察脉审症，应攻应补（根据情况选择积极疗法或等待时机），毫不可紊。毒未传变，一脏见症者，半月愈；三脏见症者，1个月愈；五脏俱受病者，50日痊愈；此皆独得之法，已经印证海内名公。疗法易于掌握，此疾易治（如果用我的方法），且不会留下紫红色疤痕；身无痛苦，交媾不染，生嗣无恙，不伐胃气元神。诚千古不易王道之圣药也——有利于人且极具天才。设或妄施汗、下、点、擦、熏、洗等药，徒速一时效验，殊不知毒伏于内，戕贼脏腑，酿成上述提到的五脏中毒，以致投药罔效。

反之，余能刻效收功，又能祛除水银之毒（通常都是市面上常见形式的水银①），使得病者终身无患。

我们的作者始终对在治疗过程中使用水银采取争论态度，他谴责使用氯化亚，但对使用二硫化物的做法却视而不见。在1717年帝国支助出版的《御纂医宗金鉴》，关于梅毒的章节里指出，当在治疗过程中使用水银的时候，病人能够恢复得相当迅速，但会造成毒素侵入骨骼，长久积淀，会出现上文我所提到的第二种和第三种中毒形式。

《疮疡经验全书》随后以学生与作者问答的形式，提供了更多关于梅毒的信息——这是中国古代作者最喜欢使用的指导交流形式。

第一个问题的答案很有意思：

或问曰："霉疮如何产生？"余曰，岭南之地卑湿而暖，霜雪不加，虫蛇既不挖洞，也不蛰伏，污秽蓄积于地，11月（冬天开始）湿毒与山瘴，相互蒸腾，诱使身体虚弱的人出现阳霉疮②，并在妓院中蔓延传染；疾病流行的原因在于气运。

或问曰："霉疮既然是气运造成，那为什么又被称为广疮？"余曰，广

---

① 根据《疮疡经验全书》原文，这里指的应是中药"轻粉"。——译者注
② 阳霉疮中的"阳"，指的是男性生殖器。——译者注

疮属于痘症，痘疮同样是古所未知。痘疮起于北方；汉代（公元前206年至220年）传入南方，被称作"胡痘"。

接下来是作者治疗第一、第二、第三种梅毒形式的医案介绍。虽然作者在当时并没有如此进行区分。我把第一种、第二种的治疗方法翻译如下。

一名学生，18岁，生活在乡下，渐渐眉发脱落，全身佝偻：病人最开始被当作风湿病而接受治疗。当检查他的脉搏时，我发现他的脉搏沉涩且缓，表明病人体内的金（肺）元素在压迫木（肝）元素，霉疮毒气是致病的根由。我随后给病人开了发药（接下来作者描述了这种药剂的10种草药成分）。

作者随后给病人开了牛黄蟾酥丸，该药丸是用牛黄、蟾毒①、麝香、乳香、硫化红汞、二硫化砷合成）。病人服用后大量出汗。

接着作者让病人服用了化毒乙字丸（这个处方包括牛黄、琥珀、桑蚕、硝酸钾、硫酸铁盐、盐、明矾和头发灰等，并且也含有前种药物中的水银和二硫化物）。同时我让病人服下了"龙胆泻肝汤"（该药包括龙胆根、大黄和其他草药）。当服用这些药10天过后，病人出现栗粒状的疮，不久即自行脱落。大约20天左右，这些毒被中和掉，头发和眉毛会重新长出来。

以下是这位皇家皮肤病医生所记录的29个医案中的第二个：

一位诗人，将广疮传染给了妻子。经过多方调治，两人都得到治愈，最起码他们是这么想象的；从此这对夫妻所生的孩子，很容易夭折，他们前来向我咨询，我告诉他们，他们的孩子都是因为广疮遗毒所致。

像这样的情况，孩子初生时没有外皮，或携带有许多疮、肿块、肤癣——这都是先天疾病。我为父亲把脉时，没有发现任何异常；他的身

---

① 这篇犀利的文章，并没有向外国人提供更多关于蟾毒的信息。获取蟾毒的方法是，用油纸包住蟾蜍头部，然后不断捶打，由此获取数量可观的分泌物。干燥后的提取物被小心地从油纸转移到1英寸到2英寸的薄圆杯中，提取物起先为乳白色，慢慢会变为黑色。质量好的蟾毒，价值堪比同重量的白银。次等蟾毒主要是从暹罗和日本进口，而中国蟾毒产地是四川，主要用来制造喷嚏剂药粉。

体系非常平和。但这种疾病却潜伏在母亲的身体中，且病情极重，由此伤害其子宫。我给他们开了"逍遥汤"（由10种植物成分组成）。

我一共开了20剂"逍遥汤"，同时又给他们开了化毒壬字丸（pill No.9，包括虎骨、淡水龟甲、硫化红汞、二硫化坤等）。

随后我又开了加味养荣丸（一种草药）。

经过我的治疗，不到一年的时间，两人喜获一子，两年以后又添一女。两个小孩在接受温和天花接种以后，从此不会再得这种疾病。

天花传入与接种技术入华

在这位皇家皮肤科学者的著作中，曾零星提及，痘症（variola）在中国最早出现于汉代（公元前206年—220年）。并且他认为是中国的世敌匈奴人传播了这种疾病，因此将其命名为"胡痘"。《东医宝鉴》（朝鲜）对此曾做过更为精确的描述，该书认为天花最早出现于周末汉初（公元前256年—前205年）。因此毫无疑问，天花最早出现（历史中首次记载）于公元前3世纪中期，且来自蒙古；但近225年后，当天花从南方再次传入中国时，中国人却将其视作一种全新的疾病。公元48年，名将马援领军讨伐武陵蛮（位于湖南省洞庭湖西南部），撤回的军队因此染上疾病，并将这种疾病称作"虏疮"，"虏疮"可能暗示俘虏是疾疫的传染源。根据一些权威书籍，如《赤水玄珠》（这是一本汇集了无数天才成果的天才治方）和《天花的正确疗法》（音译）都认定"虏疮"是中国天花的起源。看起来天花在中国因为长时间消失而被遗忘，随后又因为亚热带地区的蛮族，而再次传入中国。

最早对天花进行论述的医家是北宋（10世纪）的钱仲阳。①

接　种

科林森医生（《天花与医疗种痘的思考》）曾援引指出："中国人从6世纪开始进行接种实践"。我没有发现比上述《痘症定论》中所提到的接

---

① 当中国人想要创造一个文字来表达这种新疾病时，他们将代表疾病的"疒"与代表扁豆的"豆"结合起来，创造出了"痘"字，读音为tou，"豆"表音，另外"疒"和"豆"都具有表意功能："指一种豆状脓疱的疾病"。

种技术的更早的起源时间，该书认为这项技术最早是在宋仁宗统治时期（1023—1063），由一位尼姑所传授。在这段时期，有一位非常著名的宰相王旦，他是一位伟大的政治家和学者。天花曾经夺走他所有孩子的生命，当他在很大年纪时又有了一个儿子，这时他非常担心自己的儿子，希望自己的儿子不再感染这种疾病。因此他召开一次专门会议，与会医生都是幼儿科方面的专家，他询问这些医生是否懂得天花的治疗方法。

医生全体都表示"不敢言明于治痘，但略知治痘之法"。大臣随后将他们解散，送给每人10两银子，要求他们凭其所知，以尽其力，并要求每当有小孩患上天花时，立刻前来会诊，如果成功治愈这种疾病，则会得到丰厚的报酬。

一位来自四川的京官听说了情况，并得到拜访这位宰相的机会，于是将以下信息告诉他。在江苏，一位年轻女子宣示要远离尘世，并拒绝结婚，把自己献给佛祖，但她不剃光头，宁愿蓄发。

她漫游到峨眉山（是与释迦牟尼相关的圣地，临近西藏），住在山顶一座茅庵里。那个地区所有的女性都成为其信徒，随她斋戒、诵读经文和做善事。最近，她告诉其追随者，她被指示去传授天花接种的知识，内容包括挑选身患天花但痘较少且结痂的患者。痘必须较尖、圆形、红色、有光泽，包含青黄色稠状脓汁。痘痂放置一个月后可以使用，如果天气炎热，脱落的痘痂放置15天或20天就可以用了，冬天则需要放置40～50天，春、秋两季与此相同。取8粒干燥的痘痂和2粒棉花；然后把这两样东西放在净磁盅内研碎。种痘时，应挑选吉日，并避开凶日。在操作过程中要用一个银管，银管顶端为弧形；将粉末吹到男孩的右鼻孔里，女孩则吹入左鼻孔；种痘六天后，人会出现轻微发热的现象，并逐日加重；发热两、三天后，开始出痘，并出脓浆，最后结痂，百无一失。住在峨眉山附近的居民都接受了接种，并请求这位神医亲自种痘。当听到这些以后，宰相派人去请这位受人尊敬的隐士，她来到京城并成功地实施了种痘。她拒绝接受报酬，并且回答道："我只是一名修行之人，根本不需要任何金银丝绸。如果你能对皇帝忠心耿耿，同时又成为满朝官员的楷模，为国家稳定和地方和平做贡献，使人民安享太平，那么比起那些金银丝绸来说，这些是对我最好的馈赠。"说完之后，她便返回到圣山之中，多年之后，她告诉其随从，她并不是凡胎，她是慈悲观世音菩萨的化身，她的使命就是通过种痘来保护幼儿性命。她又说到，"我教授给你们的，你们也应该传授给其他人"。当听到这般陈述后，所有的妇女都非常崇拜她，赞扬她的正直，并问她，应该如何称呼她，她回答道："就称呼我为天姥娘娘"，她又嘱咐到：无论什么时候，只要有人向我敬香或者想我祈愿，或者请求我排忧解难，我就会从天庭显灵，化凶为吉"。说完之后，即坐化而去。自此每座官方庙宇都会供奉这位"天花女神"，有许多城市仅仅崇拜这一位神祇。很显然，事实应是西藏的僧侣在峨眉传播了天花接种技术，而西藏僧侣的知识则来自印度，印度在非常遥远的古代已经掌握了这一技术。

气　象

我要再一次向德·阿诺克斯伯爵所做的半年气象记录表示感谢（见图1）。

ABSTRACT of METEOROLOGICAL OBSERVATIONS taken at WÊNCHOW during the Half-year ended 31st March 1884.

DATE		Barometer	THERMOMETER		Humidity, 0–100	Nebulosity, 0–10	RAINFALL		REMARKS
			Diurnal Mean Temperature in Shade	Extreme Temperature in Shade			No. of Days	Total during Month	
1883.		*Inches.*	° *F.*	° *F.*				*Inches.*	
October	Max......	30.46	77.4	83	91				
	Mean	30.19	72.8	...	65.6	4.8	1	0.01	
	Min......	30.00	68.3	58	32				
	Range ...	0.46	9.1	25	59				
November	Max......	30.39	62.1	76	100				
	Mean	30.25	60.9	...	79	8.6	19	7.10	Heavy rain on 6th, 8th, and 21st.
	Min......	30.02	59.7	47	44				
	Range ...	0.37	2.4	29	56				
December	Max......	30.64	54.0	63	93				
	Mean	30.36	49.6	...	71.7	4	5	0.87	
	Min......	30.20	45.2	39	37				
	Range ...	0.44	8.8	24	56				
1884.									
January	Max......	30.55	53.6	64	100				
	Mean	30.32	50.3	...	79.7	7.7	11	1.35	
	Min......	30.05	47.0	36	40				
	Range ...	0.50	6.6	28	60				
February	Max......	30.54	49.2	65	100				
	Mean	30.30	46.1	...	79.5	6.6	13	5.54	On the 4th, snow on the hills.
	Min......	30.00	43.0	34	56				
	Range ...	0.54	6.2	31	44				
March	Max......	30.44	58.2	74	100				
	Mean	30.12	54.6	...	82.2	7.1	16	7.61	Heavy rain on 6th and 16th. 6th: moon halo. 28th: very high tide, 19 feet, being 2 feet higher than ordinary high springs.
	Min......	29.80	51.1	41	50				
	Range ...	0.64	7.1	33	50				

图1　瓯海关气象观测记录表

瓯海关《医报》（1891.04.01—1891.09.30）

劳里医生有关温州健康的报告

表1　温州地区外国居民人口统计

成年男性	成年女性	男童	女童	总计
12人	6人	2人	2人	22人

过去6个月以来，温州外国居民的健康状况都相当不错。每一名海关职员都接受过诊治。我希望江心屿上建立的新户外职员宿舍能够发挥有益的作用。目前为止，这里的每位职员几乎都得过疟疾，但他们染上毒素的原因，很有可能是之前宿舍不卫生。时间将会证明新建筑是否会更加卫生。

天气相当潮湿，雨季几乎贯穿整个4~9月。看一看气象观测记录表，就会知道雨天是如此之多。

在这段时期，有一名婴儿出生，也有一人死亡。

死亡原因是急性痢疾，病人是一名边远地区来的女传教士。她的病情相当严重，在就诊第二天就不幸去世了。

9月8日，另一位女传教士遭遇严重事故：她不慎从20~30英尺高的城墙上跌落，其手臂严重骨折。

7月份，英国皇家海军舰艇"金翅鸟"号停泊在温州，很多船员患上腹泻和热病；他们很少上岸，他们患的热病多为疟疾型。船只停泊在瓯江中流。布兰德利医生在禁止将水果带上船后，腹泻患者开始显著减少。

据说在8月和9月时，当地人中有大量人口患病，但并没有当地人到我这里来接受治疗。然而据我所听到的疾病与不断提高的死亡率信息来看，这场疾病不是霍乱就是霍乱性腹泻，极有可能是后者。我无法掌握任何可靠的关于死亡率的详尽细节，因此猜测无可避免。温州城到处弥漫着厕所的气味，因此发生疾病毫不奇怪。每条街道上都有无数的茅房和公厕，当然我明白这些厕所都相当有利可图。如今的温州与《梅威令医生有关温州卫生状况的报告》里所描述的已经大不相同。① 毫无疑问，大量增长的人口是发生改变的重要原因。温州的街道远不如我所观察到的其他城市干净，可以说相当令人厌恶，就像我已经说过的，厕所的味道在街道上弥漫，这对公共卫生必定是有害的。梅威令医生所描绘的令人舒适的海风，如今我们已经享受不到。这座被人称作"基督之城"的可怜城市，正在遭受磨难。

表 2　过去 6 个月我所观察和治疗的疾病类型

弛张热	间歇热	肝充血与胆紊乱	腹泻	湿疹
神经痛	心悸	听觉黏膜炎	脱肠	神经虚脱和衰弱
痢疾	支气管黏膜炎	扭伤导致腹股沟腺炎	腋生疱疹	痔疮
手臂哆开骨折	手掌割伤	蠕虫	子宫癌	漆中毒

我诊治了两名漆中毒患者。他们使我想起了丹毒。病人的恢复非常缓慢，治疗手段看起来都无效，我相信其他医生也会发现这一点。

另附上瓯海关气象观测记录表（见图 1）。

METEOROLOGICAL TABLE, April to September 1891.

MONTH.	Highest Reading of Barometer.	Highest Day Reading of Thermometer.	RAINFALL.		REMARKS.
			No. of Days.	Quantity.	
	Inches	*° F.*		*Inches*	
April............	30.400	79	18	6.61	
May.............	30.346	90	19	7.40	Several severe thunder-
June.............	30.056	89	16	7.77	storms occurred, but the
July.............	30.026	90	17	9.56	port has not been visited
August	30.550	93	16	15.33	by any typhoons.
September	30.450	94	12	8.91	

NOTE.—"An 'inch of rain' means a gallon of water spread over a surface of nearly 2 square feet, or 3,630 cubic feet = 100 tons upon an acre."—*Whitaker's Almanack*, 1891, p. 53.

图 1　瓯海关气象观测记录表

---

① 该报告即瓯海关《医报》（1877.10.01—1878.03.31）。——译者注

瓯海关《医报》（1891.10.01—1892.09.30）

劳里医生有关温州健康的报告
（1891.10.01—1892.03.31）

在过去6个月中，温州外国居民的健康状况相当不错；仅有几例因为气候导致的疾病发生。在2月和3月，可以看到山上覆盖了一层薄雪。过去的6个月降雨并不是太多。在过去两个月中，无论是外国居民还是当地人，患支气管黏膜炎的人都相当普遍，但目前我还没有发现流行性感冒病例。温州当地人中并没有发现严重的传染病；水痘出现过一段时间，外国居民中有两名儿童患上水痘。

意　外

"草坪网球腿"——一名狂热的网球选手，他曾参加过许多比赛，其小腿突然遭遇意外。他向其对手大声呼喊"你击中我了"，随后坐了下来，并被抬送回家。不久之后我见到了他。病人感到小腿中部相当疼痛，疼痛处按下去有塌陷感。病人的腿最后无法着地。我的结论是某些肌肉纤维（也许是跖肌）已经被撕裂。我随后对病人进行了包扎，并让病人穿了一双弹性袜，3周后病人可以在拐杖的帮助下行走。这名病人的病情与来自渥太华的鲍威尔医生于1883年7月7日在《柳叶刀》杂志上所报告的病例情况类似。受伤的人在最后都会大喊"有人击中了我"。

头盖骨骨折——患者是一名8岁的中国男孩，他从30英尺高的城墙上不慎跌落，其右边颅骨遭受骨折，右眉和右太阳穴被割伤。虽然恢复速度缓慢，但他正在康复当中。

手腕脱臼——一名海关苦力，在从码头跳到舢板上的过程中，不慎跌落，造成左手腕脱臼。意外发生后，我立刻见到了他，重新接上后，病人的情况已大为缓和。

脸部割伤——患者是一名 70 岁的中国盲人，在晚上与窃贼搏斗时，跌倒或是被甩下了狭窄的楼梯，导致其脸部严重受伤。病人下巴被撞出了一个大窟窿，左上嘴唇几乎被撕裂；左脸颊和左眉还有割伤。在仔细缝合后，伤口愈合良好，仅留有轻微畸形。

手指甲外翻——患者是一名中国男演员，在与其同伴争斗的过程中，指甲受伤。由于出现了危险的炎症，有必要将其指甲拔除。

肘关节开放性骨折——患者是一名女传教士，在我最近的报告里曾提到过她。她不慎从城墙上跌落并被送往上海接受治疗。其主治外科医生切除了她身上的死骨。随后——受伤 5 个月后——发现有必要在其肩关节处截肢。病人不久还是不幸去世。

以下是我过去一段时期所治疗过的内科与外科病例（包括外国居民和当地人），如表 1 所示。

表 1　病例列表

闭经	哮喘	支气管黏膜炎	子宫癌[*①]	痫
水痘	肝充血	肺充血	腹泻	手腕脱臼
消化不良	手指甲外翻	头盖骨骨折	淋病	脸部割伤
"草坪网球腿"	咽炎	肺结核	弛张热	

另附上瓯海关气象观测记录表（见图 1）。

METEOROLOGICAL TABLE, October 1891 to March 1892.

MONTH	BAROMETER.		THERMOMETER.		RAINFALL.	
	Highest.	Lowest.	Highest.	Lowest.	No. of Days.	Quantity.
1891.	Inches	Inches	° F.	° F.		Inches
October	30.32	29.80	81	65	18	6.18
November	30.65	29.93	76	47	4	2.21
December	30.57	29.90	67	40	12	2.64
1892.						
January	30.60	29.90	65	38	5	0.42
February	30.50	29.75	63	38	19	5.35
March	30.40	29.75	65	38	22	8.02

图 1　瓯海关气象观测记录表

---

① 由来已久的老病，病人最后在 10 月份去世，死时非常痛苦。

劳里医生有关温州健康的报告
（1892.04.01—1892.09.30）

在过去半年里，外国居民患病人数非常多，尽管这段时期并不像去年同期那样炎热，降雨也不是很多。气象观测记录表显示，降雨总量为28英寸，降雨天数为73天，而对应的1891年则为55英寸和98天。

有一例死胎、一例流产和一例死亡。

在7月和8月份，百日咳相当流行，共有5名外国儿童患上此病；除一名外，另外4名患病都非常严重，咳嗽往往会持续3个月时间。

治疗并不是很令人满意。安替比林——受到如此多人的追捧——实际上被发现并无疗效。溴化铵的疗效更好，但可能会导致溴中毒。

温州并没有出现霍乱流行。

以下是我过去6个月所治疗过的疾病类型，如表1所示。

表1　疾病类型

脑充血	慢性便秘	良性腹泻以及热带性腹泻	肩关节脱臼	急性痢疾
枪伤（取出子弹）	肝充血	白带	腰痛	弛张热
直肠水果核清除	贝壳类中毒或过敏	百日咳	蠕虫	

贝壳类中毒或过敏——患者是两名男传教士，居住在同一屋中，两人在6月2日中午与邻居一起吃了午餐。晚上8点，我被召到病人住所，发现两人都感到极为痛苦。两人从下午5点30分开始上吐下泻，并伴随剧烈

腹痛。在我离开病人时已经是很晚了，其症状还相当严重。（第二天）早上我发现两人病情都有好转，但都很虚弱，其腹部脆弱，体温略高，口腔味觉受损。我不知道具体是什么物质导致如此严重的胃部和腹部紊乱，但一顿午餐让问题立刻变得简单。我查看了两位先生的厨房和厨具，发现一切都很干净，既没有铜质厨具，也没有罐头食品。咖喱虾仁是菜单上唯一可能导致问题的菜。我的病人挨坐在一起，并互相帮忙相继加入了咖喱；有些虾并不新鲜，而他们吃了很多虾；另有一人在邻居刚放下汤匙后就立刻取来自用。聚会规模很大；在这个季节，同样的钱看起来很难购买足够的虾；因此他们（商贩）可能在里面掺了一些不新鲜的虾。包括主人在内的其他四人也吃了同样的菜，但并没有出现严重后果。在午餐与症状出现之间，也没有进餐或喝酒。

恶性热带腹泻——患者最终死亡。病人最开始是在 8 月 30 日犯病，死于 9 月 15 日；病人患病时间，包括死亡当天计算在内，共 17 天。该病情与约瑟夫·费尔爵士在《热带疾病》第 129 页所描述的情况非常类似。根据病情来看，不是痢疾就是肠道性腹泻。在 13 日，有一名病人流产，其毫无痛苦地把 4 个月大的胎儿流掉了。病人患有百日咳，为了护理自己的胎儿，再加上长期的疾病将她弄得憔悴不堪。

另附上瓯海关气象观测记录表（见图 1）。

METEOROLOGICAL TABLE, April to September 1891.

Month.	Highest Reading of Barometer.	Highest Day Reading of Thermometer.	Rainfall.		Remarks.
			No. of Days.	Quantity.	
	Inches	° F.		Inches	
April	30.400	79	18	6.61	Several severe thunderstorms occurred, but the port has not been visited by any typhoons.
May	30.346	90	19	7.40	
June	30.056	89	16	7.77	
July	30.026	90	17	9.56	
August	30.550	93	16	15.33	
September	30.450	94	12	8.91	

NOTE.—"An 'inch of rain' means a gallon of water spread over a surface of nearly 2 square feet, or 3,630 cubic feet = 100 tons upon an acre."—*Whitaker's Almanack*, 1891, p. 53.

图 1　瓯海关气象观测记录表

瓯海关《医报》（1892.10.01—1893.09.30）

劳里医生有关温州健康的报告
（1892.10.01—1893.03.31）

尽管今冬天气严寒，但温州外国居民中并没有出现严重的病例。温州已有超过 20 年的时间没有遇到过这样寒冷的天气了。中国人遭受了寒冬严酷的折磨，我相信有不少人被冻伤，虽然我直接观察到的病例只有两例。

有一人因为肠热病而死。

以下是我治疗过的疾病类型，如表 1 所示。

表 1　治疗疾病类型

断指	支气管炎	心力衰竭	慢性痢疾	肠热病
冻伤	手掌脓肿	胸膜炎	肺充血	脸部和背部刺伤

肠热病——患者是英国皇家海军舰艇"琳内特"号的一名军士长。他在 1 月 26 日登陆上岸，1 月 10 日开始生病，并于 2 月 2 日死亡。并没有对他进行解剖，但根据他临死的病症来看，一定是发生了肠道穿孔。

另附上瓯海关气象观测记录表，如图 1 所示。

图 1　瓯海关气象观测记录表

劳里医生有关温州健康的报告
（1893.04.01—1893.09.30）

在过去 6 个月里，外国居民的健康状况相当不错，但由于长时段的湿热天气，使得这个夏季相当难熬。在 9 月份，当地人患病很多，病症多为腹泻和热病。

以下是我治疗过的疾病类型，如表 1 所示。

表 1　治疗疾病类型

手部受伤	腹泻	肝淤血	痛风	阴囊切伤
弛张热	尿酸结石	蛲虫		

阴囊切伤——在 5 月份，我治疗了一个非同寻常的病例。一名当地人被抬送到我这里接受治疗。他的阴囊被切伤，且大量出血，衣服全被鲜血浸透了。据病人自己讲是由于挂衣服时不慎从墙上跌落受伤，但随后的调查证明真相并非如此。病人喝了大量黄酒后，经常会前往温州城内的一家妓院，他的伤口就是在那儿造成的。在彻底清洗过阴囊后，我发现了一个新的切伤，伤口大约有 1.25 英寸。需要缝上 5 针，以收拢伤口边缘。幸运的是，病人的阴茎并没有受伤，使用碘酒涂抹后，伤口愈合得相当不错。

另附上瓯海关气象观测记录表，如图 1 所示。

METEOROLOGICAL TABLE, April to September 1893.

MONTH.	BAROMETER.		THERMOMETER.		RAINFALL.	
	Maximum.	Minimum.	Maximum.	Minimum.	No. of Days on which Rain fell.	Quantity.
	Inches	*Inches*	*° F.*	*° F.*		*Inches*
April	30.340	29.650	74	50	18	3.53
May	30.200	29.740	81	60	13	3.31
June	30.054	29.730	87	60	17	8.40
July	29.940	29.568	91	74	11	6.05
August	30.036	29.670	90	75	15	6.17
September	30.140	29.394	93	75	19	11.11

图 1　瓯海关气象观测记录表

瓯海关《医报》（1893.10.01—1894.09.30）

劳里医生有关温州健康的报告
（1893.10.01—1894.03.31）

至 29 日，过去 6 个月，温州港与邻近地区的外国居民的总体健康状况都非常好。与去年相比，今年冬天气候温和，只是在 12 月末和 1 月初时出现严寒天气。10 月至 2 月初温州出现严重干旱，给当地人带来巨大痛苦。据说肠热病相当盛行——看看温州贫困阶层是如何绝望地尽一切可能获取水源，他们喝的水只比粪坑里的污水强一点，对于此种说法我毫不怀疑。

由于上海出现天花流行，我对一些成年人和儿童实施了种痘措施。在 1 月下旬，来自阿伯丁的霍厚福医生抵达温州，并创建了一所与偕我公会有着密切关系的医院和诊所。他的医疗服务深得温州当地人赞许，相信外科医疗必将在此地大有可为。

以下是我治疗过的严重病例，如表 1 所示。

表 1　治疗疾病类型

月经不调	败血症	支气管炎		腹泻	流行性感冒
弛张热	坠落导致肩部扭伤	急性扁桃体炎，并伴有脓症			

另附上瓯海关气象观测记录表（见图 1）。

METEOROLOGICAL TABLE, October 1893 to March 1894.

MONTH.	Highest Reading of Barometer.	THERMOMETER.		RAINFALL.	
		Highest by Day.	Highest by Night.	No. of Days on which Rain fell.	Quantity.
	Inches	°F.	°F.		*Inches*
October 1893	30.400	75	58	9	4.60
November	30.430	65	48	...	...
December	30.490	66	37	3	0.28
January 1894	30.400	57	35	13	3.09
February	30.500	64	38	9	1.30
March	30.500	68	42	17	6.62

图 1　瓯海关气象观测记录表

劳里医生有关温州健康的报告
（1894.04.01—1894.09.30）

表 1　温州地区外国居民人口统计

成年男性	成年女性	男童	女童	总计
15 人	11 人	1 人	2 人	29 人

这个夏季相当难熬，在外国居民中出现大量疾病患者，但大多数患者的病情都很轻微。7～9 月，我一共出诊 110 次。温州本地人患病较多的仍是腹泻、霍乱性腹泻、痢疾以及为数不少的疟疾。

自 4 月至 9 月，霍厚福医生在偕我公会的诊所里共诊治 3424 个内科与外科病例，其中有 2117 个病例都是首次就诊。每时每刻都有许多偏远地区缺医少药的病人来此接受治疗，对于这些人我们并无相关记录。英国新建领事馆时曾发生几起事故，霍厚福医生迅速对受伤工人进行了治疗。

以下是我过去 6 个月所观察与治疗过的疾病类型，如表 2 所示。

表 2　观察与治疗过的疾病

霍乱性腹泻	肝充血与胆错乱	结膜炎	便秘	单纯性腹泻与热带腹泻
肠内寄生虫	痛风	血尿症	痔疮	拇指割伤与手臂扭伤
弛张热	风湿热	口炎性腹泻	呕吐（怀孕）	

另附上瓯海关气象观测记录表（见图 1）。

METEOROLOGICAL TABLE, April to September 1894.

MONTH.	Highest Reading of Barometer.	Highest Day Reading of Thermometer.	RAINFALL.		REMARKS.
			No. of Days.	Quantity.	
	Inches	° F.		*Inches*	
April	30.100	75	18	7.20	
May	30.200	78	21	9.05	
June	30.000	86	16	11.05	Typhoon on the 29th June; lowest barometer 28.950.
July	29.980	89	4	0.39	
August	29.984	94	8	4.67	Typhoon on the 3rd August; lowest barometer 29.250.
September	30.130	89	10	3.34	

图 1　瓯海关气象观测记录表

瓯海关《医报》（1894.10.01—1895.09.30）

劳里医生有关温州健康的报告
（1894.10.01—1895.03.31）

在过去半年里，外国居民的健康状况非常好。有一例分娩（死产）和一例死亡记录在案。自 12 月至 1895 年 3 月，城区与郊区出现了严重的天花流行；据说死亡率非常高，首先遭难的是儿童。但在天花流行的尾声，成年人（无论男女）也都出现了天花病例。我虽然也找过其他港口的资料，但看起来几乎不可能找到关于天花死亡率的可靠信息。1882 年北海暴发腺鼠疫时，我根据调查棺材铺能够对死亡率得出可信的估计。但在温州，因为城市规模较大，这个方法看起来行不通。我在地方衙门进行了调查，但是衙门里并无官方记录，他们估计天花导致的死亡人数有 4000 人。但根据其他资料，我估计包括成年人与儿童，死亡人数应该在 2000 人。说来奇怪，12 月至 1895 年 1 月温州还出现了麻疹流行。

一名天主教遣使会牧师在照顾染上天花的信徒时也被传染。天花病情往往很复杂，但这名牧师的病情很简单，且没有并发症以及后续症状。

在 11 月份，霍厚福医生在一艘从厦门驶来的船上发现了一名腺鼠疫病例。这名患者没有被允许登陆，在船只离港后死在了船上。

上述提到的欧洲人是死于口炎性腹泻，她长期遭受该疾病的折磨。她于 1890 年在广州染上此病，同年又前往英国，在伦敦接受希恩医生的治疗。1893 年秋季她回到中国并接受上海彼得·西斯医生的治疗。1894 年 7 月她找到我寻求医治，虽然用尽了各种治疗方法，病情仍旧不断恶化，于 1895 年 2 月不幸去世。

口炎性腹泻是我处理过的最可怕的热带性疾病。病人如果救治及时，立刻送往欧洲并食用流质食品（牛奶），那么大多能够恢复良好；但正如最近我看到的这名病人，无论怎样改变居住地的气候、饮食、卫生条件以及用药，都无法阻止病情的不断恶化。

希恩医生对此疾病的研究非常具有价值。最近戴维森主编的《卫生与温暖气候疾病》（1893）一书中有一篇约瑟夫·费尔爵士所写的"热带性腹泻"的文章，该文认为口炎性腹泻归类于热带性腹泻，而汉口的贝格医生则认为它们是相同的，① 而不是不同的疾病。我的看法是，我同意肠道存在特殊的工作机理，能够使得我们的肠道不出现阳性。我认为贝格医生指出的治疗方法是正确的，但目前我们无法证明散道宁能够治疗此疾病。我曾两次对病人使用贝格医生所建议的治疗方案，剂量与方法都精确地遵照其建议执行。事实是其治疗方案的确延缓了病情的恶化，但当小肠开始萎缩后持续了非常长的时间才停止。病人出现了严重的消瘦和夜间盗汗，使我觉得很像肺结核的病症，但是口炎性腹泻这种病症中病人不会咳嗽——取而代之的是不间断的排便和舌头疼痛。

一位欧洲人还出现了产后子痫病症，尽管并不是由气候所引起，但仍值得一提。

附录——一名非初产妇原本将在三周内分娩，突然在 11 月 5 日夜出现产后子痫；随后出现了无意识的病状。在使用氯仿后，病人在第二天早晨停止了子痫的病症，但 11 月 6 日夜病情复发。11 月 7 日病情没有发作，但病人仍处于昏迷状态。在无任何帮助的情况下病人在当夜自行分娩，是一名死婴。在分娩后，病人的意识开始恢复，没有再出现惊厥。目前病人正在缓慢恢复当中。病人没有肾脏病史，9 月其腿部和脚步曾出现过浮肿，当时我认为是宫缩压的结果。没有任何迹象表明此次的惊厥是由宫缩导致，疾病是单纯的功能性紊乱或是急性癫痫所致，我在氯仿中添加了适量的三氯乙醛和溴化物。

考虑到该疾病的高死亡率，我希望能够尽快搞清楚其病理。施皮格伯格说 3~4 名得此疾病的妇女，就会有 1 人死亡。温州的霍厚福医生，在以上病例中给了我很多帮助，我很感激他。

3 名欧洲儿童出现了麻疹病症。皮疹分布多且广，异于寻常欧洲所常见的病例，病人的某些部位可以看到被跳蚤咬的痕迹。病人体温最高达到 103.2 华氏度，并且长期高烧不退。发热具有间歇性。10 天之后，皮疹消

---

① *Customs Medical Reports*，**XXXIV**.

退。开始会有瘙痒和麻刺感——病情会影响到睡眠。

以下是我过去 6 个月所观察与治疗过的疾病类型，如表 1 所示。

表 1　治疗疾病类型

结膜炎	结膜瘀斑	咳血	痔疮	淋巴腺炎	产惊
弛张热	麻疹	口炎性腹泻	扁桃体炎	痘症	

另附上瓯海关气象观测记录表（见图 1）。

METEOROLOGICAL TABLE, October 1894 to March 1895.

MONTH.	Highest Reading of Barometer.	Highest Day Reading of Thermometer.	RAINFALL		REMARKS.
			No. of Days.	Quantity.	
1894.	Inches.	° F.		Inches.	
October	30.270	84	8	3.40	
November	30.400	73	9	0.80	
December	30.540	66	8	0.64	
1895.					
January	30.450	65	13	0.91	Hail and snow, 12th January; 1 inch of snow, 14th January.
February	30.450	66	11	3.49	
March	30.480	75	14	4.21	Thunder, lightning, rain, hail, and snow, 17th March.

图 1　瓯海关气象观测记录表

霍厚福医生有关温州健康的报告
（1895. 04. 01—1895. 09. 30）

由于劳里医生已经离开温州前往欧洲，他将我留下来作为他的继任者，以完成过去半年的健康报告。外国居民的健康状况并不是很好，当地人也出现疾病盛行的情况。

虽然夏季平均气温并不是特别高，但除了偶有凉爽外，夏季持续的时间特别漫长；而空气大部分时间极端潮湿、窒闷，难以忍受。夏季让这里的外国人常常感到苦闷和乏力。干旱造成水渠与水井的水位极低，而暴雨缓解了干旱，当地人在井水匮乏时极度依赖河水作为饮用水，传染病由此借机大肆扩散，霍乱就是通过这样的方式造成大量死亡。

外国居民当中有一名新生儿和两起死亡事件。其中一名死亡的女士已经在温州生活了四年时间。她在前往上海的船上因为热射病（中暑）导致心力衰竭而去世。

另一名死者是名男婴，他的父亲是一名传教士，他因为消化不良被父亲带到温州城寻求医疗救助。男婴原本在治疗之下恢复良好，但突如其来的腹泻、腹痛和腹坠在 20 个小时后要了他的命。事实上，一所学校里的 4~5 名中国人也出现类似症状，大多数患者以暴卒告终，这明确地将罪魁祸首指向亚洲霍乱。至于这些儿童是如何感染上这种疾病的，目前还不得而知。

以下是我治疗的外国人的疾病类型，如表 1 所示。

表 1　治疗疾病类型

腹泻	弛张热	风湿性痛风	支气管黏膜炎	痛风	结膜炎
贫血	心脏脂肪变性	急性肝脏充血	急性与慢性扁桃体炎及咽炎	霍乱	耳炎

另外，我还治疗了许多患有严重疾病的中国人。

有一名中国人患有痢疾，他的职业是外国人在当地聘用的厨师。他是在其雇主离开温州后患上的痢疾，患病一两天后开始寻求医疗救助。尽管我们使用了大剂量的吐根进行治疗，但病人最后还是不幸身亡。

另有一名中国人左太阳穴内留有一枚子弹，他因为三个月前与海盗的一场冲突而受伤。子弹由前额射入，已经快要碰到大脑，随后划了一个圆，最后停在耳朵附近。我们将子弹取了出来时，太阳穴位置的血管出现了大量出血。这个连接部位因为血管十分柔软、易裂所以非常难缝合。但所幸病人最后伤口愈合得还算不错。

还有一名中国人前臂中弹，他的手臂和前臂因为火枪炸膛而严重受伤。另外我们在偕我公会的诊所还治疗过一个头皮大面积创伤的病人，以及许多患有大小疾病的中国人。

另附上瓯海关气象观测记录表（见图1）。

METEOROLOGICAL TABLE, April to September 1895.

MONTH.	Highest Reading of Barometer.	Highest Reading of Thermometer.	RAINFALL.		REMARKS.
			No. of Days.	Quantity.	
	Inches.	° *F.*		*Inches.*	
April	30.040	79	17	4.54	3rd, 4th, 7th, and 29th thunder and lightning.
May	30.300	81	24	8.25	19 days fog.
June............	30.050	92	7	2.40	10 days fog.
July	29.990	92	16	6.40	6 days thunder and lightning.
August	29.974	93	9	8.47	9 days thunder and lightning.
September.........	30.180	90	13	5.13	8 days fog. Heavy gale of wind on the 5th; lowest reading of barometer at 3 P.M., 29.368.

图 1　瓯海关气象观测记录表

瓯海关《医报》（1895.10.01—1896.03.31）

霍厚福医生有关温州健康的报告

在过去半年里，除 10 月份之外，外国居民的健康状况都相当好。

去年夏天温州全城暴发了严重的霍乱，霍乱一直持续到 10 月底；随着天气转凉，再加上暴雨重新将河渠与水井注满，病源的消退最终使得霍乱渐渐平息下来。但在这场霍乱中，共有 4 名外国人和许多中国人不幸蒙难。

此次霍乱还侵入一座教会建筑物，并夺走一名欧洲婴儿和三名中国女学生的生命。

紧接着，该建筑物里的一名传教士也染上霍乱。这名患者一出现霍乱病症，我们就对他进行了治疗。我们对于他的康复抱有巨大的期望，但猛烈的霍乱还是重创了他的身体，4 天之后病人被彻底压垮。

这名传教士死后第二天，他的妻子也不幸染疾。尽管我们进行了快速处理，但她仍在 40 个小时后去世。

我们的一位同事在一个星期天早晨染上霍乱，他在数小时内迅速衰竭，并在 24 小时后去世。

在此我还要感谢瓯海关的劳里医生，他原本被滞留在未能入港的轮船上；我还要感谢英国皇家海军舰艇"火焰之刃"号的佩尼医生，现在他们都已身处温州。这些绅士在护理与诊治工作方面，提供了极具价值的帮助。

以下是我治疗的外国人的疾病类型，如表 1 所示。

表 1　治疗疾病类型

支气管黏膜炎	疟疾	失眠	消化不良	扁桃体炎	肛门脱垂

一名女士患上严重的间歇热，并伴有肺部并发症。由于病人没有得到及时医治，当我见到她时，其病情已经相当严重，但目前恢复得还算令人

满意。

　　已经有大量中国人愿意到偕我公会诊所看病。肺病尤其是肺结核，是我们最常接触到的疾病。

　　另附上瓯海关气象观测记录表（见图1），在此要向哈林先生表示感谢！

METEOROLOGICAL TABLE, April to September 1895.

MONTH.	Highest Reading of Barometer.	Highest Reading of Thermometer.	RAINFALL.		REMARKS.
			No. of Days.	Quantity.	
	Inches.	° *F.*		*Inches.*	
April	30.040	79	17	4.54	3rd, 4th, 7th, and 29th thunder and lightning.
May	30.300	81	24	8.25	19 days fog.
June	30.050	92	7	2.40	10 days fog.
July	29.990	92	16	6.40	6 days thunder and lightning.
August	29.974	93	9	8.47	9 days thunder and lightning.
September....................	30.180	90	13	5.13	8 days fog. Heavy gale of wind on the 5th; lowest reading of barometer at 3 P.M., 29.368.

图 1　瓯海关气象观测记录表

瓯海关《医报》（1896.04.01—1896.09.30）

霍厚福医生有关温州健康的报告

过去半年来，外国居民和华人的健康状况都相当不错，仅有少数由外地输入的恶性疾病。至于天气，总是在下雨，今年夏季则比往年要来得凉爽。幸运的是，温州今年并未出现霍乱疾病，目前为止我还没有在温州见过此种疾病，腹泻倒是很普遍。

这段时期没有死亡事件发生。但有一名新生儿——这是一名男婴，他目前很健壮。由于产妇羊水过多、宫缩乏力和胎盘滞留，再加上婴儿个头很大，导致产后出血。我对产妇注射了热水与麦角，出血症状终于得到控制，这名母亲也得以迅速恢复。

今年6月，一名海关老职员被严重炸伤，并出现热射病症状。因此每当夏季时，家人就会让他到相对凉爽的地方度夏。

"普济"号轮船在温州靠岸后，船长、船员、乘务员、侍童以及两名海关职员一同在船上用餐，之后船上所有人都出现发烧与腹泻现象。一周之后，仅有两人康复。罪魁祸首很有可能是他们早先吃的冰激凌。

以下是我所治疗的疾病类型，如表1所示。

表1　治疗疾病类型

疟疾	腹泻	胃炎	结膜炎	角膜基质炎	角膜破裂
初期伤寒	口腔炎	喉炎和咽炎	哮喘（痉挛性）		

另外，也有许多中国人在偕我公会诊所得到治疗。

另附上瓯海关气象观测记录表（见图1），在此要向理船厅厅长本森先生表示感谢！

METEOROLOGICAL TABLE, April to September 1896.

MONTH.	BAROMETER.		THERMOMETER.		RAINFALL.	
	Maximum.	Minimum.	Maximum.	Minimum.	No. of Days.	Quantity.
	Inches.	Inches.	° F.	° F.		Inches.
April.............................	30.280	29.640	78	51	15	5.04
May.............................	30.266	29.650	88	60	17	3.74
June.............................	30.080	29.594	93	66	15	12.47
July.............................	29.986	29.460	93	73	13	12.93
August.............................	30.064	29.700	94	77	8	4.34
September	30.200	29.830	93	72	12	1.77

图 1　瓯海关气象观测记录表

瓯海关《医报》（1896.10.01—1897.09.30）

霍厚福医生有关温州健康的报告

去年 10 月到今年 3 月，外国居民当中并没有发生很多疾病，因此我无法写出一份内容翔实的报告。今年 3 月到 9 月，情况就没有那么好了，一些居民正在遭受小病的折磨，另外这个秋季腹泻相当流行，令人多有烦言。

今年年初时，天气非常潮湿，一直到 6 月，气候尚有凉意。之后气温也不是太热，每日最高气温很少能超过 90 华氏度。但过于潮湿的天气和频繁的降雨使得温州夏日的午后格外难熬，人们的健康状况自然因此大受影响。秋季气温突变相当常见，最高温度和最低温度常常可以相差 10 华氏度。

这段时期，在外国居民中有 1 名新生儿，另有 2 人死亡。前者是一名初产孕妇，接生从开始到结束只花了 2 个小时，整个过程相当顺利。另外两起死亡事件都发生在 9 月。一名死者为 14 个月大的女童，她患上了 1~2 天的腹泻，她的父母自己对其进行治疗。第三天时，女童的病症仍在持续且变得很虚弱，其父母开始寻求医疗救助。当日傍晚，女童拒绝进食，仅喝了一点热牛奶，两小时后开始出现疝气和绞痛的症状，体温达到 108 华氏度。无论我们采取怎样的抢救措施，次日清晨女孩还是被压垮了。这个家庭的另外两个儿童也相继患上腹泻，所幸最后都顺利康复。三个星期后，这个家庭的母亲患上痢疾，出现严重的腹泻与里急后重的病症。我让病人服用了 30 粒吐根和 15 滴忘忧草，每 8 小时服药一次，偶尔用硝酸银（稀溶液）进行鸦片灌肠和结肠灌洗。但病人难以忍受吐根和灌肠的痛苦，病情发展到第五天，症状减弱仅几小时后，这位母亲早产了一名 6 个月大的婴儿。虽然没有出血现象，但腹泻仍旧持续，病人依旧虚弱，她已经油尽灯枯。迹象显示她的心脏已经开始出现衰竭。我让病人摄入刺激剂和陈化食品，产生了一些效果。之后我对病人进行了生理盐水静脉注射，但也只取得局部效果。第七天，病人因为心脏衰竭而死。

许多居民患上腹泻，但有两人总是一再复发。在第一个病例中，我让病人使用了芳香白垩散、鸦片、铋、萨罗、儿茶，并仅摄入陈化食品，病人最后得到治愈。另外一个病人还患有肝炎和胃黏膜炎，我用矿物酸、收敛剂和铋治好了他。

以下是我所治疗的疾病类型，如表 1 所示。

表 1　治疗疾病类型

肌肉风湿症	急性腹泻	慢性腹泻	神经过敏和衰弱	荨麻疹
肌肉和神经痛	失眠	肩膀和脚踝受伤	风湿性关节炎	风湿性虹膜炎
消化不良	耳漏	生疖	消化不良	疟疾
瘙痒症	便秘	出血	天花	

进入温州港的船只上发现了天花病例，病人已经被送到上海综合医院接受治疗，目前已经康复。

另附上瓯海关气象观测记录表（见图 1），在此要向理船厅厅长表示感谢！

METEOROLOGICAL TABLE, October 1896 to September 1897.

MONTH.	BAROMETER.		THERMOMETER.		RAINFALL.	
	Highest.	Lowest.	Maximum.	Minimum.	No. of Days.	Quantity.
1896.	*Inches.*	*Inches.*	° F.	° F.		*Inches.*
October	30.390	30.000	88	63	12	8.63
November	30.440	29.882	75	55	5	1.85
December	30.720	30.134	66	29	4	0.97
1897.						
January	30.652	30.000	66	30	12	5.05
February	30.706	30.104	54	28	20	6.65
March	30.520	29.970	69	38	22	6.42
April	30.330	29.900	77	45	16	7.66
May	30.244	29.600	81	57	20	8.20
June	30.100	29.750	89	62	23	16.55
July	30.082	29.710	95	67	8	0.70
August	30.100	29.500	92	75	14	5.19
September	30.270	29.820	89	63	16	5.88

图 1　瓯海关气象观测记录表

瓯海关《医报》（1897.10.01—1898.09.30）

霍厚福医生有关温州健康的报告

除 1897 年年底之外，这段时期温州外国居民的健康状况总体上相当好。只有少数病例，而且不是很严重。

相较以往，今年夏天格外凉爽。往年 5 月和 6 月降雨会很多且天气潮湿，但今年大不一样。

令人感到最为不幸的是，外国居民中有一位受人尊敬的女士在怀孕期间因为痢疾性腹泻而去世。

10 月末，病人因为正处在怀孕期，出现直肠炎和内出血的病症后，开始寻求医疗救助。尽管我们竭尽所能进行救助，但病人仍旧出现持续性的不规律腹泻和内出血。病人病情逐渐恶化并且出现类似痢疾的病症，病人严重虚弱，最终造成悲剧。病人在 11 月 26 日早产，这名男婴只存活了 30 个小时即告死亡。之后病人病情稍有缓和，但腹泻仍旧不止。这位女士在 11 月 29 日终于被彻底压垮。

另外还有一名健康男婴出生，产妇是初产，经证实她来自海关支所。生产过程一切正常，不过相当冗长，我不得不使用氯仿对她进行麻醉。

以下是我所治疗的常规疾病类型，如表 1 所示。

表 1　治疗疾病类型

月经不调	蛔虫病	过敏性皮炎	生疖	便秘
腹泻	痛经	肠炎	轻热病	锁骨骨折
痛风	肝脏消化不良	手掌割伤	内出血	虹膜炎
喉炎	溃疡性狼疮	疟疾热	麻疹	耳漏
卵巢炎	怀孕	牛皮癣	肾绞痛	风湿病
踝关节扭伤				

由于这个冬天温州出现抢米风潮，所以我在这期间暂时离开了温州，但温州的外国人并没有被骚扰。

柯克医生在温州待了很短一段时间，在医务上给予我们很大帮助，我非常感激他在医院所做的工作。

偕我公会医院和药房已经诊治了许多中国病人，这期间还做了许多小手术。

另附上瓯海关气象观测记录表（见图1），在此要向理船厅厅长金德布拉德先生表示感谢！

METEOROLOGICAL TABLE, October 1897 to September 1898.

MONTH.	BAROMETER.		THERMOMETER.		RAINFALL.	
	Maximum.	Minimum.	Maximum.	Minimum.	No. of Days.	Quantity.
1897.	Inches.	Inches.	° F.	° F.		Inches.
October	30.384	30.052	82	54	18	5.64
November	30.544	30.100	82	40	5	1.88
December	30.654	30.150	67	33	7	1.26
1898.						
January	30.734	30.130	65	33	9	1.02
February	30.420	29.760	69	36	14	5.01
March	30.460	29.980	75	36	13	3.01
April	30.380	29.700	78	46	16	7.45
May	30.410	29.680	87	56	19	6.89
June	30.050	29.640	90	60	15	7.99
July	30.070	29.800	92	72	5	5.15
August	29.980	29.525	93	71	19	15.22
September	30.130	29.800	92	69	11	4.96

图 1 瓯海关气象观测记录表

瓯海关《医报》（1898.10.01—1899.09.30）

霍厚福医生有关温州健康的报告

温州外国居民的健康状况总体来说非常好，实在没有什么重要的事情值得报告。与其他港口相比，我想温州可能是最卫生、最清洁的地方，虽然有些季节相当潮湿且令人压抑。说到底，温州最令人感到抱怨的就是无聊（倦怠）。

温州街道大多中部会隆起，街道边缘则会铺设砖块，或是铺设巨长的花岗岩。水渠遍布街道，根据规定，污水必须排入水渠，而水渠的出口又在某地与瓯江相连。最终，一场暴雨把街道和水渠的污物全都冲入瓯江下游。

水源供给的情况相当不错，但在发生霍乱或伤寒时，井水经常会被污染。疟疾热相当普遍，但不属于恶性种类。

冬天，由于气温突变可能会使居民出现感冒或黏膜炎，但目前为止还没有发现恶性病例。1~2名居民偶尔会得热病，病人会出现打寒战的症状，但目前温州还没有被疟疾传染。

今年夏季相当炎热，初夏时相当难受；但8月两场台风之后，境况已经大大改善。

两名中国居民死于家中——一名死于心脏病和水肿，另外一人死于全身衰竭。

以下是我所治疗的疾病类型，如表1所示。

表1　治疗疾病类型

支气管黏膜炎	风湿病	神经痛	疟疾	痛风
慢性荨麻疹	消化不良	腹泻	急性胃炎	痛经
怀孕	晕厥	比目鱼肌撕裂	臀肌和腰方肌扭伤	

　　我也同样遭受锁骨骨折，伤口在锥状韧带和斜方韧带之间，但所幸伤口愈合良好。

　　另附上瓯海关气象观测记录表（见图1），在此要向理船厅厅长穆勒（Muller）先生表示感谢！

METEOROLOGICAL TABLE, October 1898 to September 1899.

MONTH.	BAROMETER.		THERMOMETER.		RAINFALL.	
	Maximum.	Minimum.	Maximum.	Minimum.	No. of Days.	Quantity.
1898.	*Inches.*	*Inches.*	° F.	° F.		*Inches.*
October	30.330	29.880	85	56	8	8.20
November	30.580	29.930	75	40	8	5.35
December	30.500	30.130	65	34	2	0.36
1899.						
January	30.500	30.100	66	34	7	1.56
February	30.500	29.900	64	35	11	3.76
March	30.500	30.000	70	40	10	1.39
April	30.350	29.800	76	41	13	4.25
May	30.300	29.850	83	57	19	10.45
June	30.170	29.700	87	64	10	3.98
July	29.975	29.490	93	72	9	2.10
August	30.030	29.650	96	72	16	10.70
September	30.200	29.850	88	64	11	5.90

图1　瓯海关气象观测记录表

瓯海关《医报》（1901.10.01—1902.09.30）

鲍理茂医生有关温州健康的报告
（1901.10.01—1902.03.31）

自去年 10 月下旬到温州以来，我已经对瓯海关的欧洲籍工作人员进行了 63 次专业探访，除一人之外，其他人都没有什么大的毛病。这名病人饱受疟疾的折磨，他在广州工作时也曾两度患上疟疾，也正是这个原因他才在去年调换到温州工作。我想可以确定的是，他并不是在温州染上的疟疾。

除海关职员外，温州的外国居民大部分是传教士，其间，他们的健康状况都相当好。有一位新生儿出生。

我在教会医院治疗了一些枪伤病人。大部分被送来的病人很快就康复，其中有一个年轻人左肺被击中。有一男子被海盗击中，导致大腿骨粉碎性骨折，他被扣留了将近一个星期才送入医院。这名男子送来时情况已经相当危急，因此我们无法保证能够治好他，朋友最后决定把他带回家。另有一男子也是因为被海盗击中，他的情况也非常严重，我们现在正在对他进行抢救，希望他能转危为安。

以下是我所治疗的疾病类型：

（1）一例恶性毒瘤，毒瘤有椰子大小，长在一个 12 岁女孩的背部，我们对其进行了切除。手术后三天，病人脉搏为 150 次/分钟，体温为 101 华氏度。从第三天开始，病人状态开始稳定，脉搏与体温都恢复正常，两星期内，伤口已经恢复。目前我们还没有找到脉搏出现异常的原因。

（2）一例脓肿病，病源不详。病人是一位 32 岁的农夫，来看病之前左臀和左大腿已经肿胀近三个月，病人的肿胀还伴随有痛感和组织硬化。病情逐步开始出现恶化。病人入院后，左臀上半部开始出现浮肿，浮肿在后部与内侧非常突出，病情已经延伸到臀沟以下。肌肤显现出暗红色，通过仔细触诊，我们基本掌握了病情的变化。整个浮肿范围大概有 6 英寸，主要沿着大腿分布，组织出现硬化，病人手指则出现类似象皮病的症状。我们对肿胀突出部位进行了切割，仅有液状脓汁溢出。在接下来的六周内，病人最初流出的脓水很多，但逐渐减少，同时硬化与肿胀现象也开始减弱。我在温州无法找到任何对丝虫性脓肿临床特点进行详细描述的文献。我怀疑丝虫性脓肿正是这个病人患病的根源所在。

（3）在中国人中，眼炎相当流行，在临床上很难将此种普通眼炎与英格兰见到的淋病性眼炎区分开。许多患者往往会在患病 2~3 个月后才接受治疗，因此导致失明。在患病初期，涂抹硝酸银能够迅速治愈此疾。

今年冬天气候相当温暖，却又异常干燥，事实上最近四个月几乎滴雨未落。最近三个月，水渠污秽不堪，井水也已干涸，所以人们只能从很远的地方买水喝；但我没有听到大量当地人出现异常染病的消息。

（1）当我对中国人使用氯仿后，病人往往会一动不动且一声不吭。在麻醉效果出现后，病人不会呕吐，并且几乎可以立刻且持续进食。这与英格兰的情况大不相同，英国病人往往会在吸入氯仿 24 小时后感到异常痛苦。

（2）我在这里治疗的大多数疟疾病例，符合教科书的精确描述，病人往往不是间歇，而是持续发烧；这种现象，据我所闻，相当普遍。在服用足量奎宁 1~3 天后，发烧病症能够得到缓解。

（3）当地蠕虫病患者数量之多，令我诧异。我治疗过的蠕虫病患者，几乎都会有胃部不适、疼痛、肠气胀痛或其他消化不良的症状；服用一剂量的散道宁能够祛除蠕虫。有一名 58 岁的妇女，开始出现痉挛症状，明显属于神经性病例；另外，她还患有消化不良症状。在服用一剂量散道宁祛除蛔虫后，痉挛病症没有复发。

另附上瓯海关气象观测记录表（见图 1），在此要向理船厅厅长南丁格尔先生表示感谢！

METEOROLOGICAL TABLE, 1901.

MONTH.	THERMOMETER.			BAROMETER.		RAINFALL.	
	Highest.	Lowest.	Mean.	Highest.	Lowest.	Days on which Rain fell.	Quantity.
	° F.	° F.	° F.	Inches.	Inches.		Inches.
January	66	39	52.5	30.400	29.970	17	3.60
February	61	27	44.0	30.590	30.090	1	0.12
March	68	36	52.0	30.525	29.900	15	2.85
April	74	45	59.5	30.375	29.680	19	9.81
May	83	57	70.0	30.300	29.750	20	7.24
June	85	64	74.5	30.010	29.650	17	8.20
July	92	69	80.5	29.954	29.700	14	7.22
August	89	74	81.5	29.990	29.210	19	14.57
September	88	67	77.5	30.220	29.220	6	3.82
October	81	60	70.5	30.400	29.900	10	6.10
November	74	44	59.0	30.490	30.100	3	0.06
December	68	34	51.0	30.557	30.015	9	1.63

图 1   瓯海关气象观测记录表

鲍理茂医生有关温州健康的报告
（1902.04.01—1902.09.30）

1902 年 7 月中旬，温州开始出现霍乱病例，但据报告称平阳县在两三个月前已经出现霍乱病例。霍乱逐步扩散，两周内几乎席卷整个城市。在 7 月末，死亡率达到最高点；8 月至 9 月上旬，每天死亡的人数开始减少。今年夏季降雨出奇地少，因此万物干涸，水源稀缺。9 月 15 日大雨下了一夜，注满了温州的部分河渠。这场倾盆大雨降下的同时，温州霍乱的死亡人数也与之同步暴增；这场传染病夺走了许多人的生命，9 月 15 日这次高峰比霍乱初现时还要凶猛。到我写这份报告为止——10 月 10 日——霍乱已经再次平息。

最为可信的估计是，温州城在这场霍乱中共有 5000 人或 6000 人丧生，如果算上属县，总共大概有 30000 人丧生。

霍乱第一波高峰平息后，温州曾出现过严重疟疾的流行，几乎遍布整个城市。居住在山上的居民与平原居民相比，虽然得霍乱的人不多，但同样遭到了疟疾的侵袭。疟疾造成的温州死亡人数也相当高。

在这段时期里，外国居民当中并没有人得霍乱，但总体健康状况低于平均水平，他们都遭受热病、腹泻、虚弱无力等病症的折磨。

瓯海关《医报》（1903.04.01—1903.09.30）

鲍理茂医生有关温州健康的报告

尽管温州与上海交流密切，但今年在本地并未出现霍乱流行。

1903年3月，温州曾出现脑脊髓膜炎流行。大多数病人是乡下人，我亲自经手观察的病人仅有2例。该疾病在平阳县的死亡率相当高，许多人在仅仅患病1天或2天后即宣告死亡。根据观察，该疾病症状与《奥斯勒医学》（第二版）中的描述非常接近。

4月至5月，又发生了严重的疟疾流行，同样造成大量患者死亡。

在最近三个月，即7月、8月和9月出现了痢疾的疾病流行。以我观察到的情况来看，吐根对大多数成年病人非常有效，但有一个小孩在服用吐根后依旧无法控制病情。

在这段时期，有1名或2名温州人染上登革热（dengue），这两人都是从宁波返回当地的，目前在宁波与上海都还没有出现登革热流行。外国人中仅有1名染上登革热，他是在抵达温州几日后开始出现症状。与去年一样温州有惊无险，逃脱了此病的魔爪。

今年偕我公会在一座山上获得了一幢别墅。此别墅海拔1200英尺，距离温州城大概1.5小时的车程。女士和孩子们会在此地度过温州最炎热的季节，以避免天气带来的憔悴和焦躁。

虽然许多舢板在温州与福州之间频繁往来，但目前为止我在温州还没有见过鼠疫病例。这里最年老的居民也没有听说过这种疾病曾在这里出现。

我在教会医院已经工作了两年，每周接诊200~300名患者，还从没见过麻风病例和伤寒热的病例。梅毒倒是非常流行：我几乎每天都能遇到淋病、淋菌性风湿病、淋菌性眼炎患者。据我接触到的情况，温州的癌症患者没有英国那么多，但恶性毒瘤的普遍程度则与英国无异。

瓯海关《医报》（1910.04.01—1910.09.30）

斯默登医生有关温州健康的报告

　　至 1910 年 9 月 30 日，这个港口的总体健康状况都非常好。温州外国居民人数一直不多，今年 3 月时有人离开温州回家度假。另外还有许多人选择在 7 月至 9 月最热的这段时间，搬到别墅区或是其他度假地消暑。出现这种现象的原因在于，虽然温州并未出现恶性疾病流行，但本地令人极端厌烦和压抑的气候条件，以及沉闷的社会气氛，外国人始终无法适应。这导致人们经常感到心神不安、头痛不止，小病小痛几乎是许多人的日常状态。

　　在肠病之中，慢性与复发性肠病最容易导致长期治疗。这两种疾病的起始阶段，通常便秘会导致浅表性结肠炎，随后会出现出血和分泌黏液的迹象以及轻微的发烧，并伴有腹部下坠和压痛的病症。看起来非常像慢性痢疾，但区别在于显微镜下检测不到阿米巴虫。

　　各种传染疾病在温州当地人中已经显著下降，鼠疫与霍乱难见踪迹，痢疾也不再那么普遍。这主要是因为夏季以来异乎寻常的大量持续降雨。

　　偕我公会医院①共有 120 张病床，医疗方面碰到较多的疾病为肺结核（极其普遍）、结膜炎、周期性痢疾（偶尔会有口炎性腹泻病例）。另外，在外科手术方面，我们做过长骨（尤其是大腿骨）坏死手术、子宫颈手术、睑内翻手术（极其常见）以及肛瘘手术。

　　散道宁是一种常规治疗药物，能够通过百里香酚提取获得。奎宁则是一种所有人都愿意使用的治疗疟疾的药物，即便是温州内地最守旧的庄稼汉，无不将奎宁奉为灵丹妙药。性病极其普遍，其中大多数是被飞沫传

---

① 1907 年偕我会与同宗的圣道会、美道会合并称为"圣道公会"（United Methodist Church，U. K.）。参见项滨、张伊凡《传教士对中国医学领域的影响：以温州"定理医院"为例》，《中华医学科研管理杂志》2012 年第 4 期，第 223 页。——译者注

染，这些无辜的受害人着实可怜。在我们所治疗的患者当中，有50%的病人是腿部与脸部出现溃烂病症。稻作农民往往会在腿部出现大面积溃烂，我们对患者施行提尔斯植皮手术，患者术后可以重新工作，疗效极好。

另附上瓯海关气象观测记录表（见图1），在此要向理船厅厅长沃克上尉表示感谢！

METEOROLOGICAL SUMMARY.

Port of Wenchow, April to September, 1910, inclusive.

MONTH.		Average Max. Temp.	Average Min. Temp.	Rainfall.
April	..	64.4° F.	54° F.	4.02 ins. on 16 days.
May	...	75.9	63.5	7.95 ins. on 18 days.
June	...	87.4	74.2	6.43 ins. on 11 days.
July	...	92.6	78.1	12.07 ins. on 13 days.
August	...	89.7	77.2	14.58 ins. on 17 days.
September	...	84.23	72.73	7.61 ins. on 9 days.

Giving an average mean temperature of 75° with rain every other day.

图1 瓯海关气象观测记录表

瓯海关《医报》（1913.10.01—1914.03.31）

安格司医生有关温州健康的报告

截止到 1914 年 3 月 31 日为止，半年以来温州没有出现重大疫情。温州最近一次出现霍乱病例，是在 1913 年的 10 月份。圣诞节期间，温州出现了天花病例；但很少有当地天花患者会向外国人寻求帮助。

外国人当中，有一名年轻的小姐患上了口炎性腹泻，她在温州已经居住了五年。患者病情已是末期，因此病人已经返回英格兰。瓯海关有一名英籍职员，添了一个男婴。

偕我会教会医院①最近很是忙碌。几乎有一半的住院病人，患的都是没有太高记述价值的溃疡和眼疾。前者多为梅毒性溃疡、外伤性溃疡和败血性溃疡，后者多为各种程度的青光眼、虹膜炎和白内障。

一些更值得记载的疾病，其中包括枪伤；许多患者是福建人，他们的伤口是海盗造成的，海盗在海上袭击了他们的民船。

腹水很常见——因为门静脉阻塞所引起的肾脏、心脏等疾病，常会（也有可能不会）伴随出现肝肿大或脾肿大；这些患者常常在抽除积水，症状缓解后，就匆忙离院，却未能做出更详尽的诊断。一名妇女，年纪在 50 岁左右，患上了腹水，住院前体重 125 斤，10 天后离院时只剩下 45 斤！

有许多例肉芽瘤病例。这种疾病通常出现在病人的下半身，患者多为成年男性。温州的肉芽瘤病例，并不符合目前通行的疾病分类；另外采取任何抗梅毒治疗手段都无效。肉芽瘤局限在皮肤和皮下组织，且表现出极端慢性的特征。在 25 名患者中，其中许多人有 10~15 年的病史。他们的病变部位，通常在大腿或臀部。肉芽瘤在初期，通常是孤立分布，约樱桃

---

① 这里指白累德医院。——译者注

核大小，明显但皮表并不可见，似乎潜藏在皮下组织。渐渐的，症状会逐渐可见，所在部位的皮肤会变得光滑；肉芽瘤此时约榛子大小，呈现蓝色。逐渐开始出现卫星症状，病变区域大概有手掌大小。病变皮肤会呈现红色，并出现溃疡。最终，病变区域可以达到手臂所能伸展的范围，真菌溃疡的范围大概有高尔夫球大小。目前还没有证据显示，此病能够自愈。切除整块病变皮肤，并配合必要的皮肤移植，能够立刻取得很好的疗效。

最近出现了一个极具教育意义的奎宁中毒病例。一名年轻人在中午时被送来看病，体温在 104 华氏度。在他的血液中检测到了疟原虫。在次日早上 9 点，病人服用了 3 剂的 10 格令硫酸奎宁液；在早上 10 点钟，因为预计病人会在两小时后打摆子，因此又让病人服用了 1 剂 12 格令奎宁。白天病人状况良好，但晚上病人诉眼前有轻微泛黑的症状。于是晚上病人又服用了 5 格令的重硫酸奎宁片；这是病人最后所服的奎宁。接下来的几天，病人出现彻底的盲症。7 天后，病人甚至很难看清自己的手指；随后病人出院，并转而接受中医治疗。4 个月后，这名病人在日光和电灯下都可以看到东西，但如果是在煤油灯下，则需要人引路。病人后来没有出现疟疾复发。药剂师否认在剂量上出现过可能的失误。

安格司 （W. B. G. Angus）
瓯海关，1914 年 4 月 20 日

瓯海关《医报》（1914.06—1915.09）

施德福医生有关温州健康的报告

1914年6月至9月：在此期间，温州外国居民的健康状况良好。6月时有一例阿米巴痢疾患者。8月时有一名斑疹伤寒患者，同时患有胆囊炎并发症。死亡人数为零。

在当地人中，梅毒与结核病例很常见。一般来医院寻求治疗的梅毒患者，都已进入梅毒第三期。骨关节结核病在当地里很流行，中国人已经知道了对这种疾病进行手术的价值，有时病人会主动要求进行切除手术。

当地有许多人患沙眼，并使许多人致盲。但很难说服中国人接受长时间的治疗，以彻底治愈沙眼。

麻风在当地并不常见。我只在当地见过麻木性麻风。

在有一段不长的时间里，我被当地各种形式的肿瘤疾病所震惊——主要是纤维瘤。

霍乱经常会在每年夏末光临这座城市，但这段时期还没有出现。最近也没有出现任何传染病。

1914年10月至1915年3月：外国居民的健康状况非常好。

针对中国人的医疗工作，有很多都需要进行手术。其中针对肿瘤、骨结核、关节结核、腺结核、眼科手术，尤其是睑内翻、瘘管、鼻窦和痔疮的手术，在所有手术中占的比例较大。

在当地乡村地区，男性中流行着某种类型的腹水病，但女性患者很少，患者并不会出现肝肿大或脾肿大的并发症。患者的肝脏有时会出现萎缩，但也非绝对。根据掌握到的病史，病人中有1/3在患上腹水之初，曾患过腹泻。血吸虫卵蛋白只能在少数病人的排泄物中找到。在有些月份中，血吸虫可能会致命，但病情也有可能会持续一整年。目前我还没有观察到病情能够持续超过18个月的血吸虫病例。

我诊断过两例钩虫病。其中一名病人还患有麻木性麻风病，这名病人是一个 19 岁的男孩。据病人的邻居讲，男孩三岁丧父，他的父亲手臂有麻木性皮损且瘫痪，足底溃烂。男孩双手的无名指和小拇指，及其手掌周围皮肤有麻木性斑块，另外左臀也有斑块。病人左手已经开始出现爪形手的症状，左轮匝肌也有麻痹现象。尺骨神经、外腓骨神经和耳大神经都在变厚。病人膝反射异常，下颌反射正常。

接下来所记述的，是一个特殊病例，这种病我只见过一次，但我没能对病人进行详细诊断。病人是一个 18 岁的男孩。右腿有条状溃疡，溃疡从足二趾根部，穿过脚背，一直延伸到内踝，然后从内踝沿着内隐静脉延伸到大腿中部。溃疡底部已经凸起，溃疡部位的直径，从数毫米到 1.5 厘米不等；有些部位的溃疡已经连成一片，其他区域的溃疡部位各自分离，一般间隔 2 ~ 3 厘米。在大腿中部以上区域，还有类似的条状溃疡区域，存在两个微发红的小瘤，这两个小瘤明显正在萎缩。根据病人口述，5 个月前患者足二趾根部，开始出现很小、坚硬、疼痛的小瘤；两个星期后，小瘤开始溃疡。类似的溃疡迅速蔓延到大腿。病人没有出现麻木或瘫痪的症状。我使用水银和砒霜进行治疗，并使用了一些当地的腐蚀剂，但并没有取得任何疗效。病人待的时间很短，没有接受足够长时间的碘化钾治疗。

风湿热在当地很少见，一年当中我只治疗过一例。

在 3 月末时，温州出现了麻疹和天花疫情。因为患上这两种传染病的中国人，并不会来医院寻求帮助，因此我常常无法获取第一手资料。但教会学校受到麻疹传染的情况除外，学校的麻疹通常都是寻常病例，且没有后续并发症。有传言说，天花流行的程度并不严重。

1915 年 4 月至 9 月：在这几个月中，规模不大的外国居民里，出现了很多病患。

4 月份时，有一名白喉病例，病人迅速接受了抗毒素治疗。一名 16 个月大的婴孩，患上了蛔虫病，胳膊上还长了脓疮，并导致持续的上吐下泻。

有一例急性中耳炎，在没有化脓的情况下，自行痊愈。

在 9 月份，有一个热病病例，病因不详，已经复发过两次，中间不发热的间隔期分别为 11 天和 12 天。随后我被请去为他看病，病人是一名中年男子，正忍受着发热和腹痛的煎熬。根据所诉病情，病人在前两天的晚上也出现过发热的情况。疼痛感会迅速平息，但发热的状况一直会持续到两天以上，体温最高超过 103 华氏度，晚上体温为 99.5 华氏度，早上体温为 100 华氏度。在发热期间，病人脉搏很快（110~130 次/分钟），但很规律；发热的症状消失后，病人会显得筋疲力尽，脉搏仍旧很快（110~120 次/分），出现二重脉。两天后，病人脉搏变缓且规律，状况大为改善。症状消失 11 天后，病人热病会复发。自从能够起床后，病人在复发前自行走了 0.25 英里的路。最近一次发作，发热持续了 3 天时间，并伴随有脉搏紊乱。发热与脉搏紊乱会同时消失。第二次复发的间隔期为 12 日。这一次复发的症状不是那么严重，也没有伴随心律不齐的状况。病情共持续 3 日。

在夏天，病人的工作是负责在户外频繁巡视水渠，但在发病的前几天，病人并没有暴露在高温下，病人第二次发病，是在因为患上膝滑膜炎而卧床数天后。病人第一次和第二次患病后，都接受了血液检查，但并没有找到螺旋体。

外国人中还有几个神经衰弱和流感病例。

医院的 100 个床位已经全满，在夏天，有时还需要增加床位。

这段时期，并没有出现大规模传染病流行。在 7 月和 8 月，出现了几个霍乱病例。在 7 月出现了几例杆菌性痢疾。

在 4 月份，我见到了一例狂犬病病例，病人是在被狗咬伤 7 周后发病。

这里有一个有价值的特殊病例值得记载，病例为急性延髓麻痹，病人是一名 34 岁的男性。某晚该男从梦中醒来，发现说话和吞咽困难。5 天后，当我见到他时，病人已经彻底无法吞咽，左右两边的软腭、脸右部和舌头右部都出现了麻痹。声带出现撕裂。病人体温为 102 华氏度，脉搏为 108 次/分钟。只能通过插入胃管，让病人服用小剂量的士的宁。病人发病一个月后，面部神经瘫痪显示出好转的迹象，又过了两个星期后，病人可以开始少量吞咽流食。再过了 4~5 天后，病人的胃管被拆除。病人发病两个月后，已经可以再次发声，又过了一个星期，病人可以在夹杂很强鼻音的情况下开口说话。虽然快速康复，暗示病人可能只是患上了癔症，但当第一次见到病人时，病人所承受的巨大痛苦，以及持续三天的高热和过速的脉搏，这些病症除了指明是延髓麻痹外，别无解释。病人没有梅毒病史，但他的妻子曾经流产，且两人在婚后三年都未能产子。

瓯海关《医报》（1916—1917）

施德福医生有关温州健康的报告

　　这段时期外国居民的健康状况都很好。没有人死亡，7月份有一名18个月大婴孩患者上了杆菌性痢疾。8月份有一名35岁的男子，被太阳晒伤；病人没有其他后遗症。

　　1917年2月，同一名病人患上了腹部隐痛，病情持续数周，某晚病人右边肋骨出现刺痛，痛感在持续10分钟后停止，该部位变得非常敏感。随后几天连续数晚，病人都出现了这样的痛感。我随后被请去为他看病。胆囊部位的区域，病人很敏感，但却也没有其他病症。病人食欲低下，感到无力，右肩感到疼痛，但也没有其他严重病症。病人说没有出现热症，也没有再出现过刺痛。病人也没有出现呕吐现象。病人看起来最有可能患的是胆结石。病人在床上躺着休息了数天，其间清淡饮食，病人感到有所好转，胆囊部位的敏感有所降低，但右肩和胆囊部位偶尔会出现阵痛。好的方面是，病人可以缓慢地做一些运动。接下来的两晚，病人睡觉时大量出汗，病人说可能有轻微发热的情况。出汗显示可能有肝脓肿的症状，我开始让病人每天注射1格令的依米丁。此后病人迅速好转，一周后病人可以恢复工作。本次治疗一共注射了7次依米丁。病人没有痢疾病史。病人恢复工作一个月后，右肩再次出现疼痛，数天后在肝脏部位出现刺痛。当我再次为他看病时，病人右肋骨腋前线下方敏感。我再次使用依米丁进行治疗，病人也迅速好转。目前病人仍在持续注射依米丁。

　　本年我接手了两次分娩：一例正常；另一例出现了胎盘前置，婴儿不幸夭折。

　　当地中国人里没有发现传染病。

　　这座城市在11月至12月间，腹泻非常普遍，同时当地还出现了严重的干旱天气。

　　1月至2月时，当地出现了天花流行，尤其是在城市的东郊。

瓯海关《医报》（1917—1918）

施德福医生有关温州健康的报告

温州的外国居民，本年总人数约为 30 人，患病情况超过往年。有幼儿患上了百日咳、风疹、支气管炎和沙眼；成年人所患疾病，9 月份有风湿病、坐骨神经痛、副伤寒，7 月份有结肠炎、慢性痢疾，10~11 月有淋病、横痃后软疮、口炎性腹泻初期，另外还有虚弱症和贫血症。这些疾病的价值，都不值得进行详细记述，除了慢性痢疾病例之外，这名病人在治疗期间出现了吐根中毒的现象。这名病人的病症，已经持续 3~4 年。起初注射吐根就能很好地缓解病症，病人的粪便中已经没有找到阿米巴虫后，病人再次注射吐根。注射后的第一周，病人出现了好转，但因为期间出现台风，病人有两天无法进行注射，病情因而再次复发。病人恢复注射吐根后，痢疾症状得到缓慢改善。注射持续了一个月，每次注射的量为 22 格令。病人痢疾在接近康复后离开了本港，但我后来从他的医疗看护口中得知，这名病人后来患上了自发性肌肉轻瘫，患病部位主要在颈部、肩部、手臂和咀嚼肌。肛门括约肌也出现了病症。在注射士的宁后，病人出现缓慢好转。

当地中国人没有出现传染病。肠道热在当地秋季相当流行，冬天则会出现许多腹泻病例。因为我几乎没有到中国患者家里进行过门诊，所以无法知道中国人所患轻型热病的确切情况，一般这种类型的病人很少会到医院来寻求治疗。

本年白累德医院共接收门诊病人 25548 人次，住院病人 1418 人次。共使用氯仿施行手术 297 人次。腹部外科手术，在当地还是一件新鲜事。以往我们无法使任何一名病人，同意施行腹部手术，但 1916 年秋季一名够胆的妇女接受了皮样卵巢肿瘤切除手术，此后我们又进行了 10 例腹部手术；其中 7 例是卵巢肿瘤，6 例成功，另外一例附着在骨盆上，很难进行安全切除；在其余的腹部手术病例中，有一名患有肝硬化（此病在当地很常见）妇女，接受了肝固定术。她在手术六个月后返回医院，此时腹部仍然需要引流（此时引流液已经只有先前的1/3），但分泌和吸收明显已经达到平衡，在3～4个月内引流液都维持在一定量。她的健康状况明显好转，并日渐长胖，但原筋膜的创口已经张大，并出现了疝突出。我决定削减创口面积。当天手术后，病人看起来排便正常，术后第三天，病人焦躁不安且开始呕吐。不幸的是，她的病情继续恶化，开始出现昏睡，随后陷入昏迷，第五天去世。很显然，这是因为两块小小的肝组织，而久拖的慢性中毒病例。这是一系列手术中唯一的死亡病例。

麻风在当地极为鲜见，但也偶尔会遇到零星患者，其中绝大多数来自瑞安县，瑞安距离此地大约半天路程。本年我见过一名患麻木性麻风的青年男性。患麻木性麻风的患者，背部、胸口和手臂皮肤会出现浅色的斑块。尺骨和腿部末端神经可能会轻微增厚。

瓯海关《医报》（1918—1919）

施德福医生有关温州健康的报告

当地气象报告详见图1。

Monthly temperature : —

	1918, Apr.	May	Jun.	July	Aug.	Sep.	Oct.	Nov.	Dec.	1919, Jan.	Feb.	Mar.
Mean	60.5	68.4	75.1	83.8	82.6	77.9	69.8	57.8	52.8	49.9	44.8	55.7
Mean Max.	66	74	80	90	89	85	76	62	57	52	50	61
Mean Min.	55	62	70	77	77	71	63	53	49	40	39	50

Rainfall :—

5.54	8.66	23.2	9.56	9.18	4.50	1.70	5.46	2.82	3.53	3.65	4.40 inches

图1　当地气象报告

医报——温州当地人口大约有10万人。

外国居民大概有30人，本年的总体健康状况不错。我所治疗过的疾病包括痢疾、疟疾、流感、淋病、支气管炎、风湿性关节炎、主动脉疾病。

中国人所患流感情况

本年在传染病方面，流行最严重的就是流感。流感暴发始于5月。全城到处是患者，病人会出现发热，并伴随咳嗽与精神萎靡的症状，但黏膜炎的症状并不明显。发热的症状持续4~5天后，病人会极度虚弱。并无流感病人死亡。随着天气逐渐临近夏季，流感病例也渐渐减少。但在9月初时，又突然出现大量恶性流感病例，且伴随有支气管炎或肺炎症状，有时还会咳血，最终病情发展为支气管肺炎。温州府其他地界几乎没有受到流感影响，有些地方完全没有流感病例。乡村地区的流感疫情，比城镇要更严重。在城镇患流感的比例在10%以下，但学校除外，学校的患病率在50%~60%，令人欣慰的是，除了一所学校有一名学生病亡外，再无死亡病例。另一方面，在许多乡村地区，流感造成了重大的损失。总体而言，根据报道，受感染的村庄起码有一半人口患病，病情是如此严重，有的村庄死亡率高达10%。许多家庭3/4的成员被夺去生命。本次流感的病情发展往往如戏剧般飞快；发病一天，甚至更短就能使人丧命。有3~4户人家，在2天内全家人都死亡。10月末，疫情才渐渐平息。此后仅有零星病例出现，且大多为轻型。

脚气病在温州并不常见，但1918年春季，当地驻守的士兵暴发了脚气病。军队中大约有12个脚气病例，所有都是干性脚气病。没有出现死亡病例。

此外，并无传染病出现。

在中国较为富裕的阶层中，新胂凡纳明①的使用相当普遍。

吐根在肝脓肿治疗中的应用

吐根在治疗肝脓肿中的巨大价值，已经一再得到证明。数天前有几个肝脓肿病例，本来已经确认要进行手术，但在仅仅注射吐根后，病人看起来已经得到缓解，即使是那些脓肿破裂看起来已经贴近皮肤的病例，也能通过注射吐根得到疗效。

垂体囊肿

以下是一个垂体囊肿的医案，病人患病时间长，此医案有其特殊价值。病人是一名36岁的男子，就医诉其病状，左眼已盲，右眼部分失明，常感到眼花和无力。他说："8年前，左眼开始出现断断续续的病状，病情渐渐发展，大约两年前，只能看清贴近鼻子前面的东西。"此后左眼完全失明。大约8年前，右眼有时也会出现症状，但病情发展较慢。目前右眼有一半失明。他的视力因此一直模糊不清（可能是垂体临时性的充血和肿胀）。5~6年前，病人开始变得性格暴躁。4~5年前，他在走路时会出现眼花，他现在的情况比过去要强一些。除两年前的一些时日，病人没有头痛症状。也没有呕吐症状。

病人在入院时，其皮下脂肪比同龄人要厚许多；尤其是腹部。如前所述，病人左眼全盲，右眼间歇性偏盲。左眼对光反射消失，间接光反射存在。左眼视神经盘比右眼暗淡。尿液中没有糖分。在使用碘化钾进行治疗一个月后，病症没有好转或变化。

---

① 抗梅毒药物，价格较为昂贵，其他港口的海关医官，一般习惯将其称为"九一四"。——译者注

第二部分

英文
文献

junks cruising after pirates abou
Chê sea coast, it seems that th
of Fukien and Tsichow are sti
erous and as savage as ever.
d is consort bound from Ningpo
w laden with rice and sundries wer
attacked near Wênchow by a cou
irates, who boarded the merchant
ving ransacked everything of valu
better, left them with twenty-fi
nd seriously wounded. Sin
have been issued by the Governor
T'an, for the capture of the pirate
te a large fleet of war junks is no
it seems to be the universal opinio

xpression, spread himself out over the
whole subject of the health, pestilence
amines, and topography of the place
Thirty-six closely printed pages have
ot sufficed to relieve him of his whole
urden of knowledge, for at the begin
ing of his paper he says that he reserve
he medical
ccasion; but
f which he h
ully have the
hat we sho
uch a trifle
He begins
district in wi
ind passing

During a fierce gale which raged at Wen
chow about a fortnight ago, several seriou
disasters occurred, attended in many case
with lost of life. Four large junks, lade
with poles, were upset and many other
dragged anchor or sustained other injuries
whilst a great number of small fishing craf
suffered a worse fate. The villagers on th
coast showed great barbarism. Instead o
ffording succour, they busied themselve
with picking up wreckage thrown ashore
In the worst cases they even wrested th
oles away from the shipwrecked people
who in their exhausted state were made t
ield the logs to the merciless people
Owing to the unusually cold weather a
Wenchow there is considerable suffering
mongst the poorer classes, who are no
rovided with extensive wardrobes, and
specially amongst those who have a pre

e sent to Ta-c
Yo-ching-hsien
pirate-robbers
used considerat
ies of both this
how. Some tim
oes plundered two
the Yu H'uan Bay
re) which caused the
to order one of his
against them. On
e of the bay the office
vessel decided to an
red a party of soldier

RIOT AT WENCHOW.

e Yungning, from Wênc
ed here on Saturday, b
culars of a riot which had
chow on the night of the
first intimation of this ri
ed up from Ningpo from information
lied by the Yungning on arrival a
port, though efforts had been made b
E H Parker British Consul and al

(FROM A CORRESP
Notice to mariners, also
ad to feminine sphere
markable Peak on the
avigators see on their
Vênchow, having only
ad never named, has no
ie denizens of Wênchow
Hart's Peak," in recogn
ices which the Inspecto
mperial Maritime Custo
y illuminating the coas
ormal recognition of the
y the Wênchowese, in pic-nic assembled
n the 22nd March, and that being th
irthday of the Emperor of Germany, nea
o the celebration of the Queen's Jubilee
nd within measurable distance of th
atal day of President Cleveland, th
ealth of those estimable rulers was drun

which a reference to Mr. Dou
's table on the opposite page rend
ent. My views elsewhere publis

Parker taking leave on a new de
ure, having first secured the last instal
t of the indemnity that the authorities
ed to pay for losses sustained by
iguers in the recent disturbances. To
be Mr. E H. Parker's success in giving
ral satisfaction to foreigners and native
orities in regard to the questions raised
ie riot to good luck, would be unjust to
accomplished officer. It was tact that
ted an amicable settlement

ing-kung, running as she a
ort of the most influential
fter trip with improved
esults, seems now to have
o that point where if more
of necessity become in
g superfluity. As has bee
the impetus given by
y means of shipment has
nt export of al
spects for tea

astation that met ou
e river of Wênchow wa
les and miles the countr
vast expanse of wate
teads and graves, an
nds crowded with cattle
frowning background
t most depressing au
We passed too quickl
by the pen. Women an
roups, doubtless talkin
ses, while the men wer
nay in their boats. In some places wher
he bridges were still standing only th
pper portion of their arches was visibl
oking like mirages—water above, belo
nd around them? Great indeed mus
ave been the downpour to have caused suc
n inundation. It was a comforting chang
o turn one's gaze from the immerse
ountry to the numberless fishermen pur
uing their calling as if no such thing
ome troubles existed. The flooded cour

Macgowa
ow recen
put down
sumption
outhwaite
ld be tra

itants of the so-called
ave put away their store-cl
ar. The rejoicings were co
ietness and decorum, the
of nastiness was eaten,
count of tomtomming and t
ulged in; in fact, everyth
accordance with "olo
Year's Eve most of the
icipal thoroughfares were
ted with coloured lamps,
re lighted in nearly all th
ty and suburbs. That this
isement did not result in
onflagration is simply miraculous,
mmunity is by all right-thinking
tributed to the special interve
ien Tien Ta Ti, the great Lord of
leaven, or some other benevole
hough here, as elsewhere, scoffers
und who point to the saturated con
verything or to some other such

o the Editor of the
NORTH-CHINA DAILY NEWS.

IR,—Although the subject of
hina was ably discussed at a lat
of the Shanghai Literary and D
iety the question was not so exha
reated as to preclude me from
nall contribution, assuming that
be unacceptable to those who
ary (but not

UNICATED.)

ically, it m
think the
mature, tha
where it u
needed;
northern C
courses, and
is doubtful
cessfully
It was urg
yed by an
of China,

R OWN CORRES

ing, on ente
d some stragg
trawropes, th

that were
ent the enemy
ug. had they resisted t
would have been as useles
A proposition that was mac
channel has been abandone
a panic was created by a
quiring every family to br
darins a basket of stones.
as secure as if they had
protection; the authorities
solicitous for their safety.
threw missiles, and others o

China, Imperial Maritime Customs, Medical Reports
(1877. 10. 01—1878. 03. 31)

CHINA.

IMPERIAL MARITIME CUSTOMS.

II.—SPECIAL SERIES: No. 2.

MEDICAL REPORTS,

FOR THE HALF-YEAR ENDED 31ST MARCH 1878.

15th Issue.

PUBLISHED BY ORDER OF
The Inspector General of Customs.

SHANGHAI:
STATISTICAL DEPARTMENT
OF THE
INSPECTORATE GENERAL.
MDCCCLXXVIII.

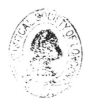

INSPECTOR GENERAL's Circular No. 19 of 1870.

INSPECTORATE GENERAL OF CUSTOMS,

PEKING, 31st *December* 1870.

SIR,

    1.—IT has been suggested to me that it would be well to take advantage of the circumstances in which the Customs Establishment is placed, to procure information with regard to disease amongst foreigners and natives in China; and I have, in consequence, come to the resolution of publishing half-yearly in collected form all that may be obtainable. If carried out to the extent hoped for, the scheme may prove highly useful to the medical profession both in China and at home, and to the public generally. I therefore look with confidence to the co-operation of the Customs Medical Officer at your port, and rely on his assisting me in this matter by framing a half-yearly report containing the result of his observations at.........upon the local peculiarities of disease, and upon diseases rarely or never encountered out of China. The facts brought forward and the opinions expressed will be arranged and published either with or without the name of the physician responsible for them, just as he may desire.

    2.—The suggestions of the Customs Medical Officers at the various ports as to the points which it would be well to have especially elucidated, will be of great value in the framing of a form which will save trouble to those members of the Medical profession, whether connected with the Customs or not, who will join in carrying out the plan proposed. Meanwhile I would particularly invite attention to—

    a.—The general health of............during the period reported on; the death rate amongst foreigners; and, as far as possible, a classification of the causes of death.

    b.—Diseases prevalent at............

    c.—General type of disease; peculiarities and complications encountered; special treatment demanded.

    d.—Relation of disease to $\left\{\begin{array}{l}\text{Season.}\\ \text{Alteration in local conditions—such as drainage, &c.}\\ \text{Alteration in climatic conditions.}\end{array}\right.$

    e.—Peculiar diseases; especially leprosy.

    f.—Epidemics $\left\{\begin{array}{l}\text{Absence or presence.}\\ \text{Causes.}\\ \text{Course and treatment.}\\ \text{Fatality.}\end{array}\right.$

Other points, of a general or special kind, will naturally suggest themselves to medical men; what I have above called attention to will serve to fix the general scope of the undertaking. I have committed to Dr. Alex. JAMIESON, of Shanghai, the charge of arranging the reports for publication, so that they may be made available in a convenient form.

MEDICAL REPORTS, NO. 15. [OCT.-MAR.,

3.—Considering the number of places at which the Customs Inspectorate has established offices, the thousands of miles north and south and east and west over which these offices are scattered, the varieties of climate, and the peculiar conditions to which, under such different circumstances, life and health are subjected, I believe the Inspectorate, aided by its Medical Officers, can do good service in the general interest in the direction indicated; and, as already stated, I rely with confidence on the support and assistance of the Medical Officer at each port in the furtherance and perfecting of this scheme. You will hand a copy of this Circular to Dr. ...., and request him, in my name, to hand to you in future, for transmission to myself half-yearly reports of the kind required, for the half-years ending 31st March and 30th September—that is, for the Winter and Summer seasons.

4.—   *   *   *   *   *

I am, &c.,

(signed)   ROBERT HART,
I. G.

THE COMMISSIONERS OF CUSTOMS,—*Newchwang,*   *Ningpo,*
                              Tientsin,   *Foochow,*
                              Chefoo,   *Tamsui,*
                              Hankow,   *Takow,*
                              Kiukiang,   *Amoy,*
                              Chinkiang,   *Swatow,* and
                              Shanghai,   *Canton.*

SHANGHAI, 30*th June* 1878.

SIR,

IN accordance with the directions of your despatch No. 6 *A* (Returns Series) of the 24th June 1871, I now forward to the Statistical Department of the Inspectorate General of Customs, the following documents :—

A.—Report on the Health of Shanghai, pp. 1-10 ;

B.—Report on the Health of Canton, pp. 11-16 ;

C.—Report on the Health of Chefoo, pp. 17-20 ;

D.—Report on the Health of Ningpo, p. 21 ;

E.—Report on the Health of Swatow, pp. 22-24 ; and

F.—Report on the Health of Amoy, pp. 25-27 ; each of these referring to the half-year ended 31st March 1878.

G.—Report on the Health of Newchwang, pp. 28-35 ; and

H.—Report on the Health of Takow and Taiwan-fu, pp. 36-37 ; each of these referring to the year ended 31st March 1878.

I.—Report on the Sanitary condition of Wênchow, pp. 38-47.

Notes on the Diseases affecting Europeans in Japan, pp. 48-80. For this valuable paper I am indebted to Dr. ELDRIDGE of Yokohama, and I have gladly inserted it as complementary to the series of Reports on disease in China.

I have the honour to be,

SIR,

Your obedient Servant,

R. ALEX. JAMIESON.

THE INSPECTOR GENERAL OF CUSTOMS,
Peking.

The Contributors to this Volume are—

R. A. JAMIESON, M.A., M.D., M.R.C.S. .... Shanghai.

F. WONG, M.D., L.R.C.S.E. .... Canton.

J. G. BRERETON, L.K.&Q.C.P., L.R.C.S.I. .... Chefoo.

J. H. MACKENZIE, M.D. .... Ningpo.

E. I. SCOTT, L.K.&Q.C.P., L.R.C.S.I. .... Swatow.

D. MANSON, M.D., CH.M. .... Amoy.

J. WATSON, M.D., L.R.C.S.E. .... Newchwang.

T. RENNIE, M.D., CH.M. .... Takow and Taiwan-fu.

W. W. MYERS, M.B., C.M. .... Wênchow.

S. ELDRIDGE, M.D. .... Yokohama.

I.—Dr. W. W. Myers's Report on the Sanitary Condition of Wênchow.

The city of Wênchow, situated in Latitude 27° 18′ 4″ 0‴ N., and Longitude 120° 38′ 28″ 50‴ E., lies on the south bank of the large and deep Ou-kiang 江 甌, about 20 miles from its mouth.

The river flows at this part west and east, between long ranges of hills to the north and south, down to the sea.

That the Chinese must possess more than an elementary acquaintance with sanitary laws the condition of this city would seem to indicate; and whereas in Peking and other cities the knowledge has for long been allowed to lie dormant and its former products to fall into ruin and disuse, here the contrary obtains. The streets, regularly laid out and closely paved, slope down on each side to drains or gutters, which in their turn communicate with the canals running through all the city. About every hundred yards are latrines and urinals which are emptied in the early mornings at regular hours. These privies, well supplied with water and their contents not allowed to remain long enough for putrefactive changes to take place, constitute a system which by itself is a most commendable advance in hygienic science. At early dawn scavengers go round, sweeping and clearing the streets and side gutters, emptying and cleaning the utensils used in the houses during the night, and collecting all rubbish and refuse, taking it away to be either destroyed by fire, or used for the fields. The canals are, as a rule, pretty full, or at anyrate by their depth able to retain a sufficient supply of water between the intervals of rain to allow for the usual evaporation. They communicate one with the other, here and there widening out into a broad sheet or small lake; and thus a steady though slow circulation is kept up. They are constantly dredged, and all vegetable or other matter is carefully collected and removed. As may be supposed, the absence of those atrocious smells consequent on decomposing organic matter usually met with on entering most other Chinese cities is strikingly noticeable in Wênchow. The inhabitants, taken as a whole, well to do and contented, are able in the great majority of cases to live in comparatively roomy and airy houses isolated from each other by high walls, and in a great many instances, spacious courtyards. To judge by the absence of all appearance of overcrowding, I am of opinion that the population is by no means excessive in proportion to the area available for its accommodation; and this notwithstanding the many plots of common, etc., scattered throughout the place.

This has been aptly styled "a cathedral city:" large and gorgeous temples abound and numerous priests and nuns luxuriate in the markedly devotional spirit shown by the people. One advantage derived from these frequently recurring Joss-houses is the large greens or open spaces generally connected therewith, where the laity, old and young, may congregate if it so please them, and inhale the fresher air, while the general atmospheric circulation and purity are also improved.

The people seem to be very careful as to the water they drink, drawing their supplies from wells dug in places as remote from habitations as possible. These are further secured by encircling walls closely cemented so as to keep out the surface drainage. As far as I have observed, this water is kept solely for potable purposes, canal water being used for washing, etc., etc. Thus the dipping of filthy vessels, and other means of contamination common elsewhere, are avoided if not prohibited. As with very rare exceptions no interments take place within the city, and for the reasons before given, decomposing vegetable or animal matter is scarcely to be met with, the water ought to be good; and this I am glad to say chemical and microscopical examination—as far as I have been able to carry it—appears to bear out.

Last year was an exceptionally wet one all over the south of China, and that we were not without our full share a glance at the hygrometric table will show. Although the days in each month on which rain actually fell in the city were not as numerous as I expected to find, still so intermingled were the rainy with the dry days, so marked the dampness of the atmosphere with rain pouring on and near the hills to north and south of us, that it is matter of surprise when going over the record to find that it rained with us on so comparatively few occasions. It seemed to all as though "wet" weather had scarcely ever ceased from June of last year until January of this. When we did have a fine clear day it was certainly most enjoyable, the summer heat, pleasantly tempered by the fresh sea-breezes which blow up the funnel-like valley directly on to the city, was scarcely felt, and speaking from my own experience, the sensible effect of temperature here contrasted most favourably with that of Shanghai and Ningpo, through both of which places I had occasion to pass on my way from and to Wênchow in July and August.

In the city the perfect system of drainage obviated many of the disadvantages of the wet season; but on Conquest Island opposite the city and in the middle of the river, where several of the residents were living, and where the meteorological instruments were kept, the damp was more palpable. Notwithstanding this, I think I may fairly assert that the great depression and languor complained of so much in most up-river places is felt here to a very limited extent if at all; but on the contrary, (thanks to the sea-breezes which have so ready access to us,) we are often conscious of an exhilarating and bracing effect, which goes far to modify other discomforts. Of course from one year's observations—and that said to be, by those best qualified to speak, an exceptional one—it would be premature to say much about climate; but I feel justified in hoping and to some extent believing that this place will be found to combine many of the sanitary advantages of a seaport with but comparatively few of the drawbacks peculiar to most riverine settlements. Of course, should the settlement be eventually fixed at or about the mouth of the river the port will then be to all intents and purposes a seaside one; but on this subject I will say something farther on.

The city may be said to be enclosed by a circle of small hills along the summits of which the walls run. The ground within these is considerably elevated above the river and therefore disaster or flooding from tide or freshet is unknown in Wênchow. On the plain extending from the base of the large hills forming the south side of the valley up to the walls of the city, rice is largely cultivated, the means for irrigation and transport being afforded by numerous canals.

Shut out from the city as these are, no injurious effects from malaria or other causes are to be met with or indeed looked for. Throughout the city are many good double-storied houses which with a few additions (*e.g.* glass windows, extra flooring, etc.,) may be readily converted into comfortable and healthy abodes. Rents too are remarkably low, which is another advantage, although I presume the natives would not be long in finding this out were the demand sufficient to warrant consideration of the matter.

On our arrival here we felt the want of beef very much, as that sold in the market for Chinese consumption is of the most objectionable kind, being generally procured from the carcases of animals that have died from disease or been slaughtered in anticipation of the event. After some little time, however, the community were able to arrange with a Chinese compradore to kill regularly, the animal being submitted to medical inspection before, and the beef after, slaughter. We have thus been getting tolerably good and at anyrate healthy meat; and as the butcher now and then varies the programme by killing a sheep, we feel much more satisfied on this score than at first seemed probable. In the cooler weather goat-mutton is to be had; and this is by no means a bad substitute for the other, forming a pleasant change in the bill of fare. Geese, fowls, eggs, ducks and vegetables are plentiful; and, could one get over long cherished prejudice, the pork ought to be found good, as the pigs are as a rule kept in styes, and are carefully fed and properly cared for.

When I add that all the above are cheap, the commissariat of the place will not be thought badly of.

From a medical point of view, I can only note the general good health which has prevailed among the foreign residents, but seeing that the community has been and is so small, no great inference can be drawn from this fact, especially after so short an experience, though it ought to be mentioned that the 26 residents here on the 31st of December, as also the diminished number of 23 present on the 31st March include five ladies and three children, the youngest of the latter being 18 months and the eldest 4 years and 6 months old.

Although I have made strenuous efforts to get up a native practice I cannot say that I have met with the success I hoped for. The Chinese seem as yet shy of coming under foreign treatment, and entertain most peculiar and contradictory notions as to its capabilities. On the one hand, they appear to think that in certain cases death is no bar to foreign skill, and on the other they profess to believe in the superiority of their own doctors in cases where the appearances are not so desperate.

Ague from country districts came occasionally under notice. Ophthalmia, and in fact most eye-diseases, are very common, especially catarrh and pannus. Small-pox does not seem to be more rife than the fact of vaccination not being practised would lead one to expect. Last summer, in common with most places in China, cholera prevailed for a short time, about ten days or a fortnight. Little or no treatment appeared to be adopted. The prevalent symptoms were the initiatory passage of one or two rice-watery stools, followed by collapse, *i.e.* surface coldness, slight cramps, often suppression of urine, no or very little vomiting, and in from 6 to 24 hours sudden death. Opium-smokers almost certainly died. The symptoms, however, were peculiarly undemonstrative to external observation, the patient frequently appearing to rally, and in many cases the fatal termination was not preceded by an appreciable relapse. Purging and vomiting, except to the limited extent mentioned, was very rare; but the mortality amongst the attacked was very great. I had a strong impression that attempts at rational treatment would have brought about different results, at least in a great many cases; but nothing seemed to be tried. As soon as the native doctor made out the nature of the case he departed and the domestic offices for the dying or dead commenced.

The visitation was by no means spread over the whole city, but confined to a few streets chiefly in one quarter. To obtain anything like regular statistics was of course impossible, but it seems very probable that the minimum death-rate was 10 per diem, running up for two days to 35, when it again fell to 10, and soon the unpleasant visitor left. To the wonderful sanitary condition of the place I unhesitatingly attribute the limitation of the onslaught and stay of the epidemic; and I was glad to observe that some attempt at disinfection by cleansing the rooms, burning the bed and body clothes, etc., was made. Again, the bodies were immediately coffined and removed to some remote place, generally outside the walls. I treated three patients, one of whom died. I found chloral hydrate hypodermically in conjunction with other remedies, such as friction, heat, etc., most useful. Nitrite of amyl gave no results as far as I had an opportunity of observing. The subject of the fatal attack was a confirmed opium-smoker, and so pertinacious was he, that after rallying during my temporary absence he insisted on having a pipe. No bad symptom that I could observe set in; the temperature kept at about 99°, and I left him about 3 A.M. At 8 A.M. a messenger came to tell me that he was all right. Desiring to see him myself, however, I returned with the man, and found him just dying or dead. He had sat up to drink some milk, when he suddenly fell back dead. The relatives had all along insisted to me on the certainty of his death, as he was so great an opium-smoker. Whether they tried to justify their predictions by an unlimited supply of the drug during my absence I cannot say; but if they did it was not for want of earnest warning, or strenuous promises on their part to refrain from giving him any.

Elephantiasis I have seen once or twice, but I am not in a position at present to speak as to the frequency of its occurrence or otherwise. Skin diseases are very general, scabies being the most common. Enthetic disease is very plentiful; the ecclesiastical tendencies of the place seeming to favour its spread, as the nuns are merely prostitutes and are as a rule diseased. Their favours are largely sought notwithstanding a comparatively high fee and the general knowledge of their infected state. There are about 40 convents besides several brothels containing avowed prostitutes, and it is stated that domestic morality stands very low, many married woman being notoriously dissolute. The wide spread of syphilis is by all this easily accounted for.

Opium-poisoning cases at certain periods of the year are common, and on the occasions where my aid has been sought the subjects have been generally insensible. I have been able, however, by means of atropine and strychnine, after washing out the stomach well with cold water, to resuscitate the greater number of those treated. The Chinese remedies most in vogue here are: first, the contents of the adjacent urinal or fluid from a latrine; next, the warm blood as it spurts from the recently incised throat of a sheep, goat or fowl. In ignorance of this last mode of procedure, the first few discharges from the stomach-pump are apt to cause alarm. Unaccountable as it may appear, the above would-be emetics generally fail to bring about the desired result.

Perhaps it will be as well to say a word or two about the sanitary conditions of the various sites which have been proposed for the foreign concession. These are as follows:—

(a) The piece of ground to the east of the city offered to Mr. DAVENPORT for selection;

(b) The pagoda hill opposite the city proposed by Mr. H. E. HOBSON; and

(c) The plot beyond the anchorage or lower Customs station.

I believe Conquest Island, a small piece of land lying in the middle of the river opposite the city, and at present affording site for one large temple and two pagodas has been suggested; but I assume only mentioned to be discarded. Supposing the port ever worthy of any fixed concession or settlement, one ordinary merchant (should he be able to buy up the temple, demolish it and erect his house and godowns in the place where it stands) might perhaps by dint of considerable trouble and large outlay make himself comfortable. Or supposing godowns could be located elsewhere, then perhaps at most two or three dwelling-houses might find space. However, as it is not only probable but I suppose certain that the Chinese would scout the idea of giving up a temple that is revered as this one is, Conquest Island even with its temple and pagodas demolished would be miserably inadequate for the purpose, should the increase of this port render a concession necessary, or its size and position of importance.

Had this been a port like Ningpo with only flat marshy ground to choose from, and had the pressing necessity of being close to the city put all other considerations in the background, then perhaps—could no thicker mud be attainable—the first site might be forced on our acceptance; and by means of unlimited pile-driving and interminable contributions of rubble a foundation sufficiently hard to support houses, for say one or two years, might be obtained. It might also be so raised that, except at spring tides, fluid of less consistence than slush could be kept away; but seeing that this is about the only piece of ground in Wênchow which presents such marked disadvantages I cannot see why it should be taken. I am aware that the greater part, if not the whole of it, belongs to one or two of the officials; but this is scarcely reason sufficient for putting foreigners to the pecuniary outlay which the formation of the settlement, loss of time whilst down from miasmatic disease, medical and funeral expenses would surely entail. True, a very good sanitarium might be established in the adjacent city; but though this might avert for some time the last item of expenditure, still it would scarcely amount to a saving in the long run. If low, flat ground *must* be taken on this side of the river, then a little farther back, or lower down, some could be got that is at least above high-water mark; although by so choosing foreigners would be unnecessarily tempting a state of unhealthiness that might be easily avoided by taking up some equally accessible and more elevated spot.

Pagoda Hill (b) was proposed by Mr. HOBSON, and certainly from a sanitary point of view this would appear to combine all that could be desired. It is in the direct line of the sea breezes in summer, while sheltered in winter. Good views could be got from at least three sides, and the houses could be built on good, dry gravel foundations. The only drawback would be the distance from the city, as this hill is on the opposite (north) bank of the river, which latter is at this point about $\frac{1}{2}$ to $\frac{3}{4}$ of a mile wide. Again, steamers or sailing ships would have to lie at the city side, as the anchorage is not so favourable on the other.

The aforesaid two sites have been proposed on the supposition that it is necessary for the foreign settlement to be as close to the city as possible. Now, if this means close to the native merchants and their hongs it will scarcely apply to Wênchow at present, for the simple reason that there are none. Almost all the trade is connected with the districts more or less far back in the interior of the country, *i.e.* tea and other articles for export, piece goods, opium, oil, etc., etc., for import. The people proper of Wênchow city are by no means given to extensive or speculative trade, and as a consequence, the junks go to all the places along the river and coast which happen to be near the greatest body of consumers. Of course, were foreigners to come here and establish steamer lines and other means of inducing trade, the city could and would eventually be made the point of contact; but the intermediary native merchants would be all men from other parts to whom Wênchow city only became a residence because of the necessity set up by foreigners. Thus they no less than foreigners would be settlers, with this exception, that their movements would be dependent on those of foreigners. Now, seeing that in most cases cargo going inward, and especially that coming for shipment (markedly teas) actually has in most cases to diverge from the anchorage in order to reach the city, and that the concentration of trade at this last or other places is so to speak dependent on the presence of foreigners, it would appear that practically the desire of merchants to be as close as possible to those with whom they wish to do business could be met by the establishment of a settlement at the mouth of the river, while the inconvenience to shipping necessarily attending a location higher up would be entirely obviated. I have often heard it said that this was the mistake made at Foochow, and the resulting upper and lower settlements regretted as constant sources of inconvenience. That it is not essential to the prospects of trade for the settlement to be close to the city is, I believe, shown by that at Yingtze, some miles below Newchwang.

Supposing then that the mercantile obstacles to forming the settlement at the mouth of the river are not insuperable, the sanitary advantages are immeasurably great. At this point the hills come close to the water-side, and at the extreme and seaward point of the south bank slope directly down to it. There are one or two smaller hills which intervene between those behind and the river-side, and than these no finer sites for building good, dry, healthy houses could be found. The water frontage, well above high-water mark, would be excellent for godowns, and the largest vessels could lie within 100 yards of the bank. Being close to the sea, a settlement here would to all intents and purposes be a marine one; the conformation of the hills and the proximity of the sea would render it cool in summer, and the shelter afforded by the hills would prevent its being unduly exposed in winter. Connected by deep canals and good roads with the country in the back, and with the city 8 or 10 miles off, the facilities for landing, shipping and transporting goods would be unusually great, while the opportunities for making one of the healthiest settlements in the south of China would be very marked. On the adjacent hills and in the numerous valleys there is fine scenery of all kinds, and charming walks. With but comparatively small outlay, riding and even driving roads might be made. In a word, should the port of Wênchow ever assume the commercial standing to which its geographical position entitles it, a foreign settlement at Jar Point ought to be all that could be desired.

ABSTRACT of METEOROLOGICAL OBSERVATIONS taken by the CUSTOMS,

Latitude 27° 18′ 41″ 0‴ North,

DATE.	BAROMETER.		THERMOMETERS.				HYGROMETER.					
			Dry Bulb.		Wet Bulb.		Temperature of Dew-point computed.		Elastic force of Vapour.		Humidity o—1.	
	9.30 A.M.	3.30 P.M.	9.30 A.M.	3.30 P.M.	9.30 A.M.	3.30 P.M.	9.30 A.M.	3.30 P.M.	9.30 A.M.	3.30 P.M.	9.30 A.M.	3.30 P.M.
APRIL:—	inches.	inches.	° F.	° F.	° F.	° F.	° F.	° F.				
Max......	30·07	29·95	75·	79·	73·	74·	71.6	70·5	·774	·745	·965	·882
Mean.....	29·91	29·89	69·90	71·8	68·5	69·63	67·4	67·84	·670	·680	·917	·873
Min.......	29·79	29·75	65·	67·	64·	65·	64·	63·4	·596	·583	·889	·752
MAY:—												
Max......	30·08	30·05	78·	78·	72·	74·	67·8	71·2	·680	·763	·874	·896
Mean.....	29·93	29·92	71·64	72·3	68·7	69·2	66·34	66·72	·645	·654	·834	·829
Min.......	29·79	29·78	64·	65.	62·	63·	60·2	61·4	·575	·544	·709	·796
JUNE:—												
Max......	30·04	29·97	84·	89·	81·	81·	78·9	76·2	·987	·902	·992	·882
Mean.....	29·85	29·84	77·4	78·2	74·3	74·7	72·13	72·25	·787	·789	·839	·818
Min.......	29·67	29·68	68·	69·	67·	67·	66·2	65·4	·643	·625	·838	·660
JULY:—												
Max......	30·00	29·98	88·	91·	82·	83·	78·4	78·2	·970	·964	·941	·942
Mean.....	29·72	29·79	82·2	82·6	79·1	78·87	76·93	76·25	·924	·902	·838	·810
Min.......	29·64	29·59	77·	75·	75·	74·	73·6	73·3	·827	·819	·828	·662
AUGUST:—												
Max......	30·07	30·05	85·	90·	82·	85· .	79·9	82·0	1·019	1·092	·847	·775
Mean.....	29·85	29·82	80·8	83·6	77·7	79·2	75·53	76·12	1·222	·899	·840	·681
Min.......	29·62	29.62	76·	76·	73·	74·	70·9	72·6	·755	·800	·820	·480
SEPTEMBER:—												
Max......	30·19	30·15	84·	86·	79·	81·	75·5	77·5	·882	·942	·939	·828
Mean.....	30·05	29·99	75·43	76·87	73·	74·07	71·29	72·01	763	·784	·868	·851
Min.......	29·90	29·85	67·	68·	66·	65·	65·2	62·6	·621	·567	·757	·758
OCTOBER:—												
Max......	30·44	30·39	75·	80·	71·	74·	68·2	69·8	·689	·728	·794	·711
Mean.....	30·21	30·16	67·2	72·9	62·2	66·3	58·20	61·22	·485	·540	·728	·686
Min.......	30·06	29·95	56·	62·	48·	52·	40.0	43·0	·247	·277	·550	·497

WÊNCHOW, for the ELEVEN MONTHS ended 28th February 1878.

Longitude 120° 38′ 28″ 50‴ East.

Self-registering Thermometers.		Rain in 24 Hours.	Wind.				Clouds.		No. of days in each month on which no rain or snow fell.
Maximum in Air.	Minimum in Air.		Force as per Naval Scale.		Summary of Direction.		0—10.		
9.30 A.M.	9.30 A.M.	Inches.	9.30 A.M.	3.30 P.M.	9.30 A.M.	3.30 P.M.	9.30 A.M.	3.30 P.M.	
° F.	° F.								
83·	73·		2·	2·			2 at 10 / 1 ,, 9 / 2 ,, 8 / 2 ,, 7 / 1 ,, 5 / 1 ,, 4 / 2 ,, 0	5 at 10 / 2 ,, 9 / 2 ,, 3 / 1 ,, 0	6
75·17	67·04		·8	1·090					
68·	57·		·000	·000					
84·	73·		4·	4·			11 at 10 / 4 ,, 8 / 3 ,, 7 / 4 ,, 5 / 2 ,, 4 / 3 ,, 3 / 3 ,, 1	6 at 10 / 1 ,, 9 / 3 ,, 8 / 6 ,, 7 / 1 ,, 6 / 5 ,, 4 / 3 ,, 3 / 2 ,, 0	21
74·98	68·29		·758	1·111					
67·	59·		·000	·000					
91·	83·		2·5	3·			11 at 10 / 6 ,, 8 / 1 ,, 7 / 1 ,, 6 / 1 ,, 5 / 1 ,, 3 / 5 ,, 0	10 at 10 / 5 ,, 8 / 2 ,, 6 / 1 ,, 5 / 1 ,, 3 / 5 ,, 0	16
75·6	74·05		·425	·783					
69·	66·		·000	·000					
94·	88·		7·	3·			3 at 10 / 9 ,, 8 / 5 ,, 7 / 2 ,, 6 / 3 ,, 5 / 3 ,, 4 / 1 ,, 3 / 1 ,, 1 / 1 ,, 0	3 at 10 / 2 ,, 9 / 5 ,, 8 / 3 ,, 7 / 3 ,, 6 / 3 ,, 5 / 4 ,, 4 / 4 ,, 3 / 1 ,, 1 / 1 ,, 0	21
85·64	79·24		·427	·895					
76·	74·		·000	·000					
90·	88·		2·	3·			1 at 10 / 6 ,, 9 / 3 ,, 8 / 3 ,, 7 / 6 ,, 6 / 7 ,, 4 / 5 ,, 3 / 3 ,, 1 / 1 ,, 0	5 at 10 / 8 ,, 8 / 3 ,, 7 / 3 ,, 6 / 3 ,, 5 / 8 ,, 4 / 8 ,, 3 / 1 ,, 2 / 1 ,, 1	21
87·63	77·79		·580	·870					
76·	70·		·000	·000					
93·	79·	2·	2·	2·			11 at 10 / 1 ,, 9 / 5 ,, 8 / 1 ,, 7 / 4 ,, 6 / 4 ,, 4 / 3 ,, 4 / 2 ,, 3	11 at 10 / 1 ,, 9 / 3 ,, 8 / 4 ,, 7 / 4 ,, 6 / 4 ,, 4 / 1 ,, 4 / 1 ,, 3 / 1 ,, 2	17
81·60	71·80	1·272	·4	·566					
71·	66·	·000	·000	·000					
86·	70·	1·1	2·	4·			3 at 10 / 2 ,, 9 / 1 ,, 8 / 3 ,, 6 / 7 ,, 4 / 6 ,, 3 / 2 ,, 2 / 4 ,, 1	4 at 10 / 5 ,, 9 / 3 ,, 8 / 2 ,, 7 / 1 ,, 6 / 1 ,, 5 / 1 ,, 3 / 5 ,, 0	25
77·26	62·13	·475	·838	1·					
67·	50·	·000	·000	·000					

In default of a Rain-guage no observations were taken.

8

MEDICAL REPORTS, NO. 15.   [OCT.-MAR,

DATE.	BAROMETER.		THERMOMETER.				HYGROMETER.					
			Dry Bulb.		Wet Bulb.		Temperature of Dew-point computed.		Elastic force of Vapour.		Humidity 0—1.	
	9.30 A.M.	3.30 P.M.	9.30 A.M.	3.30 P.M.	9.30 A.M.	3.30 P.M.	9.30 A.M.	3.30 P.M.	9.30 A.M.	3.30 P.M.	9.30 A.M.	3.30 P.M.
NOVEMBER:—	inches.	inches.	° F.	° F.	° F.	° F.	° F.	° F.				
Max.......	30·57	30·44	69·	77·	67·	73·	65·4	70·2	·625	·733	·882	·796
Mean.....	30·29	30·21	60·7	64·3	58·	61·1	55·57	58·22	·441	·485	·830	·805
Min.......	30·01	29·92	49·	52·	46·	49·	42·7	46·0	·274	·310	·789	·799
DECEMBER:—												
Max.......	30·44	30·50	62·	71·	61·	69·	60·1	67·4	·519	·670	·935	·883
Mean.....	30·21	30·20	52·2	56·7	50·1	54·2	48·	51·70	·335	·384	·856	·834
Min.......	29·99	29·86	41·	43·	38·	41·	34·1	38·6	·196	·234	·760	·844
1878.												
JANUARY:—												
Max.....	30·62	30·53	53·3	62·	53·	58·	52·70	54·4	·402	·423	·987	·850
Mean.....	30·70	30·57	40·45	44·79	38·54	41·98	31·45	38·60	·176	·234	·701	·790
Min......	29·99	29·79	29·	32·	28·	31·	24·4	28·7	·126	·154	·738	·762
FEBRUARY:—												
Max......	30·57	30·51	53· .	56·	52·	55·	51·	54·	·374	·417	·930	·928
Mean.....	30·33	30·29	43·27	45·94	41·88	43·63	40·21	40·85	·249	·255	·896	·805
Min......	30·07	29·99	36·	39·	33·	37·	28·5	34·4	·153	·199	·721	·642

Instruments placed in verandah facing S. on Conquest Island.

REMARKS.

Dew-point, Elastic force of Vapour, and Humidity computed from the Greenwich factors published in 1856.

The readings for April commenced on the afternoon of the 19th, those for February ceased for all the instruments except the Barometer on the 18th, and those of the latter on the 13th when it was unfortunately broken.

The following record of observations made during the typhoon of the 3rd July 1877, may be of interest:—

At 9.30 A.M. the force of wind was estimated at 7 of the Naval Scale, from which hour the storm increased up to some time between 11 and 12 o'clock noon, when it began to moderate, and by 3.30 P.M. had quite abated. The wind, which kept steadily at East during the continuance of the gale, had come round to South at 3.30 P.M. The following is the note made for the day:—" Forenoon blowing terrifically "and rain coming down in torrents ; about noon began to moderate and clear off, afterwards gentle breeze with drizzling rain."

Readings of Barometer, July 3rd 1877.

Inches.		Inches.		Inches.		Inches.	
6 A.M.	29·65	10 A.M.	29·34	1 P.M.	29·40	5 P.M.	29·55
7 ,,	29·61	11 ,,	29·20	2 ,,	29·45	6 ,,	29·64
8 ,,	29·55	11.30 ,,	29·10	3 ,,	29·50	7 ,,	29·70
9 ,,	29·47	Noon	29·22	4 ,,	29·52	8 ,,	29·75

Self-registering Thermometers.		Rain in 24 Hours.	Wind.				Clouds.		No. of days in each month on which no rain or snow fell.
Maximum in Air.	Minimum in Air.		Force as per Naval Scale.		Summary of Direction.		0—10.		
9.30 A.M.	9.30 A.M.	Inches.	9.30 A.M.	3.30 P.M.	9.30 A.M.	3.30 P.M.	9.30 A.M.	3.30 P.M.	
° F.	° F.								
82·	66·	·3	4·	4·			13 at 10 3 „ 9 6 „ 8 3 „ 7 3 „ 5 1 „ 4 2 „ 3 1 „ 2 1 „ 0	16 at 10 2 „ 9 2 „ 8 2 „ 7 1 „ 5 3 „ 4 2 „ 3 1 „ 2 1 „ 1	
67·57	56·57	·18	1·333	1·366					17
52·	48·	·000	·000	·000					
73·	59·	1·1	5·	5·			11 at 10 4 „ 9 3 „ 8 4 „ 7 2 „ 5 1 „ 4 4 „ 0	13 at 10 2 „ 9 5 „ 8 1 „ 7 3 „ 5 1 „ 4 2 „ 3 1 „ 1 1 „ 0	
57·47	47·10	·428	1·310	1·379					19
47·5	36·	·000	·000	·000					
54·	51·5	·5	4·	4·			12 at 10 5 „ 8 3 „ 7 1 „ 5 4 „ 3 1 „ 1 2 „ 0	17 at 10 5 „ 8 1 „ 7 3 „ 4 1 „ 5 1 „ 3 1 „ 1 2 „ 0	
44·48	36·88	·242	1·709	1·903					22
35·	27·	·000	·000	·000					
68·	46·5	·9	4·	4·			15 at 10 6 „ 8 4 „ 7 2 „ 0	14 at 10 2 „ 9 8 „ 8 1 „ 7 1 „ 6 1 „ 3 1 „ 0	
48·47	38·91	·46	·875	1·125					16
41·5	35·	·000	·000	·000					

Rain Guage 4 feet above ground.

Naval Scale for estimating force of wind, from Col. Sir H. James's *Instructions;* app. p. 31.

Pressure in lb. per sq. ft.

0 Denotes calm.

1 Light air just sufficient to give steerage way. .... ¼

2 Light breeze........ with which a well-conditioned man-of-war under all sail and clean full would go in smooth water from
- 1 to 2 knots 1
- 3 to 4 knots 2¼
- 5 to 6 knots 4

3 Gentle breeze ......

4 Moderate breeze ...

5 Fresh breeze......... in which the same ship could just carry close hauled
- Royals, etc................................ 6¼
- Single-reefs and top-gallant sails 9
- Double-reefs, jib, etc. 12¼
- Triple-reefs, courses, etc. 16
- Close-reefs and courses 20¼

6 Stormy breeze ......

7 Moderate gale ......

8 Fresh gale.........

9 Strong gale ....

10 Whole gale .... with which she could only bear
- Close-reefed main topsail and reefed foresail. } 25

11 Storm .... with which she would be reduced to
- Storm stay-sails 30¼

12 Hurricane............ to which she could show ......
- No canvas 36

China, Imperial Maritime Customs, Medical Reports
（1878. 04. 01—1879. 03. 31）

CHINA.

IMPERIAL MARITIME CUSTOMS.

II.—SPECIAL SERIES: No. 2.

MEDICAL REPORTS,

FOR THE HALF-YEAR ENDED 30TH SEPTEMBER 1879.

18th Issue.

PUBLISHED BY ORDER OF

The Inspector General of Customs.

SHANGHAI:
STATISTICAL DEPARTMENT
OF THE
INSPECTORATE GENERAL.

MDCCCLXXX.

INSPECTORATE GENERAL OF CUSTOMS,

PEKING, 31st *December* 1870.

SIR,

1.—IT has been suggested to me that it would be well to take advantage of the circum-stances in which the Customs Establishment is placed, to procure information with regard to disease amongst foreigners and natives in China; and I have, in consequence, come to the resolution of publishing half-yearly in collected form all that may be obtainable. If carried out to the extent hoped for, the scheme may prove highly useful to the medical profession both in China and at home, and to the public generally. I therefore look with confidence to the co-opera-tion of the Customs Medical Officer at your port, and rely on his assisting me in this matter by framing a half-yearly report containing the result of his observations at.........upon the local peculiarities of disease, and upon diseases rarely or never encountered out of China. The facts brought forward and the opinions expressed will be arranged and published either with or without the name of the physician responsible for them, just as he may desire.

2.—The suggestions of the Customs Medical Officers at the various ports as to the points which it would be well to have especially elucidated, will be of great value in the framing of a form which will save trouble to those members of the Medical profession, whether connected with the Customs or not, who will join in carrying out the plan proposed. Meanwhile I would particularly invite attention to—

a.—The general health of............during the period reported on; the death rate amongst foreigners; and, as far as possible, a classification of the causes of death.

b.—Diseases prevalent at............

c.—General type of disease; peculiarities and complications encountered; special treatment demanded.

d.—Relation of disease to { Season. Alteration in local conditions—such as drainage, &c. Alteration in climatic conditions.

e.—Peculiar diseases; especially leprosy.

f.—Epidemics { Absence or presence. Causes. Course and treatment. Fatality.

Other points, of a general or special kind, will naturally suggest themselves to medical men; what I have above called attention to will serve to fix the general scope of the undertaking. I have committed to Dr. ALEX. JAMIESON, of Shanghai, the charge of arranging the reports for publication, so that they may be made available in a convenient form.

3.—Considering the number of places at which the Customs Inspectorate has established offices, the thousands of miles north and south and east and west over which these offices are scattered, the varieties of climate, and the peculiar conditions to which, under such different circumstances, life and health are subjected, I believe the Inspectorate, aided by its Medical Officers, can do good service in the general interest in the direction indicated; and, as already stated, I rely with confidence on the support and assistance of the Medical Officer at each port in the furtherance and perfecting of this scheme. You will hand a copy of this Circular to Dr. ...., and request him, in my name, to hand to you in future, for transmission to myself, half-yearly reports of the kind required, for the half-years ending 31st March and 30th September—that is, for the Winter and Summer seasons.

4.—   *   *   *   *   *

I am, &c.,

(signed)   ROBERT HART,
I. G.

THE COMMISSIONERS OF CUSTOMS,—*Newchwang*, *Ningpo*,
Tientsin, *Foochow*,
Chefoo, *Tamsui*,
Hankow, *Takow*,
Kiukiang, *Amoy*,
Chinkiang, *Swatow*, and
Shanghai, *Canton*.

SHANGHAI, 1st June 1880.

SIR,

In accordance with the directions of your Despatch No. 6 *A* (Returns Series) of the 24th June 1871, I now forward to the Statistical Department of the Inspectorate General of Customs, the following documents :—

Cholera Epidemics in Japan, pp. 1-30.

A.—Additional Notes on Filaria Sanguinis Hominis and Filaria Disease at Amoy, pp. 31-51.

B.—Lithotomy Statistics from Canton Native Hospital, pp. 52-55.

C.—Report on the Health of Canton for the half-year ended 30th September 1879, pp. 56, 57.

D.—Report on the Health of Amoy for the year ended 30th September 1879, pp. 58, 59.

E.—Report on the Sanitary Condition of Wênchow for the year ended 31st March 1879, pp. 60-63.

F.—Report on the Health of Tamsui and Kelung for the year ended 30th September 1879, p. 64.

G.—Report on Health Conditions in Foochow, pp. 65-70.

H.—Report on the Health of Chefoo, pp. 71-74 ;

I.—Report on the Health of Swatow, pp. 75-79 ;

K.—Report on the Health of Shanghai, pp. 80-82 ; each of these referring to the half-year ended 30th September 1879.

I have the honour to be,

SIR,

Your obedient Servant,

R. ALEX. JAMIESON.

THE INSPECTOR GENERAL OF CUSTOMS,
PEKING.

The Contributors to this Volume are—

D. B. Simmons, M.D. .... Yokohama, Japan.

P. Manson, M.D., CH.M. .... Amoy.

Flemming Carrow, M.D. .... Canton.

W. W. Myers, M.B., CH.M. .... Wênchow.

B. S. Ringer, M.R.C.S., L.S.A. .... Tamsui and Kelung.

J. A. Stewart, M.D. .... Foochow.

J. G. Brereton, L.K.&Q.C.P., L.R.C.S.I. .... Chefoo.

E. I. Scott, L.K.&Q.C.P., L.R.C.S.I. .... Swatow.

R. A. Jamieson, M.A., M.D., M.R.C.S. .... Shanghai.

E.—Dr. MYERS's Report on the Sanitary Condition of Wênchow for the Year
ended 31st March 1879.

IN my previous report * I have described at length the main features of the port from a
sanitary point of view; but little, therefore, remains for me to detail when writing about so small
a foreign community as that resident here. I would, before going further, mention that the
latitude of the city should read thus: lat. 28° 1′ 30″ 0‴ N., the longitude previously printed
being correct.

There was a visitation of cholera in August 1878, during which two Europeans were
attacked, one fatally. The first case took place on board H.M.S. *Nassau*, and I was requested by
my friend Dr. GRAHAM, R.N., to see it with him.

Briefly, I may state that most of the remedies usually adopted were tried, but that the
ultimate result seemed to be most influenced by resort to dry heat. This we accomplished in
the manner carried out by Captain COCKER, of the *Fei-Hoo*, viz., placing the patient between
the boilers. He was thus kept in a temperature of about 120°, and allowed to drink freely of
iced water. Reaction soon set in, and when the ship went to sea next morning the man
was rapidly convalescing.

The second and fatal case was at first much less formidable in appearance, but as it
occurred in the person of a lady, nine days after her confinement, to which disadvantage were
added certain other unfavourable conditions, the result was not so unexpected as would have been
otherwise the case.

The epidemic did not last long, nor did the Chinese public generally appear to suffer to
the same extent as in the previous year, though the utter absence of all treatment—in the case
of natives—undoubtedly tended, on this occasion as on last, to swell the mortality rate.

A second death took place during the year in an imported case. The patient was brought
to Wênchow in the last stages of exhaustion from miasmatic toxæmia, and never rallied. She
was stated to have been living in a miserable house, surrounded by ditches and drains, in an
inland city, where good food was rarely procurable. During the last month of her illness she
voided large quantities of biliary sediment. The organs (with the exception of the spleen, which
was remarkably atrophied, being scarcely larger than a very small hen's egg) were normal.

The health of the foreign community generally has been very good, and quite in keeping
with what one would expect from such excellent climatic conditions as usually obtain at this port.
Two births took place. One child, however, was still-born. The labour in this case, though most
gravely complicated and protracted, presented nothing worthy of further special reference. The
mother made a rapid and complete recovery.

It now only remains for me to pass on to the last section of this report—the meteorological.

* Customs *Medical Reports*, xv, 38.

ABSTRACT of METEOROLOGICAL OBSERVATIONS taken at WÊNCHOW from 19th April 1878 to 31st March 1879.

DATE.	BAROMETER.		THERMOMETERS.				HYGROMETER.						SELF-REGISTERING THERMOMETERS.				RAIN IN 24 HOURS.
			Dry Bulb.		Wet Bulb.		Temperature of Dew-Point computed.		Elastic Force of Vapour.		Humidity, 0—1.		Maximum in Air.		Minimum in Air.		
	9.30 A.M.	3.30 P.M.	9.30 A.M.	3.30 P.M.	9.30 A.M.	3.30 P.M.	9.30 A.M.	3.30 P.M.	9.30 A.M.	3.30 P.M.	9.30 A.M.	3.30 P.M.	9.30 A.M.	3.30 P.M.	9.30 A.M.	3.30 P.M.	
1878.	Inches.	Inches.	°F.	°F.	°F.	°F.	°F.	°F.					°F.	°F.	°F.	°F.	Inches.
APRIL:—																	
Max.			69.	70.	68.	68.5	67.2	67.30	.666	.716	.969	.976	75.		70.5		1.
Mean			64.4	63.6	60.8	62.6	61.37	60.72	.551	.542	.899	.908	65.3		56.1		.3
Min.			58.	58.	57.	55.	55.1	55.4	.446	.439	.683	.766	58.		53.		.000
MAY:—																	
Max.			87.	86.	80.5	79.	76.6	84.8	.862	1.195	.969	.986	88.5		80.		.8
Mean	No barometer.	No barometer.	76.5	75.8	72.6	71.8	70.61	71.24	.754	.825	.832	.856	79.1		69.8		.2
Min.			66.	68.	64.	62.	62.8	60.8	.572	.533	.710	.716	70.7		63.		.000
JUNE:—																	
Max.			89.	88.	82.	83.	80.0	80.8	1.044	1.044	.945	.946	89.1		82.2		1.4
Mean			79.9	79.4	76.5	75.	76.86	73.17	.820	.809	.797	.816	81.5		75.1		.4
Min.			72.	71.	69.	67.	64.8	62.2	.613	.560	.577	.630	74.7		67.5		.000
JULY:—																	
Max.	30.02	29.98	91.	94.5	84.	88.	81.9	86.2	1.089	1.250	.778	.847	84.		85.5		.4
Mean	29.88	29.78	87.2	88.9	82.1	85.1	78.8	79.3	.984	1.000	.763	.734	90.2		82.		.2
Min.	29.56	29.62	82.5	79.	78.5	77.	74.4	74.0	.850	.837	.766	.771	84.6		76.7		.000
AUGUST:—																	
Max.	30.04	30.05	93.	93.	84.5	86.5	83.8	85.7	1.158	1.230	.962	.990	97.		84.7		2.8
Mean	29.89	29.86	87.7	84.4	81.1	80.1	76.2	76.7	.919	.928	.757	.771	88.5		79.9		.7
Min.	29.76	29.75	70.	70.5	69.	69.5	71.5	72.0	.689	.701	.541	.593	77.		70.		.000
SEPTEMBER:—																	
Max.	30.57	30.50	89.	85.	84.	81.	78.9	78.4	.987	.971	.847	.964	92.7		82.		.8
Mean	29.95	29.88	81.9	78.5	76.3	74.9	75.	72.4	.868	.795	.797	.816	85.1		75.1		.4
Min.	29.44	29.30	73.	72.	68.	67.	63.8	63.0	.592	.576	.710	.642	74.2		68.		.000
OCTOBER:—																	
Max.	30.38	30.34	84.	84.	79.5	77.	76.35	74.6	.906	.842	.803	.878	92.		81.5		.6
Mean	30.18	30.22	72.4	71.57	68.	67.69	56.84	60.21	.442	.521	.397	.447	75-77		65.9		.4
Min.	29.99	29.98	59.	59.	49.	52.	40.	45.7	.246	.307	.364	.405	60.5		51.5		.2
NOVEMBER:—																	
Max.	30.46	30.45	77.	70.	71.	65.	66.8	61.0	.657	.536	.696	.731	79.		69.		1.4
Mean	30.30	30.30	62.8	62.	57.26	56.	55.50	50.6	.441	.368	.670	.657	66.3		55.		.567
Min.	30.15	30.15	55.	56.	48.	49.	45.0	45.2	.299	.335	.690	.716	61.		45.		.000
DECEMBER:—																	
Max.	30.52	30.52	74.	72.	67.	67.	62.1	63.0	.557	.576	.663	.734	75.		62.		1.6
Mean	30.31	30.29	57.4	53.4	48.7	48.4	44.0	45.2	.288	.301	.608	.635	57.9		45.6		.63
Min.	30.05	30.04	40.	38.	35.	31.	28.5	21.2	.153	.109	.616	.475	42.		28.		.000
1879.																	
JANUARY:—																	
Max.	30.54	30.53	67.	57.	62.	55.	58.0	53.2	.482	.406	.740	.871	68.		52.5		1.7
Mean	30.20	30.18	49.9	50.5	46.	43.4	38.2	39.2	.231	.159	.641	.843	54.3		41.		.284
Min.	30.14	30.04	37.	36.	34.	34	29.8	31.0	.163	.173	.728	.816	42.		30.		.000
FEBRUARY:—																	
Max.	30.46	30.46	70.	64.	63.	63.	57.4	62.1	.472	.558	.630	.919	73.		57.5		—
Mean	30.24	30.22	56.8	52.1	51.7	49.8	46.6	47.5	.318	.329	.620	.843	55.7		44.6		—
Min.	29.88	29.83	38.5	42.	34.	38.	27.0	33.2	.143	.200	.611	.749	45.		33.		—
MARCH:—																	
Max.	30.50	30.44	70.	68.	66.	62.	62.8	55.4	.572	.439	.780	.715	74.		61.		2.5
Mean	30.19	30.17	55.3	51.6	51.3	47.8	47.3	44.0	.326	.288	.744	.680	58.47		46.2		.6
Min.	29.80	29.84	42.	45.	38.5	41.	28.0	36.2	.149	.214	.558	.640	45.		38.		.000

Note (under Maximum in Air, 3.30 P.M. column): Readings from this instrument taken once only in 24 hours.

Note (under Minimum in Air, 3.30 P.M. column): Readings from this instrument taken once only in 24 hours.

MEAN ABSTRACT of READINGS taken during period from April 1877 to February 1878, and that from April 1878 to February 1879 inclusive.

	BAROMETER		THERMOMETERS				HYGROMETER						SELF-REGISTERING THERMOMETERS			
			Dry Bulb.		Wet Bulb.		Temperature of Dew-point computed.		Elastic Force of Vapour.		Humidity, 0—1.		Maximum in Air.		Minimum in Air.	
	9.30 A.M.	3.30 P.M.	9.30 A.M.	3.30 P.M.	9.30 A.M.	3.30 P.M.	9.30 A.M.	3.30 P.M.	9.30 A.M.	3.30 P.M.	9.30 A.M.	3.30 P.M.	9.30 A.M.	3.30 P.M.	9.30 A.M.	3.30 P.M.
	Inch.	Inch.	°F.	°F.	°F.	°F.	°F.	°F.					°F.	°F.	°F.	°F.
Highest point attained by any instrument in each period, viz.:— 9 months of 1877 and 2 of 1878...	Nov. 30.57	Dec. 30.50	July 88.	July 91.	July 82.	Aug. 85.	Aug. 79.9	Aug. 82.	Aug. 1.222	Aug. 1.092	June .992	July .942	July 94.5	...	July 88.	...
9 „ „ 1878 and 2 of 1879...	Jan. 30.62	Jan. 30.53	Aug. 93.	July 94.	Aug. 84.5	Aug. 88.	Aug. 83.8	July 86.2	Aug. 1.158	July 1.250	Jan. .987	Aug. .990	Aug. 97.*	...	July 85.	...
From April 1877 to February 1878 (inclusive):—																
The mean max.	30.28	30.23	74.2	78.	70.2	73.3	68.1	70.1	.720	.762	.917	.852	81.8	...	70.6	...
„ „ mean	30.09	30.06	65.5	68.1	62.9	64.8	60.2	61.9	.609	.601	.832	.798	69.6	...	61.8	...
„ „ min.	29.87	29.79	57.	58.9	54.5	55.2	51.8	53.5	.456	.474	.764	.695	60.9	...	53.4	...
„ „ range	.41	.44	17.2	19.1	15.7	18.1	10.3	16.6	.264	.288	.153	.157	20.9	...	17.2	...
From April 1878 to February 1879 (inclusive):—																
The mean max.	30.37	30.35	80.	78.5	77.	67.5	71.7	72.4	.807	.848	.818	.893	83.	...	73.4	...
„ „ mean	30.15	30.08	70.2	69.	65.6	65.	61.8	60.6	.565	.598	.707	.757	72.7	...	62.7	...
„ „ min.	29.87	29.84	59.2	59.	55.	54.7	51.2	55.9	.436	.434	.636	.662	62.7	...	53.8	...
„ „ range	.50	.49	20.8	19.5	22.	12.8	20.5	16.5	.371	.414	.182	.231	20.3	...	19.6	...

* 1 day.

N.B.—As during the greater part of 1877 there was no gauge available at the port, the rainfall has been omitted from the above table. It must also be recollected that during the first three months of the second period the barometer was not kept, hence the averages given for this period, and relating to that instrument, are only for eight months, and must therefore be taken for what they are worth, as indicating the mean atmospheric pressure of the second epoch when contrasted with the preceding one.

The Customs, to whom I lent my instruments during the previous year, ceased to take observations after February 1878, returning the instruments to me. I thereupon continued the readings myself, with the exception of those from the winds and clouds; nor were these obtainable from the Customs, hence this year's record is in this respect less complete than that of last.

In order to prevent misunderstanding, I may mention that the Assistant-in-Charge must have been misinformed when he speaks of the instruments as being "indifferent" (*see* Trade Reports for 1877). I can only say that they were obtained from one of the best makers at home, and have always been found accurate when compared with those standards I have from time to time been able to get hold of. I have reason to believe that the fact of there being a "correction for index error" supplied with the thermometers led to the supposition of their imperfection. I need scarcely remind those familiar with meteorological observation that this correction is necessary to all instruments, but that this does not detract from the confidence that they merit.

As this is the last report I shall be in a position to write on Wênchow, I have thought that an abstract of the general tables, contrasting the period from April 1877 to February 1878 with that from April 1878 to February 1879 might chance to be useful or interesting. It will be seen that I have omitted March in both years; but this I have been obliged to do, as the instruments were changing hands and situation at that time, and so the observations were temporarily interrupted. I have only to add that the dew-point, elastic force of vapour, and humidity are computed from the Greenwich factors published in 1857; that the instruments were placed under shade in the open air within the city; that they faced south; and that the rain-gauge was placed 4 feet above the ground.

China, Imperial Maritime Customs, Medical Reports
(1881. 04. 01—1881. 09. 30)

CHINA.

IMPERIAL MARITIME CUSTOMS.

II.—SPECIAL SERIES: No. 2.

MEDICAL REPORTS,

FOR THE HALF-YEAR ENDED 30TH SEPTEMBER 1881.

22nd Issue.

PUBLISHED BY ORDER OF

The Inspector General of Customs.

SHANGHAI:
STATISTICAL DEPARTMENT
OF THE
INSPECTORATE GENERAL.

MDCCCLXXXII.

INSPECTOR GENERAL'S CIRCULAR No. 19 OF 1870.

INSPECTORATE GENERAL OF CUSTOMS,

PEKING, 31st December 1870.

SIR,

1.—IT has been suggested to me that it would be well to take advantage of the circumstances in which the Customs Establishment is placed, to procure information with regard to disease amongst foreigners and natives in China; and I have, in consequence, come to the resolution of publishing half-yearly in collected form all that may be obtainable. If carried out to the extent hoped for, the scheme may prove highly useful to the medical profession both in China and at home, and to the public generally. I therefore look with confidence to the co-operation of the Customs Medical Officer at your port, and rely on his assisting me in this matter by framing a half-yearly report containing the result of his observations at..................upon the local peculiarities of disease, and upon diseases rarely or never encountered out of China. The facts brought forward and the opinions expressed will be arranged and published either with or without the name of the physician responsible for them, just as he may desire.

2.—The suggestions of the Customs Medical Officers at the various ports as to the points which it would be well to have especially elucidated, will be of great value in the framing of a form which will save trouble to those members of the Medical profession, whether connected with the Customs or not, who will join in carrying out the plan proposed. Meanwhile I would particularly invite attention to—

    a.—The general health of....................during the period reported on; the death rate amongst foreigners; and, as far as possible, a classification of the causes of death.

    b.—Diseases prevalent at...........................

    c.—General type of disease; peculiarities and complications encountered; special treatment demanded.

    d.—Relation of disease to $\begin{cases} \text{Season.} \\ \text{Alteration in local conditions—such as drainage, \&c.} \\ \text{Alteration in climatic conditions.} \end{cases}$

    e.—Peculiar diseases; especially leprosy.

    f.—Epidemics $\begin{cases} \text{Absence or presence.} \\ \text{Causes.} \\ \text{Course and treatment.} \\ \text{Fatality.} \end{cases}$

Other points, of a general or special kind, will naturally suggest themselves to medical men; what I have above called attention to will serve to fix the general scope of the undertaking. I have committed to Dr. ALEX. JAMIESON, of Shanghai, the charge of arranging the Reports for publication, so that they may be made available in a convenient form.

3.—Considering the number of places at which the Customs Inspectorate has established offices, the thousands of miles north and south and east and west over which these offices are scattered, the varieties of climate, and the peculiar conditions to which, under such different circumstances, life and health are subjected, I believe the Inspectorate, aided by its Medical Officers, can do good service in the general interest in the direction indicated; and, as already stated, I rely with confidence on the support and assistance of the Medical Officer at each port in the furtherance and perfecting of this scheme. You will hand a copy of this Circular to Dr. ...., and request him, in my name, to hand to you in future, for transmission to myself, half-yearly Reports of the kind required, for the half-years ending 31st March and 30th September—that is, for the Winter and Summer seasons.

4—   *   *   *   *   *

I am, &c.,

(signed)   ROBERT HART,

I. G.

THE COMMISSIONERS OF CUSTOMS,—*Newchwang,   Ningpo,*

                                                 Tientsin,   Foochow,

                                                 Chefoo,   Tamsui,

                                                 Hankow,   Takow,

                                                 Kiukiang,   Amoy,

                                                 Chinkiang,   Swatow, and

                                                 Shanghai,   Canton.

SHANGHAI, *1st March 1882.*

SIR,

  IN accordance with the directions of your Despatch No. 6 *A* (Returns Series) of the 24th June 1871, I now forward to the Statistical Department of the Inspectorate General of Customs, the following documents :—

  Report on the Health of Amoy, pp. 1–3;

  Report on the Health of Swatow, pp. 4, 5;

  Report on the Health of Hoihow, pp. 6–10;

  Report on the Health of Chefoo, pp. 11, 12;

  Report on the Health of Ningpo, p. 13;

  Report on the Health of Wênchow, pp. 14–50;

  Report on the Health of Shanghai, pp. 51–54 ; each of these referring to the half-year ended 30th September 1881.

  Special articles on—

   Distoma Ringeri and Parasitical Hæmoptysis, pp. 55–62.

   The Periodicity of Filarial Migrations to and from the Circulation, pp. 63–68.

  An Appendix of translations and notes relating to recent pathological investigations, which are of special interest to medical practitioners in China, pp. 69–104.

I have the honour to be,

SIR,

Your obedient Servant,

R. ALEX. JAMIESON.

THE INSPECTOR GENERAL OF CUSTOMS,
  PEKING.

The Contributors to this Volume are:—

P. MANSON, M.D., CH.M. .... Amoy.

J. POLLOCK, L.K.&Q.C.P., L.R.C.S.I. .... Swatow.

E. A. ALDRIDGE, L.K.&Q.C.P. .... Hoihow.

J. G. BRERETON, L.K.&Q.C.P., L.R.C.S.I. .... Chefoo.

W. A. HENDERSON, L.R.C.P.Ed. .... Ningpo.

D. J. MACGOWAN, M.D. .... Wênchow.

R. A. JAMIESON, M.A., M.D., M.R.C.S. .... Shanghai.

For everything enclosed within square brackets [　], the Compiler is responsible.

Dr. MACGOWAN's Report on the Health of Wênchow for the Half-year ended 30th September 1881.

INASMUCH as the period of residence of foreigners at Wênchow scarcely numbers in the aggregate threescore years and ten, information touching the influence of the climate on their health is of insufficient importance to be placed on record, it is presumable that a degree of discursiveness in this Report will be pardonable.

Reserving for another occasion the subject of medical topography, it will suffice to state that Wênchow is a departmental city containing a population of between 80,000 and 90,000, with tributary districts swelling that number to 500,000. It is situated 15 miles from the sea, on the right bank of the Pungcha or Ou* river, having its source in the mountains which separate the south-western corner of Chêhkiang province, the province of Fukien, near the source of the Tsientang and Min rivers; those mountains and those of the coast forming part of the Nanshan of RICHTHOFEN. The mountains, or hills rather, of the coast presented at no remote period, at their junction with the sea, a series of deep bays, which have become filled up by alluvial deposits forming a dead level to the very basis of the heights which the waters formerly laved, the hills rising abruptly from the valleys, and, where isolated, presenting the appearance of islands. What were once marshes now constitute a chief portion of the province for a great distance inland. This paludal region is begirt, except seaward, with pine-clad mountains, but has been long reclaimed, and is a very fertile rice country.

Owing to its oranographical surroundings, Wênchow has a greater number of rainy days and a greater rainfall than any port in the empire, *malgré* the deforestization, which here, as in the United States, does not seem to have had any hygrometric effect. It has a distinct rainy season, extending from the middle of May to September, and during the other months of the year rainy days are of frequent occurrence; nevertheless, for foreigners it is probably the healthiest portion of China. Its summer heat is mitigated by the rains and sea breezes, the thermometer seldom remaining long in the nineties, and in winter it rarely indicates the freezing point. A Northern invalid who has been over-stimulated by ozone, positive electricity, hydrogen superoxide in the air, or whatever causes peculiarity of climate north of the Yangtze, may here inhale an admirable alterative, while invalids from the South, who require a Northern winter, may here escape the Arctic blasts which in higher latitudes pierce him as if he were gossamer. In fine, Wênchow possesses the climate of Nice without a *mistral*. In summer the tourist may cruise among beautiful islands and fish to his heart's content; in winter he may scale Alpine heights of illimitable extent, not needing to traverse a plain between this and the "Roof of the World;" and if endowed with requisite qualities, become a mighty hunter before the people, who here suffer from ravages by tigers, animals which are as troublesome here as they are under

* 甌 Ou; this is the name formerly applied to the entire region. It is now classical for Wênchow; etymologically, *Tuileries.*

the equator or on the banks of the Amoor. Unfortunately, this port, so attractive to the invalid, is uninviting to patients, because for such there is no suitable accommodation. This is a delightful resort for those only who can "rough it."

An indication of the climate of Wênchow is furnished by its flora. It is the northern limit of the bastard banyan *(Ficus pyrifolia)*, but still maintaining its tropical magnificence; and the coir palm *(Chamærops excelsa)*, which here attains its highest latitude as an industrial product, meet chestnuts and dwarf oaks of the North; and it is at this overlapping of zones that a peculiar species of orange flourishes, the well-known Wênchow bitter orange, a delicious stomachic, fit to be designated the mild cinchona orange. The bitter principle is contained in the membrane which subdivides the pulp; the pulp itself is sweet.

This hasty glance represents the aspect of the region when in repose; but it is subject to floods from the mountains and cyclones from the ocean, storms that lay waste the fertile fields, and by their destructive agency occasion famine and pestilence. Records of these most violent of physical disturbances are to be found in local gazetteers, and as the phenomena are interesting to meteorology, I subjoin a list which comprises a period of over 15 centuries, and includes the maritime portions of Chêhkiang and part of Fukien. First, however, it is fit to premise a few explanatory remarks on the sources of that information.

Every province, every department, and almost every district in the Empire has a great pile of volumes which are denominated topographies, but as they relate to geography, public works, buildings and temples, physical phenomena, natural history, biography, manners and customs, matters fiscal and military, to annals and the like, "gazetteer" appears a more suitable term, although to some, "miscellanies" may seem preferable. The earlier records of these gazetteers are collated from general history and local traditions. At a later period, when local registers came to be kept at yamêns, these and the ana of scholars and families furnished the matter of which they are composed. It is not often, however, that the public archives are well kept, and the gentry, when they undertake to get up a new edition, are obliged to supplement material from their own records. A century or more will sometimes elapse between editions, and generally it will be found that the new ones have eliminated, as not worth perpetuating, information which foreigners—the statistician, for example—would greatly prize, a fact to be noted in connexion with the subjoined lists. Another explanation is requisite to the right comprehension of the tables. When facts on any subject are derived from a district gazetteer, they will be found more numerous than when they are furnished by the departmental or the provincial volumes. A list of epidemics, for instance, furnished by a district gazetteer will appear more formidable than when a departmental work has been drawn from. If defective, the records are never inaccurate; what are registered as facts were actual occurrences or appearances, although sometimes misinterpreted, as in cases of certain physical phenomena.

Record of Storms, Floods, Droughts and Famines in the Departments of Chüanchow, Foochow, Wênchow, and Ningpo, situated approximately between latitude N. 24° 40′ and N. 30° 02′, and longitude E. 118° 50′ and E. 121° 22′.

Abbreviations.—S.W., storm wave ; Ty., typhoon ; St., storm ; Fl., flood ; Fa., famine ; Dr., drought ; Sp., spring ; Su., summer ; A., autumn.

A.D.	Moon.	Chüanchow.	Foochow.	Wênchow.	Ningpo.	A.D.	Moon.	Chüanchow.	Foochow.	Wênchow.	Ningpo.
291	4	...	...	S.W.	...	1216	...	...	Dr.	...	Dr.
293	6	...	...	St., S.W.	...	1217	...	...	Fl.	...	...
304	...	...	...	Fa.	...	1217	...	...	Ty.	...	...
480	4	...	...	...	...	1220	...	...	...	...	Dr.
648	8	St., S.W.	...	...	...	1221	...	...	Fa.	...	...
663	7	...	...	S.W.	...	1222	...	...	Dr.	Dr.	...
674	6	...	...	Fa.	...	1224	A.	Fl.	...	...	...
684	6	...	...	St., S.W.	...	1233	3	...	...	Fl.	...
689	7	...	...	Fl.	...	1233	8	...	...	Fl.	...
768	A.	...	Fl.	...	...	1240	6	...	Dr.	...	...
783	6	...	...	Dr.	...	1241	...	...	Dr.	...	...
784	8	S.W.	...	...	...	1240	6	...	...	...	...
791	...	...	...	...	Dr.	1246	...	...	Fl.	...	...
797	4	...	Fl.	...	...	1248	...	...	Fl.	...	...
840	...	...	...	...	Fa.	1352	...	...	Dr.	...	...
841	...	...	...	...	...	1295	...	...	Dr.	...	...
984	8	S.W.	...	...	...	1297	...	...	...	Fa.	...
1004	...	...	Ty.	...	...	1278	6	...	Fa.	Fl.	...
1001	8	...	...	Ty.	...	1279	...	...	Fa.	...	...
1005	8	...	Ty.	...	...	1291	6	...	...	...	...
1029	...	...	Fl.	...	...	1293	6	Dr.	...	...	...
1066	8	St., Fl	...	...	...	1297	7	Fl.	...	S.W.	...
1067	6	St., S.W.	...	...	...	1308	...	St.	...	S.W.	Fa.
1093	A.	...	...	...	Dr., Fa.	1324	...	St.	...	...	Fa.
1094	...	...	...	...	Fa.	1330	...	...	...	...	Fl.
1101	...	...	Dr.	...	...	1332	...	...	...	...	Fa.
1110	...	...	Dr.	...	...	1333	...	Fl.	...	Fl.	...
1126	...	...	...	St.	...	1343	A.	...	...	St.	...
1130	A.	...	...	...	...	1344	...	...	...	...	Fa.
1133	1	...	Fa., Fl.	...	...	1345	...	...	...	Fa.	...
1134	9-10	...	Fl.	...	...	1346	S.	...	...	...	Dr.
1135	5	St., Fl	Fl.	...	...	1347	...	...	...	St., S.W.	...
1149	...	...	...	...	...	1349	...	...	...	...	...
1150	...	...	...	Fa.	Fa.	1350	7	...	...	Fa.	Dr.
1152	...	...	...	S.	...	1354	...	3 Tides	...	Fa.	...
1159	...	...	...	S.	...	1356	6	...	St.	...	...
1160	7	...	Fl.	...	...	1357	...	...	...	S.W.	...
1163	...	...	...	Fa.	Fa.	1363	8	...	...	S.W.	...
1165	...	...	...	Fa.	Fa.	1367	...	St.	...	...	...
1166	8-17	...	...	S.W.	...	1376	7	...	...	S.W.	...
1171	5	...	Dr.	Fl.	...	1377	...	Fl.	...	...	...
1171	6	...	...	Dr.	...	1381	6	Fl.	...	...	...
1174	...	...	...	...	Fa.	1389	...	...	...	Fa., Dr.	...
1178	5	...	...	Fl.	S.	1399	...	Fl.	...	...	...
1179	6	...	...	S.	Dr.	1417	...	Fa.	...	...	...
1180	Su.	...	...	Fl.	...	1426	...	...	...	...	Ty.
1183	...	...	...	...	Dr.	1432	6	...	...	...	Ty.
1185	...	...	...	...	Dr.	1446	5	Fl.	...	...	Dr., Fa.
1188	...	...	Dr.	...	Dr.	1449	...	...	...	...	Fa.
1189	...	...	Fl.	...	...	1456	...	Dr.	...	...	...
1192	4	...	Fl.	...	...	1457	S.	...	...	...	Dr.
1195	A.	...	...	...	Ty.	1459	...	Dr.	...	...	...
1195	A.	...	...	...	Fa.	1467	1	...	...	Fl.	...
1203	6-7	...	...	...	...	1478	...	...	...	...	...
1205	...	...	Dr.	...	...	1479	...	Fa.	...	...	Fl.
1210	1	...	Fl.	...	...	1480	...	...	...	...	S.W.

RECORD of STORMS, FLOODS, DROUGHTS and FAMINES—*continued.*

A.D.	Moon.	Chüan-chow.	Foochow.	Wênchow.	Ningpo.	A.D.	Moon.	Chüan-chow.	Foochow.	Wênchow.	Ningpo.
1481	...	...	...	...	...	1624	A.	...	...	...	Dr.
1483	8	...	St.	...	...	1627	7	...	...	...	Fl., Dr.
1486	Sp. to Su.	Fl.	...	...	...	1628	S.	...	...	...	Fl., Fa.
1487	9	...	...	...	Dr.	1628	7	...	...	...	St.
1489	Sp.	Dr.	...	...	...	1633	...	...	...	...	Dr., Fa.
1490	6	...	...	St.	...	1635	...	...	...	...	Dr., Fa.
1491	...	...	...	Fa.	...	1637	6	...	...	...	St., Dr.
1493	...	...	...	...	S.W.	1638	...	...	...	...	St., Fl.
1494	7	St.	...	...	...	1639	...	...	...	...	Dr., Fa.
1499	4	Fl.	...	...	...	1640	S.	...	...	...	St.
1500	12	Dr.	...	...	...	1640	8	St.	...	...	...
1502	...	Dr.	...	...	...	1641	...	...	...	...	Fa.
1504	9	Fl.	...	...	...	1642	...	...	...	...	Dr., Fa.
1505	...	...	...	...	Fa.	1647	...	...	...	...	Dr.
1509	...	...	...	...	Dr., Fa.	1649	8	Fa.	...	...	...
1514	...	...	...	...	Dr., Fl.	1650	9	St.	...	...	Dr.
1512	...	...	...	...	Dr.	1651	...	...	...	Ty.	...
1513	...	...	...	Fa.	Fa.	1653	A.	...	...	...	Dr.
1514	...	Dr., Fa.	...	Fa.	...	1654	A.	...	...	...	Dr.
1529	8	St.	...	...	...	1656	6	...	...	...	St.
1524	...	...	...	...	St., S.W.	1655	...	...	...	...	Fa.
1525	...	...	...	...	Ty., Fa.	1658	5	...	...	...	St.
1527	...	...	...	Dr., Fa.	Fa.	1660	7	...	...	Ty.	...
1535	8	...	...	...	St.	1662	A.	Ty.	Fl.	...	...
1536	...	...	Dr., St.	...	...	1664	A.	Fl.	...	...	...
1538	...	...	...	...	S.W.	1665	6	Fl.	...	...	...
1540	...	...	...	...	S.W.	1666	...	Dr.	...	...	...
1542	Sp.	...	...	St.	...	1668	...	...	...	...	St.
1542	A.	...	...	Dr.	...	1669	7	...	...	Fl.	...
1546	...	Dr., Fa.	...	Fa.	Fa., Dr.	1670	...	Dr.	...	...	...
1548	...	...	...	St.	...	1671	...	Dr.	...	Fa.	...
1555	9	...	...	St.	...	1672	...	...	...	...	Dr.
1558	7-8	...	...	St.	Dr.	1674	8	...	...	...	Fl.
1562	...	...	...	St.	...	1675	6	...	...	Fl.	...
1569	7	...	...	St.	...	1676	A.	...	...	...	Dr.
1570	...	...	...	...	Fl.	1677	4	Fa.	...	...	Fl.
1575	6	St.	...	St.	...	1679	8	...	...	...	St.
1576	...	...	...	St., Dr.	S.W.	1680	...	Fa.	...	...	...
1579	5	...	Fl.	...	...	1681	A.	Dr.	...	Fl.	...
1585	7	...	...	...	Fl.	1682	...	...	...	...	Dr.
1586	...	...	...	...	Fa., Dr.	1683	4	...	...	Fl.	Fl., Dr., Fa.
1587	6	...	...	...	S.W.	1684	...	...	...	Dr.	...
1589	7	...	...	...	St., Fa.	1686	...	...	...	...	Dr.
1592	8	...	Fl.	...	...	1688	5	Fl.	...	...	...
1595	5	St.	...	...	...	1690	...	...	...	S.W.	Dr., Fa.
1597	8	Ty.	Ty.	...	...	1692	...	S.W.	...	...	Dr., Fa.
1599	...	...	...	...	Fl.	1694	...	...	...	...	Fa.
1601	...	Fl., Ty.	...	Ty.	...	1698	...	...	...	...	Fl.
1602	6	Fl.	...	...	...	1699	4	St.	...	...	...
1603	9	Fl.	...	...	...	1700	9	...	...	Fl.	...
1604	8	Ty.	...	...	...	1702	...	...	...	...	Dr., Fa.
1607	8	Fa.	...	...	...	1704	8	Dr.	...	Dr.	...
1608	5-6	Ty.	...	Dr., St.	...	1707	S.	...	...	...	...
1609	5	...	...	Fa.	Fa.	1711	...	...	...	...	...
1610	5	...	...	Fl.	Fl.	1713	S.	Fl.	...	...	...
1612	...	...	...	...	Fl.	1714	...	Fl.	...	...	...
1614	A.	Dr.	...	Ty., Fa.	...	1718	6	...	...	...	...
1615	S.	3 Tides.	...	...	...	1719	8	Fl.	...	...	...
1615	A.	...	...	Fl.	...	1721	5	...	Dr.	...	...
1616	8	Fl.	...	...	...	1722	...	...	...	...	Dr., Fa.
1617	...	Fa.	...	...	...	1723	6	Ty.	...	...	Dr., F.
1618	...	Fa.	...	...	Dr.	1724	7	...	...	...	Dr.
1620	S.	S.W.	...	...	...	1725	6-7	Fl.	Fl.	...	...
1621	6	...	...	...	Dr.	1729	7-8	...	St.	...	Fl.

RECORD of STORMS, FLOODS, DROUGHTS and FAMINES—*continued.*

A.D.	Moon.	Chüan-chow.	Foochow.	Wênchow.	Ningpo.	A.D.	Moon.	Chüan-chow.	Foochow.	Wênchow.	Ningpo.
1729	A.	Dr.	...	...	Dr.	1809	...	...	...	...	Fa.
1731	7	Fl.	...	...	...	1810	...	...	...	Ty.	...
1734	7	...	·	St.	...	1814	...	...	...	Fl., Dr.	...
1738	9	...	...	Fl.	...	1818	...	...	...	...	S.W.
1739	...	...	...	Dr.	...	1819	3	...	...	St.	...
1741	...	...	...	Dr.	...	1819	6	...	...	St.	...
1745	7	...	...	...	S.W.	1820	6	...	...	St.	Dr.
1747	A.	...	...	...	Dr.	1821	A.	...	...	Ty.	...
1749	...	St.	...	...	...	1823	Sp.	...	...	St.	...
1752	...	...	...	...	Fa.	1832	...	...	...	Dr.	...
1753	...	St.	...	...	Dr.	1834	...	...	...	...	Fa.
1756	8	...	·	...	Fl	1835	Su.	...	...	Fa., Ty., Dr.	...
1758	...	Fl., Dr., Fa.	...	...	...	1836	6	...	...	Dr., S.W.	...
1759	...	Fl.	...	...	Fl	1839	7	...	...	Fl.	...
1760	A.	...	...	...	Fl	1844	8	...	...	St.	St., Fl.
1762	...	Fl.	...	...	...	1847	7	...	...	Ty.	...
1769	6	...	...	...	St.	1848	...	...	...	...	Dr.
1772	A.	...	...	...	Fl	1849	4	...	...	St.	...
1796	5-6	...	...	Dr.	...	1853	8	...	...	...	St.
1796	8	...	...	Fa.	...	1854	6	...	...	St.	...
1799	...	...	...	...	Dr., Fa.	1856	7	...	...	Ty.	...
1801	6	...	...	Ty.	...	1858	8	...	...	Ty.	...
1805	5	...	...	Ty.	...						

Of the above-named ports, only Chüanchow is situated on the sea, the others being at tide distant.

Wênchow and Ningpo are fuller, because district gazetteers have been consulted, the others being from departmental gazetteers ; those, moreover, are of recent date, these are a century and a half old.

By "famine" nothing more in many cases is meant than local dearths, and none are stated to have been attended with cannibalism, but the poor were often driven to child-selling.*

Floods are recorded only when they are remarkable for violence, extent and destructiveness, and present no peculiar appearance, as elsewhere, they overleap barriers, submerge towns, furrow the face of the earth, and destroy crops and life. The suddenness of their rush, particularly when they are the result of waterspouts or pent-up subterranean reservoirs, causes them to be referred to supernatural agency. The gyratory waterspout is considered to be a dragon, and it is likely that it gave rise to belief in such a monster ; while water suddenly rushing from the ground is attributed to an embryotic dragon which is formed in an egg, the product of that aërial being and a serpent, the breaking of the egg causing the flood.

By "storm wave" is meant what the records style "overflow of the sea."

The two cases of a "third tide in a day," so designated, are not to be confounded with the periodical bore or egre, but are exceptional phenomena. According to the *Hsing Pau*, that phenomenon was witnessed at Shanghai 28th October 1880. It was neap tide, low water

* Of the 35 famines recorded by WANG FÊNGCHOW (鳳洲 綱鑑坌編, an abbreviated history), occurring between A.D. 153 and 1640, six were attended by cannibalism, in two of which parents ate their children, and children ate their parents. For an account of *Droughts and Famines in China*, A.D. 620 to 1643, by A. HOSIE, M.A., H.B.M.'s China Consular Service, *vide Journal of the N.-C.B., Royal Asiatic Society.*

at 0.15, a short time before which the supplementary tide appeared. A strong N.E. gale was reported as blowing off the coast on the day previous; the wave may have been due to that cause, but such gales are of common occurrence, while "third tides" are rare. The last, according to the same paper, having taken place in 1851. The earliest of those recorded in the Shanghai gazetteer took place on the 23rd day of the 6th month A.D. 1357, when "towards dawn the sea rose suddenly, causing great alarm, as it was not the time for high water; at the proper high water time it again rose, so that it was known that the first rise was not the tide. In the canal and lakes near Pinchiang and Kiahsing the waters suddenly rose some 4 or 5 feet."* The subsequent occurrence of "third tides," to wit, 1634, 8th month; 1642, 8th month; 1648, 7th month, 21st day; 1661, 7th month, 26th day; 1662, 7th month; 1719, 9th month, 19th day; 1754, 8th month; 1778, 8th month, are given without remark. Occurring as they did during the typhoon season, they may have been storms which, having spent their force, were unobserved, but the cause of some of these oscillations, like the first named, must be sought for elsewhere. Although data are wanting for their co-ordination with earthquakes or submarine volcanic action, it is reasonable to infer that they are co-related, having their source in the volcanic chain which girdles the entire coast of Eastern Asia.†

To submarine volcanic commotion may probably be attributed a phenomenon that was observed in the summer of 1166 on the coast near Wênchow. For three days the sea made a noise and presented the appearance of coagulated milk, in the form of the perforated coin in common use, meaning apparently foaming eddies. It was preceded by a flood emitted by a serpent, which was found to be 10 feet long.

The climatologist who desires to compare the coast with an inland region on the same latitude will find the gazetteer of Chichau full of information. That department is west of and coterminous with Wênchow, and is wholly mountainous, but of no great altitude. Its "calamitous records" for the 352 years following 1511 show:—Storms, 5; floods, 49; famines, 19; droughts, 44.‡

* "Note on Cosmical Phenomena observed in the Neighbourhood of Shanghai during the past 13 Centuries," *Journal of the N.-C.B., Royal Asiatic Society.* Read 23rd December 1858, by D. J. MACGOWAN, M.D.

† Analogous to the abnormal waves that flood the China coast are those which impinge on Tungking :—"Un phénomène surprenant est que quelquefois la marée, après avoir descendu pendant environ trois quarts d'heure, remonte subitement et les canaux qui les autres jours ne sont pas navigables à marée basse, le sont pendant tout le cours de la journée.

"Il y a quelques années sur une des côtes du Tunkin est survenu un événement très extraordinaire. On a entendu un bruit effrayant plus fort que celui que peut produire la plus fort canonnade ; et ce bruit a été suivi d'une violente irruption de la mer, qui s'est avancée jusqu'à plus de deux lieues dans l'intérieur des terres, y a porté des arbres déracinés et des débris de bâtiments, et au bout de douze ou quinze heures s'est retirée dans son lit, ayant noyé nombre d'hommes et d'animaux et détruit plusieurs villages. Ce même phénomène avait eu lieu environ cinquante ans auparavant."—*Exposé statistique du Tunkin, de la Cochinchine, du Camboge, du Tsiampa, du Laos, du Lac Tho, sur la relation de M. de la* BISSACHÈRE, *Missionaire dans le Tunkin* : Londres, MDCCCXL.

‡ The same record furnishes a singular instance of suspended animation and a restoration by a stroke of lightning. In the year 1650 a child three years of age died and was interred in the garden of his parents near the city of Suichang. "A stroke of thunder" (it is thunder, not lightning, in China, that does harm) "struck the grave, and the boy was restored to life." How long he had been entombed or how the grave was constructed is not stated. It is probable that if all the facts of the case were known, they would confirm Dr. RICHARDSON's view that when blood does not become pectous, but remains in an aqueous condition, life may be retained to an indefinite period. It is painful to add that the child, so marvellously preserved, was soon after immolated by his father. A malicious neighbour gave out that the boy was, in fact, a "son of thunder," and that the parent was dirilict in not reporting the case to the magistrate ; whereupon, in terror, the father killed the poor boy.

In the foregoing record the term "storms" often includes typhoons or cyclones the central portions of which passed at a distance.

Disastrous storms and typhoons (only of a disastrous character are included) appear to average 16 in a century.

Chinese coastlanders and mariners are good prognosticators of storms. "When a solar halo, variegated like the rainbow, is visible, the appearance is styled 'typhoon mother'; then dogs and fowls are voiceless, and there is sure to be a spiral or whirlwind." It is a "crazy wind that blows from all quarters in summer and autumn." The Wênchow supplemental gazetteer says there is a grass the joints of which indicate the approach of a typhoon; it is called the "knowing wind grass."*

From the time of Yu the Great to the present, China has been heroically struggling to defend herself against constantly recurring disasters of flood; her rivers, notably the Yellow River, "China's sorrow," have tasked the skill of her engineers, and proved a drain to her resources. Has not the time arrived when she may obtain some scientific basis for ascertaining the hydrological and meteorological conditions which are the cause of her chronic ailment? What has been done for investigation of floods of the Mississippi,† which has been the model of Mr. GORDON on the Irrawaddy; measurements prolonged over considerable time, and in varying conditions; systematic investigation of velocity and flood discharge at different points, and the quantity of sediment held in suspension at different depths, are extremely desirable for all those rivers or portions of rivers which are seats of foreign commerce. Systematic observations with the rain gauge and thermometer over as much of the drainage areas as practicable, all having reference to future hydraulic works, and for comparison with observations now making in India and Burmah to discover a connexion or co-existence with phases of flood, drought and famine between that and this portion of the continent. It is still a moot question if there are cycles of famine and drought, and also on what the meteorological conditions depend, and their concurrence with the presence or absence of solar spots and their recurrence in undecennial periods. It would not be difficult, moreover, for the Customs department to pursue investigation of the waters of the rivers and coasts for the elucidation of biological and physical problems connected with the Chinese fisheries.

The meteorological observations which have been carried on for several years by the Imperial Maritime Customs by direction of the Inspector General have put the student of that science in possession of valuable data which in due time will be turned to practical account. Only one thing is wanted in order to render future observations in China as useful as they have recently become in America and Europe. The want in question is simultaneity in observation, in accordance with the request of the International Congress which met at Vienna in September 1879, to wit, "It is desirable with a view to their exchange that at least one uniform observation, of such character as to be suited for the preparation of synoptic charts, be taken and recorded daily and simultaneously at as many stations as are practicable throughout the world." This

---

* For a meteorological record of observations, for a period of 11 months, see Customs *Medical Reports*, May 1878, by Dr. MYERS.

† HUMPHREY and ABBOT, *Reports on the Mississippi*: Washington, 1861-1879. *Reports on the Irrawaddy*: ROBERT GORDON, Rangoon, 1879, 1880.

request has been almost universally complied with, and now the globe is photographed, as it were, its atmospheric condition being taken at the same moment of actual (not local) time. It is only by simultaneous observations that the actual fluctuations and the cyclonic and anti-cyclonic movements of the aërial ocean can be accurately noted. Père DECHEVRENS, Superintendent of the Sicawei Observatory, informs me that prior to January last he sent to the Chief Signal Officer of the United States army at Washington his observations made at 8.49 local time, corresponding to 7.35 A.M. Washington time, but that a modification of the time for simultaneous observation was requested, and since the 1st January meteorological observations have been taken 35 minutes earlier, or at 8.14 P.M. Sicawei mean time. To that change the International Meteorological Committee appointed by the Congress of Vienna has given its adhesion, and 0.8 P.M. Washington time is the instant for making observations in China, when it is decreed that the Customs shall fall into line. So extensive is the area occupied by Customs observers that their adhesion to the plan of simultaneous international observations, particularly if three daily observations are made, will be hailed with satisfaction by the scientific world, and eventually by the mercantile world as well, inasmuch as mariners are perplexed by observations made in cyclones that do not correspond with the teachings of accepted authorities on the laws of storms. They do not find that the centre of a storm always bears eight points from the direction of the wind, nor that the barometer always falls towards the centre, or always rises on receding from the storm centre. The tracks of storms laid down in charts of the China Sea require further investigation, having been made on insufficient data. A renewed collocation of the meteorological phenomena is a desideratum. Further, it remains to be demonstrated that the whole current of a storm ascends from its centre. In a word, the whole subject of the storms of this coast demands the attention alike of the navigator and the scientist. It is with no satisfaction that I give expression to doubts respecting the rules laid down by REDFIELD, REID, and PIDDINGTON, for in 1853 I published in Chinese a précis of what they had written on the subject.* The brochure was republished in Japan by the Prince of SATSUMA. I would fain recall it for elimination and modification. It may seem chimerical to propose the establishment of a meteorological observatory at each of the Customs stations, but the proposition is alike feasible and desirable, apparatus neither costly nor complicated, such as has been described by Dr. DRAPER, Superintendent of the New York Meteorological Observatory,—no photographic recording barometer being required,— a "dollar clock" forming the most intricate portion of the apparatus.† The average annual expense of American signal stations is about $300, exclusive of soldiers' pay and telegraphic messages, but as the observations there made are comprehensive and complicated, a much smaller sum would suffice for Customs meteorological observations.‡ For example, observations made in the interests of agriculture for forecasting the weather, investigations in magnetism, atmospheric electricity, anemometry and actinometry might be dispensed with as being but remotely connected with Customs or mercantile concerns. Investigations on solar radiation and

* 航海金針 寧波 Ningpo: Published at the expense of J. C. BOWRING, Esquire.

† For a description of Dr. DRAPER's instruments, vide Scientific American, Supplement, 3rd January 1880.

‡ General HAZEN's Report of the Signal Corps for 1881: Washington.

the absorption of the sun's heat by the atmosphere would lead to trustworthy predictions of periods of drought and scarcity, and have bearings which affect commerce hardly less than agriculture, and not very indirectly Customs revenue. In conclusion, I beg leave to suggest the adoption of the metric system by Customs observers, seeing that it must ultimately be extended to China.*

If quest be made for average specimens of the Chinese race, this beautiful, fertile, and densely-peopled region will not furnish examples, the inhabitants comparing disadvantageously with those of adjacent portions of the Empire, being physically and intellectually inferior. They are of delicate frame, insignificant physiognomy, and microcephalic—small-brained. Fewer attain to 70 years of age here than in coterminous departments, and, as in southern Chêhkiang generally, it is seldom that scholars succeed at the provincial examinations. They are simple, friendly, and law-abiding, but are charged by their countrymen as being particularly salacious. They are greatly addicted to temple attendance, and are evidently deteriorated descendants of a devout race; nowhere are temples and pagodas, monasteries and nunneries, so numerous. The religious orders are credited with contributing greatly to the perpetuation and dissemination of a contagious disorder, which accounts for their inferior physique; and as they are now largely addicted to the use of opium, there is little prospect of physical melioration.

Situated as it is on a reclaimed marsh reticulated by canals, and almost on a level with its sluggish waters, Wênchow cannot but be the abode of intermittent fever. Every spring, to some extent, and in autumn that disease prevails, affecting betimes half of the inhabitants of a village. It appears in protean form, but generally of mild type, except to new-comers, who, after acclimatisation, do not regard it with dread. Labourers and other impoverished people who cannot afford to purchase medicines lie down on the ground when seized by a fit, and after the paroxysm is over revert to their toil, and so they live until in the course of years the poison ceases to affect them; but the anæmia and debility that ensue render them an easy prey to other maladies, and they are not long-lived. Quotidian and tertian are light and transient, amenable to treatment, and disappearing on the advent of cool weather. Tertians, which are the prevailing form, assume sometimes the quartan type, becoming chronic and incurable, continuous for a year or two and then terminating fatally.

At first sight the prevalence of ague at the close of summer and in early autumn might seem due to the condition of the rice-fields. The early and the late rice are planted in May at the same time, side by side in alternate plots. The former, ripening in August, is then harvested, the latter then having attained but half its growth. A moiety of the still submerged soil being no longer shaded, is exposed to the fierce solar rays, and soon after agues begin to appear. We may not therefore conclude, however, that the poison has its genesis in rice-fields, inasmuch as those most competent to judge, the inhabitants, exonerate their fields

* Of more importance than thermometrical and barometrical observations in Formosa would be a seismological record—earthquakes in that island being about as frequent as in Japan or Luzon—its seismal area including the coast.

Valuable information on the migration of birds was recently obtained from lighthouses on the east coast of Scotland in compliance with the printed forms that were addressed to them by Messrs. BROWN and CORDAUX. As on the American coast it is found on the European, that birds dash themselves against lighthouses; might not the *phares* of this coast be utilised in this manner？

from any agency in the matter. The question must be considered *sub judice*. From time immemorial Chinese physicians have been aware of the value of arsenic in the treatment of ague, but they refrain from administering it internally, their pharmaceutical knowledge not enabling them to prepare it in doses sufficiently attenuated to be unattended with danger.

Perhaps no country has suffered more from epidemic diseases than China, and certainly there is no country whose annals contain such a continuous record of calamities of that nature, consisting mainly of notices of enteric fevers, observations on which come down from proto-historic times. More than a score of centuries before HIPPOCRATES wrote of "critical days," HWANGTI, the "Yellow Emperor," is represented as referring to the same subject,—crises in disease and the natural tendency which the body has to cure itself by critical evacuations at certain periods,—in a conversation on physiology and pathology which he held with C'HIPE, his physician and minister; and since the dawn of authorship there has been a succession of medical writers, but no caste existed to hand down the earliest observations—no Asclepiades to record the cures, nor healing temples, or material for evolving an HIPPOCRATES; yet the preserved works display great acumen and powers of observation, and the careful perusal of Chinese medical works must elicit many interesting, if not valuable, facts, but that is not now feasible. In the meantime fragmentary contributions to Chinese medical history will not be unacceptable. A work that is in the hands of every practitioner, entitled *Essay on Epidemics*, discloses the curious fact that, according to the author, physicians in China had for 1,400 years proceeded in the treatment of epidemic fevers on a wrong course, which caused frightful loss of life during all that period. The work is from the pen of WU YUHSIN (吳 有 性　瘟 疫 論), a physician of Soochow, who wrote his book in 1641, but it circulated in manuscript form only until 1508, when some public-spirited scholars contributed for its publication. The edition before me appeared in 1852.*

According to Dr. WU, erroneous views respecting the etiology of fever prevailed from the period of the TSIN (265 A.D.) down to his day. The profession had fallen into the mistake of regarding epidemic fever as caused by, like ordinary continuous fever, vicissitudes of the seasons, instead of ascribing them to a specific poison (厲 氣). At the period of his writing, the provinces of Chêhkiang, Kiangsu, Shantung, and Chihli suffered from a fearful epidemic, but he affirms that the mortality was not due to the pestilence, but to the wrong treatment to which the unfortunate patients were subjected. "Morbific cold" (傷 寒) is a generic term for fever, perhaps best expressed by *Febris synocha*. The cold of winter engenders the miasm, which enters the pores of the skin; it is non-contagious, and prevails every year,† while the poison of epidemic fevers is taken in at the mouth and nostrils, and is communicable. In the former, sudorifics are indicated, in the latter, discutients. With the exception of this great medical reformer, there has been no writer on epidemics that I can discover, after searching various catalogues. No one can write the medical history of China without reading Dr. WU on "epidemics." There is one paragraph in his work which I translate for the benefit of those

---

* [Dates as in MS.]

† The earliest known work on fever is the 傷 寒 論 by 漢 張 機, who may have flourished any time between B.C. 200 and A.D. 200. He has had numerous successors.

foreign residents in China who may be unaware of the perils of out-door exercise on an empty stomach—a matter that does not seem to have attracted the attention of physicians until modern times. This cotemporary of the illustrious HARVEY says, of three men encountering morning malaria, one whose stomach is empty will sicken and die, the other who has imbibed spirits will suffer a disease, while the third, who has well breakfasted, escapes unscathed. *

Subjoined is a list of epidemics that have ravaged this province during the ages that have intervened since the recording of such phenomena commenced. It is from the provincial gazetteer, and from those of a majority of the departments and from several districts; so far as it goes it is accurate, but, as already remarked, those publications present innumerable lacunæ.

RECORD of EPIDEMICS in the PROVINCE of CHÊHKIANG.

A.D.	Moon.	———	A.D.	Moon.	———
95	4	Hsianhsing districts.	1333	3	Preceded by a flood.
758	...	Preceded by drought and flood.	1334	...	Western part; preceded by drought and famine.
783	...	Preceded by drought and flood.			
791	Autumn	Western part of the province; preceded by drought.	1361	Summer	Shaohsing, two districts.
			1363	...	Shaohsing, two districts.
806	Summer	Eastern part of the province.	1385	...	
829	Spring	Western part of the province.	1403	7	Shaohsing, two districts.
833	Summer	Hangchow and west.	1414	7	Throughout Hangchow, Hsianhsing and Ningpo.
870	...	The entire province.			
1001	..	Entire province.	1417	5	Kinhua; epidemic, leprosy.
1195	...	Hsianhsing; preceded by famine.	1435	Winter	Hsianhsing, Ningpo and Taichow.
1131	6	Hsianhsing and western part of province; preceded by famine.	1443	...	Ningpo and Taichow; preceded by drought.
			1446	3	Hsianhsing.
1144	...	Hangchow.	1463	...	Hsianhsing; for 2 years.
1147	Autumn	Hangchow.	1480-1	...	Kiahsing; preceded by floods.
1165	...	Linan and Yuyow; preceded by famine.	1493	...	Huchow; preceded by floods.
1173	Sum., Aut.	Hangchow.	1510	...	Huchow; preceded by floods.
1182	4	Hangchow and Linan.	1511	...	Pingwu. Reappeared next year.
1188	Spring	Hangchow.	1512	Spr., Sum.	
1194	6	Western part.	1513	...	Wênchow.
1195	3	Linan, Hsianhsing; preceded by famine.	1516	5	Yuyow and Hsianhsing; preceded by drought.
1196	5	Hangchow.	1526	Summer	Wênchow; preceded by drought.
1197	3	Hangchow.	1546	„	Kiahsing; preceded by drought.
1199	Summer	Linan.	1547	...	Epidemic leprosy over several districts, preceded by unprecedented rains.
1204	5	Hangchow.	1589	...	
1208	...	Yuyow; preceded by drought.	1589	...	Chichau; preceded by floods and famine.
1210	Summer	Linan.	1590	...	Hsiaoshan, a district of Hsianhsing; epidemic leprosy, its reappearance.
1211	„	Hangchow.			
1212	2	Hangchow.	1591	...	Epidemic leprosy in Changhua district, Hangchow.
1275	4	Hangchow.			
1284	7	Hsianhsing.	1622	...	Ningpo.
1304	Spring	Hsianhsing, Ningpo and Taichow.	1624	Summer	Ningpo; preceded by drought and famine.
1305	7	Hsianhsing; preceded by famine.	1628	...	Ningpo.
1308	7	Hangchow, Yuyow and Ningpo; preceded by drought and famine.	1634	...	Chichow.

* Dr. WU quotes from the *Shanghan* (HAN period) certain interesting etymological facts, which show how some characters have been built up, the examples all relating to the healing art. This, for example, is the genesis of 瘟疫. Fever was originally written 温病, abnormal heat disease. Subsequently the 氵 was dropt and 疒 substituted, forming the present character. In like manner 疫 was formerly written 徭役, persons pressed into temporary service as menials of Government offices (villein socage), because epidemics also penetrated everywhere, affecting every house alike; but subsequently 役 was placed under, 疒 minus the radical, being used as a phonetic 疫. Lexicographers, therefore, are slightly at fault in describing the latter character as composed of disease and a javelin; it is made up of disease and socage abbreviated.

RECORD of EPIDEMICS in the PROVINCE of CHÊHKIANG—*continued.*

A.D.	Moon.	——	A.D.	Moon.	——
1641	6	Hangchow, and year succeeding.	1718	6	Siangshan.
1652	Autumn	Ningpo.	1757	...	Pinghu.
1660	Sum. & Aut.	Wênchow.	1806	...	Wênchow; small-pox.
1673	Sum. & Aut.	Siangshan.	1811	..	Ningpo; small-pox.
1678	...	Lishui.	1820	Autumn	Wênchow and Ningpo; Asiatic cholera.
1680	...	Pinghu.	1821	...	Wênchow and Ningpo.
1681	...	Ningpo.	1834	Autumn	Ningpo.
1710	...	Siangshan.	1835	Spr., Aut.	„ with dearth.
1715	...	Taichow, preceded by famine.	1864	8, 9	Ningpo.

The above is a bald but not untrustworthy record. With few exceptions, the epidemics were probably of an enteric character, but as the term by which they are designated means "diseases which affect everyone at the same time," the list comprehends numerous maladies. It relates to epidemics of a single province. Generally the epidemics named were sequels of droughts, floods, famines or civil war.

With regard to epidemics in Chêhkiang, it may be remarked they were of more frequent occurrence in the maritime regions of the province than in the hilly portions. Many of them seem to have had a limited area.

The mode of transmission of the *materies morbi* is given in only one case. In 1638 an epidemic was conveyed from Hangchow to Tungyang by female children who—a pestilence raging there—were deprived of relatives, and purchased for sale at the neighbouring city; the germ was therefore not air-borne but brought in clothes. In the toxicological chapter of the *Péntsao*, old clothes are included as poisons.

The utility of naming the particular form of an epidemic seems to have occurred to recent compilers of gazetteers, for they mention small-pox and Asiatic cholera. The same thought happily occurred to a few of their remote predecessors, and thus an interesting fact has been transmitted—the existence of an epidemic form of leprosy. It is on record that in the year 1417, in the department of Kinhua, on the Chientang river, an epidemic of leprosy (癘 風) prevailed, and also that the same malady sprang up in 1589 in the department of Shaohsing, and that the greater portion of its districts suffered, and, again, that it prevailed during the following year in Changhwa, a district in the coterminous department of Hangchow.

Concerning the contâgion as it appeared early in the fourteenth century nothing is reported; that of 1558 and following year sprang up after a period of protracted and unexampled rains,—an autumn and winter rainfall extending through more than three months. During the year that this disease prevailed in the northern part of the province, there was an epidemic at Chüchau, it appears by reference to the foregoing list, and after heavy rains, but of its nature there is no record. This sudden and apparently unprecedented outbreak of an epidemic contagious form of leprosy is remarkable from the fact that the disease is seldom met with in Chêhkiang, and never, perhaps, in the northern part of the province. Fukien to the south, and yet more in Canton, further south, are the seats of that loathsome and hideous malady. Shaohsing is remarkable, however, for the prevalence of elephantiasis of the leg; perhaps there is no part of the world which suffers to like extent from that disease—due probably, with other causes, to its low situation, being elevated but a yard or so above tide water. It appears to be the epidemic form of leprosy that SHEN LANGCHUNG describes (沈 朗 仲 病 横 彙 論). The skin becomes scaly and dies; boils and ugly ulcers appear in the flesh, engendering worms; the cartilage of the nose inflames and falls off, as do also the finger-nails; the perspiration has a fishy stench; the hair and eyebrows disappear, the vision fails, and the voice becomes husky and inaudible. Therapeutic measures are futile except in mild cases. I expect to be able ere long to extend the inquiry to the Empire at large, for the purpose partly of examining the ground on which, as alleged, the "black death" of the middle ages originated in China—a besom of destruction which swept from the East over Europe to the shores of the Atlantic.

It is in local, not in general, works that full information is to be found; the search therefore involves considerable toil.* All that the abbreviated history of WANG FICHOU (凰 洲 綱 鑑) records on the subject is soon told, and it is subjoined as a contribution towards the general subject. Epidemics are named in the foregoing work as having occurred in the years of our Lord 52, 1054, 1275, 1279, 1308, 1313, 1564, 1583, 1589, 1642, and 1644, when the history comes to a close.

Wênchow has had its full share of cholera ravages, the study of which at this date affords no information to the pathologist, but as a history of that epidemic in China is a desideratum, I submit the following contribution, first reminding the reader that epidemiologists in India are not in accord concerning the origin of cholera, very high authorities affirming that it is purely of Indian origin, and that it originated in the Gangetic Delta in 1813, while other not less eminent authorities find evidence of its anterior prevalence in other parts of the East, citing in support thereof Sanskrit, Greek and Arabian authors, showing that after periods of quiescence it reappears—at intervals sometimes of a century or more. But what is of more moment, these opposing etiological views, which prevail not in India only, but in Europe and America, indicate diverse measures for averting the disease and for limiting the area of its ravages, a contagious malady obviously demanding to be met by different sanitary, if not different remedial, management than a non-contagious disease. Some hold that "all the phenomena are explained by contagion communicated from person to person by a germ from the excreta of cholera patients, that water is the channel through which cholera poison is generally conveyed. Others find in local influences full explanation of the phenomena, holding that the disease is not communicable from person to person, that the poison is air-borne, travelling in obedience to certain fixed laws, and affected by atmospheric and telluric conditions, and, when finding a fit nidus, there developing the epidemic, and that there is no enteric or specific poison in water to produce it, although they insist on purity of water and sanatory regulations generally."

The voluminous medical literature of China and the records of remarkable occurrences found in gazetteers might be expected to throw much light on these controverted subjects, particularly on the first or historical question, but the result of my investigations thus far afford

* As chapters on an 祥 異 that are found in *hsien* and *fu* gazetteers are more to be desired and more difficult to obtain, I beg assistance—that is, the copying out of those chapters; due acknowledgment shall be made for aid in that or any other form.

only a slender contribution to the moot points,—nothing that can be considered approximately decisive,—albeit I must confess that hitherto my inquiries have been restricted to a small portion of this almost boundless field of research. The Malacca Chinese were the first to suffer from Asiatic or Indian cholera, the epidemic having reached the Straits in 1819 by way, it is believed, of Siam. In May or June of the year following it appeared in Wênchow, and about the same time at Ningpo. A septuagenarian who remembers its ravages gives a ghastly account of the city as it then appeared,—a narrative which tradition confirms, and corroborated by written and oral accounts of its first appearance at Ningpo. It then obtained the name by which it is now popularly known here, the "crab-claw disease." Attacks of the disease were so sudden and fatal that people were stricken down and died in the streets. The "symptoms," to employ the expression of a French pathologist, "commenced with death." There is but one account of this form of cholera that I can hear of; it is a monograph, the work of a physician of the city of Chiahsing. That writer says that the disease first appeared in Kiahsing (on the borders of Chêhkiang and Kiangsu) in 1821, and was regarded as *sui generis*, and received the designation of "contracting of the tendons of the leg" disease (脚 筋 吊　吊 脚 疹), which physicians treated as ordinary cholera, the "sudden vomiting and purging" disease (霍 亂), and as a consequence they did not save one patient in a hundred. Ordinary cholera is ascribed to "accumulated heat," which requires a cooling regimen. Our author regarded it as the result of accumulated cold, which, like excess of heat, disturbs the harmony naturally subsisting between the dual powers of the system, and accordingly prescribed warming remedies, a mode of combating the enemy which of necessity became universal. The disease again prevailed in the two years following with unabated virulence, and since that period it has been of frequent occurrence throughout the Empire, notably in Chêhkiang in 1860.* Scarcely a summer passes without the occurrence of numerous marked cases of this migratory contagion appearing in one part of the country or another;† it is now recognised as endemic. In this part of China, what has been styled "dry cholera" is common in hot weather, and is called *sha* (痧), a term that includes colic, sunstroke, heat apoplexy and various disorders that make their attack suddenly. At Canton it is more frequent than elsewhere; the Cantonese affirm that *sha* has prevailed among them from time immemorial, which may explain their belief that they have always had Asiatic cholera among them. It may be regarded now as endemic in this part of China as well, making its appearance even in winter. During the past winter various villages on the Pootung side of Shanghai district suffered from Indian cholera; the only difference which the epidemic

---

* According to CLEYER (*Cholera Epidemic of 1873 in the United States*), "cholera appeared in China in 1669, coming probably from Malacca," and GENTIL, in his *Voyage aux Indes Orientales*, states that it prevailed in China soon after its appearance in Coromandel in 1769. These authorities are quoted by Dr. D. B. SIMMONS in his elaborate article on "Cholera Epidemics in Japan" (I.M. Customs *Medical Reports*, September 1879). What sources of information those writers possessed does not appear. I know not what degree of importance should be attached to their statements. Besides Dr. SIMMONS, the subject has been discussed by Dr. JOHN DUDGEON in the Customs *Medical Reports* for September 1872. Unfortunately, I am at present unable to consult that paper, which doubtless contains information that I might have turned to good account. Dr. PATRICK MANSON devotes several pages to Asiatic cholera in China in the Customs *Medical Reports* for September 1877. The September number of the *Chinese Repository* for 1843 contains a paper on cholera at Ningpo, and the August number 1851 has also a few paragraphs from myself on the same subject.

† The latest cholera visitation at this port is recorded in Mr. Commissioner MACKEY's Wênchow Trade Report for 1878. It prevailed during August and September of that year, and was extremely virulent.

presented from the summer form appearing to be that it was less rapidly fatal, the disease continuing three days before its fatal termination.* The reason assigned by the Chinese for this untimely visitation was that, owing to a protracted drought, the canal waters had become polluted. (While, however, the natives attribute epidemics to droughts, they also say that a protracted and excessive rainfall is often followed by an epidemic. With regard to fever and ague and the weather, they affirm that disease prevails chiefly when a season is unusually windy.) Undoubtedly Indian cholera was regarded in the north of China as a new disease, but it is quite possible, nevertheless, that it was only a reappearance after a period of quiescence, and some of the epidemics named in the subjoined record may have been epidemic cholera. We know that the register of epidemics in recent works includes the cholera visitations. A reference to a medical treatise which is more in circulation than any other† names contraction of the tendons as an occasional symptom in ordinary endemic cholera, but Dr. WU states that while there is a resemblance they are nevertheless distinct diseases. He might have adduced in evidence that while no one regards the "sudden vomiting and purging disease" as communicable from person to person, the new disease is regarded as contagious—a thing, however, held by many as true of fever and ague. The sum of the information that I have been able to gather tends to show that Indian or epidemic cholera is new to China, and that it is not due to an enteric poison communicable from person to person, but to air-borne germs; that it is influenced by atmospheric and telluric conditions, and, consequently, that quarantine regulations to ward off invasion from the migratory foe are futile—a conclusion diametrically opposed to the opinions of Drs. SIMMONS and MANSON, opinions formed by painstaking observers after recent inquiries on cholera visitations in Japan and China. No measures that I can hear of have ever been taken by Chinese authorities of the nature of quarantine to ward off infection.‡ Dr. SIMMONS incidentally alludes, loc. cit., to an epidemic of measles immediately preceding one of cholera, those affected by the former being attacked before recovery by the latter, which reminds me of what I wrote in 1851 on the same subject. "During the autumn of 1848 (when cholera was somewhat prevalent), rubeola prevailed epidemically at Ningpo; it did not assume a malignant form, nevertheless fatal cases were not rare. The epidemic prevailed in the maritime districts of the east coast of China and through the entire Pacific coast till it reached the Samoyedes, among whom it was particularly fatal. A Russian captain reported: 'we had throughout all our colonies th measles, and great numbers of the inhabitants were taken off. Some of our islands in th Aleutian chain lost most of their population. In Sitka, amongst a population of 600, we had in one month 80 deaths, if not more; nearly all, except the Europeans, were sick, so that all the town was in sorrow from fear and dread.' The islands of the Pacific suffered from the same disease (all Micronesia), and at the Sandwich Islands it was very destructive amongst the aboriginal inhabitants. In China it affected both natives and foreigners. It is remarkable that whilst rubeola was traversing this region of the earth from the Tropic of Cancer to the Frigid Zone, cholera was pursuing a western course from the Volga to the Mississippi."§

* 申 報, 19th February 1881.
† 醫 宗 必 讀, A.D. 1637.
‡ Articles on cholera are contained in the Customs *Medical Reports* from Dr. DUDGEON.
§ *Chinese Repository*, August 1851.

Perhaps Dr. SIMMONS may obtain information respecting the surging of this wave of rubeola in the islands of the Rising Sun.

Besides the epidemic above named as occurring last winter and spring at Shanghai, there appeared concurrently epidemics of measles and small-pox, the former in the coterminous department of Soochow, the latter at Nanchang, in the neighbouring province of Kiangsi. "Everywhere throughout the Soochow region children were attacked by measles, not of the ordinary mild form, but of a virulent type—nine cases out of every ten presenting dangerous symptoms." The reason assigned for the unusual severity of the disease was the drought of the winter, followed by a rainy, snowy spring. The small-pox at Nanchang was characterised by symptoms of extreme violence at the early stage, and of their sudden subsidence, leaving the disease to pursue a quiet course to convalescence.* Throngs of grateful parents presented thanks at the shrine of the small-pox god for the recovery of their children. The synchronous prevalence of cholera, small-pox and measles in places almost contiguous is a noteworthy epidemiological phenomenon. As a contribution to the epidemiology of China, I subjoin a list of epidemics which have devastated this province, the most disastrous only being chronicled— probably but half the number that have prevailed, as I have before me only five gazetteers out of the 11 which comprehend the province.

In default of narratives from books on the subject of epidemics, an account chiselled on a mural monument in the "Temple of the Five Supernals" (五 靈 廟), demons of pestilence of this city, will perhaps make amends for their meagreness. It appears from that record that for several tens of years preceding, Wênchow suffered every spring and summer from a contagious malady, the mere symptoms of which caused the patient to be shunned by his nearest relations, who sent them to vacant temples, supplying them there with cold victuals. No one ventured out by night lest a pestilential demon might be encountered, and great distress consequently prevailed. In the year 1579 a magistrate took up the matter, summoning men of age and experience to counsel him. Some of these suggested the free distribution of medicines, others the interment of the unburied dead, and others a grand demonstration to propitiate the five demons which caused the malady, by which they might be exorcised and retire to the river bank. The magistrate took a more comprehensive view of the needs of the situation. Favouring sumptuary and spiritual measures to combat the evil, he read the people a homily—first, on the five cardinal relations (that between Emperor and people, that between father and son, the conjugal and fraternal relations and that between friends); secondly, on the five elements (water, fire, wood, metal and earth); thirdly, on the five flavours (salt, bitter, sour, acid and sweet); fourthly, on the five viscera (the heart, liver, stomach, lungs and kidneys); and fifthly, on the five (?) passions (joy, anger, grief, fear, love, hatred, desire). The gist of this quincuncial discourse was in its application—a reformation in manners, food, and in life generally, was what he considered as requisite for sanatory improvement. All those measures, at least those proposed by the elders, were adopted, and, in addition, the erection of a special temple to the five demons of epidemics was decided on (hitherto those supernals were merely honoured by shrines in various temples). With such zeal was the plan of a temple acted on that it was run up in a month, and a substantial structure it is. Magistrates gave the fines of their courts, the rich gave of their

* 申 報, 12th February 1881.

hoards, and the people contributed free labour to the undertaking, endowing the temple with land to defray the expense of incense for ever. It is gratifying to read that the worthy magistrate was able to felicitate himself on the disappearance of the plague.

At the risk of being tedious, I add a paragraph respecting the demons of plague, belief in whom controls official as well as popular action when disease of any kind is rife. In the sixth year of KAUTSU (A.D. 591) reports of an apparition in the sky reached the Emperor; it consisted of "five mighty ones" (五 力 士). His Majesty consulted his minister, inquiring whether the appearance of the gods was a calamitous or felicitous omen, and received in reply the information that the "mighty ones" were Heaven-sent demons, agents of the five epidemics, to wit, those of spring, summer, autumn, winter and pestilences in general; the minister gave also the names and surnames of the demons as if they were those of characters once known among men. They were robed respectively in green, white, red, black and yellow; each held a utensil, hammer, ladle, sword, etc. "What," inquired the Emperor, "can be done to avert calamity?" "Nothing," was the response; "it is Heaven-sent, and there is no resource." That year a great epidemic scourged the entire nation. On the 27th of the 6th month the Emperor ordered the erection of a temple and sacrifices to be made to the demons, on each of whom he conferred the military title of general. During that dynasty, the SUI, and that of the TANG, temples were dedicated to ceremonies for averting the pestilential wrath of these "mighty ones," now styled "supernaturals."

In wealthy cities—Ningpo, for example,—the demons of epidemics are borne in processions of an imposing character, every guild and precinct contributing to render them magnificent, one feature of which is the appearance on a car of young girls, who seem to form portions of lotus-flowers, being sustained in the air by iron rods dexterously passing through a trouser leg, imparting a fairy-like aspect to the pageant. Occurring as this festival does in hot weather, its observance itself is often a source of sudden disease.

In this city, devotees who take part in processions that are designed to ward off pestilences subject themselves to painful proofs of their earnest zeal. They march for many weary miles with vases of burning incense suspended by hooks from the flesh of their arms, their arms being sustained in a horizontal position by a rod extending obliquely from the hip to the hand. According to the latest local gazetteer, worship at the Temple of the Demons of Pestilence does not now suffice to ward off the diseases to which the city is described as being particularly exposed, owing to atmospheric vicissitudes, albeit it is the most cleanly city in the Empire.

It is due to the school of CONFUCIUS to state that many of its disciples endeavour to dissuade the populace from the degrading feticism into which they are plunged, particularly in matters of hygiene. Such is the statesman who recently acted as governor of Kiangsu; he shut up monasteries, turned the monks adrift, and secularised their ill-gotten property. Such also was CHANG TZÜCHI, a Minister of State under the southern SUNG, who whilom was magistrate of Changchau, in Kiangsu. In the year 1295 an epidemic ravished the city, nine houses in every ten suffering from the scourge. In vain he strove to mitigate and check the malady by establishing a dispensary and furnishing medicines gratuitously. No one applied for relief; all who needed help for themselves or friends repaired to the Temple of the Demons of Pestilence, where sacerdotal exorcists sold charms and amulets and employed imposing incantations as the sole means proper for averting or curing the prevailing epidemic, and who deprecated the use of medicines; on hearing which the magistrate himself visited the temple, and seeing a row of images of hideous aspect on either side of a grim-visaged central monster, and witnessing the fanatical mummeries by which the multitude were deluded, he ordered the arrest and imprisonment of all concerned; then, providing fortifying viands and stimulating potations to his soldiers, to proceed forthwith to smash the images and to level the temple with the ground, a work which the military accomplished before they became well sobered and capable of understanding the sacrilegious character of their mission. Meanwhile the magistrate ordered the flagellation of the monks, and sent them back into the world. While the townspeople were all wondering what form of judgment the outraged gods would inflict on the daring iconoclast, the Emperor summoned him to a secretariat in the Civil Board at the capital (吏 部 郎 中). Unfortunately, rulers of that stamp have neither imitators nor successors. Naturally, the medical profession is arrayed against the impostures of the priesthood, yet they recognise the need of supernatural aid for success in their vocation, and, in concert with the general public, invoke the assistance of departed practitioners of the healing art, several of whom have been canonised; and hence temples to the *Yo wang*, or Princes of Medicine, are everywhere to be found, being styled by foreigners temples of the "Æsculapius of China," although in all Chinese history there is no personage bearing the characteristics of the reputed son of Apollo. "Medicine Prince" is a title of several medical notabilities, none of whom were regular practitioners nor writers, but successful charlatans rather, one of them being a foreign adventurer. The earliest of those to whom temples of medicine were erected was PIEN CH'IAO, who flourished in the reign of WE LIH (B.C. 468–440). He was a native of the Ching state (Kaifung-fu), but his family belonged to the state of Lu, for which reason he was styled the Lu physician (扁 鵲 秦 越 人 盧 醫). Originally he kept a hostelry, but having met a spirit who induced him to take a certain medicine daily for a month, on the assurance that by doing so he would become spiritualised, the effect of which was that he was able to see through a stone wall, and consequently by his vision penetrate the human system and observe the viscera. Thus he became an adept in diagnosis, and the most obscure disorders gave way to his therapeutic skill. The Prince of Tsin, TING KUNG, had for prime minister a man of boundless wealth who, in the 11th year of TING KUNG, suffered from an illness that baffled the skill of the court physician, and the Doctor of Lu was sent for. He found that the patient had been unconscious for five days, but in less than three days consciousness was restored by the medicines which PIEN CH'IAO administered. The patient recovered and rewarded the doctor by a gift of 20,000 *mow* of land. The distinction thus attained he did not live to enjoy, for the court physician procured his assassination. PIEN CH'IAO is credited with anatomical knowledge obtained by dissection, and with the theory of the pulse, which, like a work attributed to him on acupuncturation and the use of moxa (扁 鵲 神 應 針 灸 玉 龍 經), may be taken as apocryphal. Certain it is that that work, according to the catalogue *raisonné* of the Imperial Library, was composed during the Yuan period.*

* The authorities quoted in MAYERS' *Manual* err greatly as regards the period when PIEN CH'IAO lived and the place of his birth, that is, assuming the correctness of the 鳳 洲 綱 鑑.

In 738 there appeared in the capital a singularly attired foreigner; he wore a velvety robe and a gauze cap; he was peculiarly shod, and bore a staff; attached to his girdle were calabashes, several tens in number, containing medicines, which he freely distributed to the ailing. His fame reached the palace, and the Emperor sent for the foreigner, who announced himself as an "obtained doctrine" (*teh-tao*) man from India. His Majesty was so gratified with him that he ordered his portrait to be taken, and conferred on him the title of Medicine Prince. His name was WEIKU. A Fukien miscellany (閩雜記) names a Medicine Prince Temple or Temple of PIEN CH'IAO, also called Temple of Dr. LU. Another says that the medicine prince, or *pusa*, was WEIKU, who came from Sumatra. Probably he had made himself famous in that island after quitting India before coming to China. He is described as having *teh-tao*, the Buddhist term for one who has entered Nirvana. He was not a Buddhist, however, yet a man of lofty religious character, but whether Brahmin or Mussulman does not appear. When the usurping Empress WU, in the latter part of the 7th century, swayed the black-haired race, a Taoist practitioner of medicine named WEI SHENCHÜN became very celebrated by his austerities as a monk and by the cures that he effected. He was constantly attended by a black dog called "Black Dragon," and obtained by popular acclamation the title of medicine prince, or king. In pictures and images of the canonised doctor, his familiar the black dog is also represented, reminding one of the canine familiar of Western classical and mediæval times. Tradition has it that SIMON MAGUS and other ancient practitioners of the black art and charlatanry in general were attended by black dogs. CORNELIUS AGRIPPA, the famous practitioner and philosopher of the 16th century, had a familiar, what HUDIBRAS calls a "Stygian pug," the doctor's "tutor and cur which read to the occult philosopher." The idea never seems to have taken root in China. WEI SHENCHÜN would probably have been soon forgotten but for the circumstance that a great Minister of State under the SUNG sway had during a severe illness a vision of WEI SHENCHÜN, who was attended with a black dog, as when in the flesh. The spirit directed the boy to swallow a pill, which he did, when a flow of perspiration followed, and the patient was quickly convalescent. The child, when he came to be a ruler, caused a picture of that prince of medicine to be taken, to which he sacrificed, and thus WEI CHÜN again became famous. Soochow boasts a medical pantheon. Formerly the edifice was consecrated to the three Emperors FU HI, SHEN MING, and HWANG, semi-mythic rulers. Subsequently the image of YU the Great was added, all four being honoured for their medical knowledge, and in 1692 a prefect ordered the effigies of K'I PEH, LUI KUNG, PEH KAU, KWEI YUCHÜ, HSIAO YÜ, and HSIAO, and changed the name to the one which it now bears, "Temple of the Healing Kings."* Thus it is clear that these temples cannot be considered as consecrated to a Chinese Æsculapius.

According to the teaching of alchemy, hartall—arsenic bisulphide—is prophylactic against malarious and demoniacal influences. Infinitesimal doses of which are taken with cinnabar in a little liquor on the 5th day of the 5th moon—Dragon festival; in the case of children the powder is smeared on the forehead.

Epidemic frenzies come under the consideration of the physiologist, and demand his attention as a branch of what is termed State medicine, information on which cannot but be

---

*The greater portion of the above is culled from numerous authors cited in the 集說詮眞積編 黃伯祿斐默氏: Shanghai, 1860.

useful to administrators of public affairs. I submit a few paragraphs on the subject, which, if valueless to professional readers, will be found not devoid of interest to laymen. In 1876 there appeared a monograph entitled *Précis of Anthelmintics* (治蠱撮要), an anonymous work by a benevolent, public-spirited gentleman of Changchau, Kiangsi. It was called forth by an event which must be fresh in the memory of foreign residents,—the panic that existed respecting supernatural clipping of queues,*—and had for its object the diffusion of useful knowledge on the calamitous visitation, the treatment of sufferers and suppression of sorcery, the cause of the mental and physical distress that then prevailed over a large portion of the Empire, besides which the volume unfolds the arcana of ancient theurgic lore on this recondite matter. That production and personal observation form the basis of the following account of the remarkable delusion by which the Empire for many months was strangely infatuated. Little is to be gleaned from the work respecting previous epidemics of the same nature; it, however, gives dates of such periods of frenzy that have occurred in his part of the country as found recorded in local gazetteers. They occurred in the following order, in the years of our Lord 1464 and the following year, 1529, 1596, 1657 and 1753. The earlier period named shows that the delusion was nearly concurrent with the beginning of witch-mania in Europe, or the date of the bull of INNOCENT VIII. Happily, the delusions in China were not intensified by religious fury, and women have seldom been regarded as addicted to sorcery, although they are etymologically implicated. *Yao*, magical, elf, bewitching, and the like, is composed of "woman" and "winning." An author of the middle of the 17th century is quoted, who gives an account of the epidemic of 1657, occasioned by wizards from the north of the Yangtze, who appeared at Chingkiang and Changchau. They possessed the power of fascinating or enchanting men whom they met abroad, so that simply calling them by name they were enabled to allure them to another city and sell them by a sort of "hypnotising," a process somewhat analogous to influences of the "evil eye," although neither this world-wide superstition nor the myth of the fascinating power of serpents or basilisks seems to have prevailed in Eastern Asia. The hypnotised being sold by their captors through Soochow and Changchau brokers led to the suppression of the practice; the brokers were severely punished, and the sorcerers quitted Changchau for Hangchau, where also they operated. For about a week, however, Changchau was troubled by spiritual manifestations which agitated the entire community. No one attempted to sleep by night, owing to numerous weird phenomena; rafters and tiles of houses shook with fearful noises, vapourish phantoms were observed, having a frowsy smell, these at times being the size of a peck measure, and suddenly expanding to the size of a house, being, in fact, black demons assuming various shapes, as, for example, that of a fox with an enormously distended mouth, and eyes like stars, or transforming into the figure of a horse or dog. These shadowy ogres entered houses and smothered people to death, or scratched and clawed them till blood flowed. Attempts were made to smite them with swords, but the swordsmen merely succeeded in hacking themselves. Of only one thing were these agents of sorcerers afraid,—that was noise. By the continued beating of gongs, of

* The "paper men" and queue-cutting craze evoked an Imperial decree (*Peking Gazette*, 15th October 1876), also a report from the Governor of Chêhkiang (*Peking Gazette*, 9th November 1876), in which documents it appears that the Government regarded the excitement as being aimed at Christian missions.

metal or wooden implements, and by shouting, from sunset to sunrise, the magical apparitions were kept out of houses, and in seven days they entirely disappeared. At that time, and previously, the population had suffered from effigies of men drawn on paper, which being enchanted and scattered became a source of great annoyance, particularly by clipping portions of queues; the hair being conveyed to the sorcerers, gave them power over the lives of the despoiled. Doctor CHOU had with him a temporary lodger who announced that he would sell charms to break all spells of that kind. He sold them cheaply and had many purchasers, but some malicious persons gave out that he himself was a sorcerer; a mob seized him, took him to the magistrate, by whom he was tortured for a confession till he died. Our author states that he himself doubted the truth of traditions which described the machinations of sorcerers, but the prevailing epidemic convinced him that the evils had not been exaggerated, for since the rise of the existing panic he had ocular demonstration of an apparition of a *yao*, a bewitching demon. Its eyes were like flashing mirrors; the phantom vanished, however, as soon as he had recourse to incantation, a recitation of a well-known spell-breaking rhyme. Consequently, he took up the subject and searched for plans that had been found efficacious in former visitations of the same nature; these he supplements with formulæ of his own and those of other modern investigators. The title that he adopts for his work, *An Account of Anthelmintics*, or worm remedies, is drawn from ancient and meturgico-medical writers, who describe seven different kinds of parasites or "venomous worms" that prey on the human system and which are not amenable to ordinary treatment, but require supernatural measures, united with articles of the materia medica, as antidotes. The agents employed by sorcerers are likened to those worms, and hence the combating agents are styled vermifuges. It appears that Kwangtung and Kwangsi are most noted for worm-poisoning.

Charmed bits of paper representing men are scattered by sorcerers, which are vehicles for sending out their ghostly emissaries. When by any means these spirits gain admission to a dwelling, they begin to injure the inmates, most commonly by clipping bits of a queue; the hair thus coming into the possession of the sorcerer, he can summon at will the soul or spirit of his victim, which he employs ever after as a servile demon, or "familiar," according to mediæval parlance,—the victim, of course, dying by the loss of his spirit. Sometimes the demons which are sent on the charmed paper thrust needles into the bodies of the victims, and at other times seal or stamp their skin by discoloured spots. At other times the demon personates a pedlar and palms off charmed commodities, victims being tempted to become purchasers by the extreme cheapness of the article. It was in this way that a Changchau man fell a victim to demons. He purchased a pair of scissors, and the same night cut his own throat with the charmed implement; and a man in Kiukiang came to grief by purchasing an enchanted melon. At night he heard some one calling him by name; he rose, but could see no one; at daylight he found himself bereft of all his hair.

Another mode of bringing people under demoniacal influence by sorcerers or practitioners of the black art is through the agency of animals—rats, bats, sparrows, butterflies, beetles, centipedes,—anything, in fact, that has life can be employed for their maleficent schemes.

The first symptom of invasion of the occult malady is pain in the stomach; after this the virus is diffused through the system. In children a few days suffice for that end; in adults it often takes 100 days before effecting specific results, and sometimes even two or three years elapse before the case terminates fatally.

In treating the disease recourse must be had to drugs and to counter-incantations. Loadstone pills, because of their power of attraction, constitute the chief means of cure, other medicines being employed as adjuvants, according to peculiarities in the case. Purgatives and emetics perform an important *rôle;* if they dislodge hairs, pigs' bristles or bamboo shavings, the patient will recover. When it is found that a person has lost a portion of his queue, an inch or two of the remainder is to be clipped off obliquely and soaked in a cloaca for a period of 80 days. Communication by aura between the hair in possession of the sorcerer and the patient is entirely severed. Most reliance, however, is placed on incantations, and anathemas that come stamped with authority; and on the occurrence of a craze epidemic, the interposition of the legally constituted custodians of public and secular interests is invoked by terrified communities. The epidemic of 1876 elicited a proclamation from the Governor of Kiangsu. If His Excellency regarded the matter as an illusion, it would not have been politic at that time to have attempted to enlighten the people; for in doing so they would have regarded him as possessed also by a malignant demon. After descanting on the pestiferous and disturbing mischief worked by the paper effigies, he proceeds to give directions for combating the evil. First, he publishes a charm composed of characters of his own invention (𧰼𧰼𧰼𧰼𧰼𧰼𧰼 𧰼𧰼𧰼𧰼𧰼𧰼𧰼𧰼𧰼𧰼), which was designed for posting over the doors of dwellings or wearing as an amulet,—it is understood that their meaning can be comprehended only by the demons against whom the cabalistic effusion is directed; and next he gives a form of anathema attributed to LAU TZ', the founder of the Taoist sect (6th century B.C., apotheosised A.D. 666 as Great Supreme), which he directs to be chanted while copying it on yellow paper with blood from the crest of a cock and vermilion, and then to be burnt, and the ashes swallowed. The words are arranged trimetrically and read, " Imprecation of the Great Supreme. In the name of All-powerful Heaven and All-efficient Earth, let demon ogres be decapitated and their spirits exterminated; let them not tarry for a day nor suffered to return to life. Begone, ye demons! I gulp your substance—whether ye be paper or blood, be ye transformed into dust! I [the supplicant] humbly trust that the Great Supreme will instantly command you according to his decrees." Minute directions are given concerning the mode of writing the charm, its incineration and swallowing. In conclusion, the Governor assures the people that the authorities are fully competent to cope with the evil and to combat all machinations against the souls of the people and the stability of the State.

Fortified by secular interposition, the people sought and obtained the intervention of the Supreme Pontiff of Taoism. This hereditary potentate, who is sometimes designated the " Taoist Pope," is supposed to exercise authority over demons (by demon in China the word is to be understood, not in a mediæval, but in a classical sense), appears on occasions like the present in an official capacity; he met the current emergency by the reissue of a charm or amulet which he had used against a cholera epidemic in 1862. There was scarcely a house door that was not protected by the charm, hardly an individual who did not wear the amulet under cap or in sleeve. In times of excitement, particularly when disease is rife, every house door will be found to have a charm, and foreigners may thereby know that the public mind is in a state of ferment either from bodily or mental suffering. They are subjoined, as they may be easily recognised, and their recognition sometimes proves serviceable.

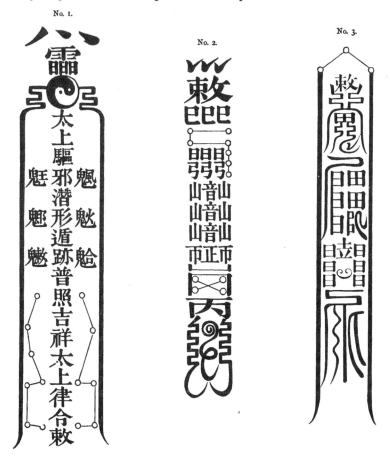

No. 1.

No. 2.

No. 3.

No. 1 is from the Great Supreme, a talisman to be used at all times (the others on special occasions). It is headed by three mystic dots and an unauthorised character employed esoterically. The central characters read, "Behest of the Great Extreme for driving off pestiferous influences, their vanishing from his diffused felicitous astral effulgence!" Astrology is made to play a part in the form of constellations, circumpolar and other stars. The gist of the charm is supposed to be in the six demon characters on the sides, which, it is said, mean urgent and imperative commands. No. 2 is from the Supreme Pontiff, Exorcist and Augur-

General, and is to be worn as an amulet. No. 3 is from the same functionary, and is for posting on doors; the figures are known only to the initiated, our author not having fathomed their mysterious depths. The promulgator of these is named CHANG, and has for his official designation, "Heavenly Teacher." He is a simple-minded, unpretentious character, and so mistrusts his power in ordinary diseases that he consults me through messengers concerning his ailments. I made the acquaintance of his holiness when he was on a visit to the Faithful of the Coast, from his seat, Dragon-Tiger Mountain, Kwangsin, Kiangsi. In his palace are innumerable sealed jars in which captured or exorcised demons are imprisoned. Besides the duty of bottling the imps of the country, he makes appointments of tutelar guardians in every palladium temple in the Empire. By his potent magic wand this master wizard wields dominion over the spirits of the universe, protecting the State from their mischievous acts, and families from their malevolence.

Our author, after enumerating a large number of the innumerable arts by which sorcerers afflict their victims, states that they are to be met by means both foul and fair; the former being the employment of unmentionable filthy rags, dogs' blood, and whatever is nasty; the latter consists in the use of orthodox writings, the recitation of which is deterrent and exorcising. The first chapter of the *Great Learning* or of the *Due Medium*, or the 64 diagrams of the *Book of Changes*, or the ever-cherished verses of the martyred patriot, T'IEN FÊNGCHOU, also a well-known jingling gibberish, as an imprecation. The classics are believed to possess talismanic virtue in protecting dwellings from all terrene and supermundane noxious agents, and when a house is constructed a box containing copies of the *Four Books* and the *Five Classics*. By these means, combined with carrying hartall and other medicines in the belt, hanging up branches of the peach tree in the house, by noises from gongs, drums, fireworks, or otherwise, demons may be driven off.

The epidemic which called forth the book under consideration continued for about eight months, from Canton to regions north of the Yangtze and as far west as the lake provinces. It was surmised at the time, and fully established afterwards, that the panic was the concerted work of secret seditious societies having revolutionary aims. A few myrmidons in each large city sufficed to create a stir by deftly clipping the queues of the unwary, and then announcing in places of public resort that they themselves had suffered in the same mysterious way. When a few well-attested cases occurred, the cause, by common consent, was referred to paper men set loose by sorcerers, and then if one suffered from nightmare, or found a blotch on his skin, or had an attack of colic, the cause was attributed to sorcery. In a word, everything that went wrong in a city, death from apoplexy or suicide, the loss of some article, or any unusual noise or dream, a phantom,—all were supposed to be the work of the invisible enemy; while some, from the mere pleasure of attracting attention and becoming objects of remark, fabricated sensational stories until a form of cerebral disease was induced in weak persons, which contributed further to fan the flame of wild superstition.

Having disposed of the therapeutic portion of his essay, our author proceeds to counsel prophylactic measures. The agents of sorcerers infest opium-dens, tea-shops, and are to be seen lounging at temples or hiding in forests, hills or caverns. Let all suspicious persons be sought out by the gentry and elders, apprehended, and sent to the magistracy. Here, however, he interposes a needful caution, inasmuch as he hears that the criminal class band together as sorcerer-hunters, and plunder travellers on pretext of searching for proofs of connexion with those dreaded men, dexterously sticking needles of foreign manufacture on the person under search, and then exacting blackmail, which the sufferer ordinarily submits to. Soon after he meets with another sorcerer-hunting party, who, finding him penniless, take his clothes and his life as well. This is no fancy sketch, for it is well known that transactions of that kind took place subsequent to the publication of the *Anthelmintic*. Nor were the murderers ruffians only; well-meaning but panic-stricken villagers seized and executed travelling merchants under the belief that self-protection necessitated summary proceedings. It is much to the credit of the common people that, under the frenzy that seized them, they almost invariably took the suspected to the yamêns for judicial examination. Our author affords a glimpse of the character of judicial examination of persons suspected of complicity with sorcerers. In Hupeh an emissary was brought to trial, and it was found that under torture—trial in such cases includes torture—nothing could extort confession, nor even a cry or moan; but when some charmed plasters were removed from his armpits and the soles of his feet, and when a loathsome emetic was poured down his throat, he cried out and vomited forth the truth, admitting that a sorcerer paid him $1 for every tuft of hair that he cut, half that sum for sticking needles, and something less for stamping skins—in a word, the miserable wretch admitted all that the inquisitors sought to establish. In this way it was discovered that sorcerers direct their emissaries to reconnoitre the premises by day disguised as priests, beggars or pedlars, of places to which the paper men are to be conveyed at night, the paper men bearing the spirits of the emissaries. In view of the above, it is directed that when one awakens at night suffering from a sense of suffocation, he is to seize a dish-cloth and press it down on the spot where the missive is supposed to be, to hold it fast until someone goes out in search of the sorcery agent, who will be found sleeping in some adjacent house. On rousing the sleeper he will be found stupefied from the absence of his spirit; held under the dish-cloth he may then be easily led to the magistrate. In this manner five miscreants were seized at Wuhsi.

At Ningkuo, in Anhwei, enemies of the mission there pointed to a chapel as a place whence paper effigies of men were dispersed, and leading a mob, showed them a basketful of the effigies as proof, they themselves having placed them here. The populace became so exasperated that violence and loss of life followed. The leader hastened to the capital to get authority for further proceedings, but was cast into prison by the Governor, from which time the excitement subsided.

Widespread panics like that of 1876 are not of frequent occurrence, but crazes in a limited area are not uncommon, showing that the section of the Penal Code which provides punishment for persons found guilty of originating false rumours is necessary for the public safety. Two instances of local panics may be adduced, as they resulted from early foreign intercourse. At Ningpo, soon after the opening of the port, a single lady was in the habit of taking early walks on the city walls, a portent that needed explanation. She was not a maniac let loose, as was testified by her immediate neighbours, who stated that her only aberration consisted in going out of the way to do good. It was finally decided that she went on the ramparts to scatter paper men for bewitching and subjugating the inhabitants. To neutralise her magic the entire population engaged the whole of several successive nights in gong and drum beating, firing off crackers, and shouting, by which the spell was broken and security ensured.

Sometimes it will be found that a wily scoundrel sets a town in a ferment to accomplish some sinister object.   An instance of this sort occurred at Wênchow several years before the port was open for trade.   A literary graduate who devoted himself to fomenting disputes and espousing cases of litigants—a man of great force of character, who lived by his wits, was regarded as an oracle in foreign affairs, who was more feared than respected, who was inextricably involved in financial affairs—announced confidentially to all he met that he had discovered there was a calamity impending over the city, the precise nature of which he was unable to ascertain, but this much was certain, a fleet of vessels filled with foreign women, of hideous mien, with long carrotty beards, would soon be found at the mouth of the river.   If particulars were wanted, they might be wormed out of the only foreign resident, a missionary, to whom this scalawag referred all whom it concerned.   The consequence of this was that the missionary was shunned as if he were a leper.   In truth, there was something mysterious about the foreigner, a man of herculean frame and commanding mien, sustaining himself with a pair of wands.   People had not yet fully made the acquaintance of that estimable gentleman, whom they now love, but regarded the crutches which sustained him, he having lost a leg, as capable of turning the city upside down.   Before the ferment had time to subside, the graduate received information that the hecates had arrived at the mouth of the river, when he declared that for his part he had done his duty by the public, and now he would see to the safety of his family and take them up-country, and let the red-haired hecates catch the hindmost.   Before he was well off with all his belongings, the quay was rendered impassable by piles of effects of every description, which the well-to-do were conveying to boats, with wives, concubines, children, and domestics.   Business was suspended, shops were closed, people stood aghast and were paralysed; they appealed to the authorities.   The Taotai sent for the missionary, assuring him that he was displeased by the popular exhibition, and forthwith he issued a soothing proclamation, which quickly allayed the commotion.   It was not long before the facts of the case transpired,— that the whole affair was a ruse by the graduate, who could not otherwise get out of town. Everyone smiled except his ill-starred creditors.

At the present time, according to a native correspondent of the *Shên Pau*, two medical sorcerers are exercising a powerful sway over a large portion of country bordering the Great Lake.   They are dames, but assume and are accorded the tile of unmarried women, implying that they are a sort of fairy.   By charms they secure exemption from diseases, and by incantations they inflict disease on those who decline paying for the promised immunity.   They have obtained such an ascendancy that when an illness occurs it is ascribed to their vindictiveness, and their aid is invoked.   There are none so poor as not to be taxed—a dollar or so per annum,— the rich paying a hundred or more dollars.   They employ several tens of men in collecting fees, and these myrmidons have become so exacting that their depredations are likened to those of robbers, and represented as more destructive than fire or flood.

These glimpses at the everyday life of the people show the need that exists for the means now in use for their enlightenment.   In the diffusion of correct views regarding the seen and the unseen universe, the periodical press is a most important agency, and the demand for newspapers is an earnest that the clouds of superstition and ignorance, which are sources of manifest weakness to the Empire, will be gradually dissipated; gradually, not quickly, for, as the West knows too well, a period of dark and dreary ages is not susceptible of rapid change.

These glimpses at the social life of the Chinese disclose much suffering through ignorance and superstition, yet they do not seem to have been afflicted with delusions so disastrous as the witch-mania of our dark and dreary ages, which, it is computed, caused 9,000,000 persons to perish at the stake. Happily, the means which gradually enlightened and emancipated our progenitors are now in active operation throughout the land, diffusing correct views both of the seen and unseen worlds, the periodical press being among the most promising.

The recent discovery by DA SILVA LIMA of Brazil of the existence in that country of the Indian disease beriberi, and its later discovery in Japan by Dr. SIMMONS, show that that malady has a wider range than was supposed. On turning to certain translations that I made from the Chinese, and from late verbal inquiries, I find that beriberi is well known under the designation "malarial leg"—*kioh-k'i*, the same word which the Japanese pronounce *kakké* (脚氣). Not being familiar with the characteristics of the Indian malady, it did not occur to me that the Chinese malady and the Indian were identical until I read Dr. SIMMONS' paper on "Kakké" in Japan.

Inquiry into the literature of malarial leg ascends to the misty and undefined period when the semi-mythic and proto-historic narratives of China interlace; it necessitates a critical study of Chinese archæology, subjects which are hardly germane to a medical report. This much, however, is relevant. A disease named *kioh-k'i* or *chiao-ch'i* is described in the *Neiching* (內經), or rather in the 靈樞經, doubtless the oldest medical treatise extant,—a work attributed to HWANGTI, B.C. 2697,—although it has no claims to antiquity much, if any, beyond the period of the early CHOU or the sources whence CONFUCIUS compiled his annals. According to a writer quoted by SHÊN LANGCHUNG in his work on *Etiology* (沈朗仲病機彙論), the "chüeh" (厥) (a word meaning stone-throwing implement, which contrivance was probably named after the disease) is the "malarial leg," which during the HAN dynasties was called the "slow wind disease," and that in the SUNG sway it obtained its present designation; but the description does not apply to this disease at all,—it means a sort of syncope. It was also during that period that the earliest known monograph appeared on the subject, *Generalisation of the Treatment of Malarial Leg,** a work long lost, but named in the Imperial Catalogue and described or copied into the great work of YUNG LOH. It is in two volumes or chapters, the last containing 46 prescriptions. Since the SUNG the disease is found described in all systematic treatises on the healing art. Two forms of the malady are recognised, which correspond with *beriberi hydrops* and *beriberi atrophia*, and, as the name of the disease indicates, their etiological views accord with those of Western observers. "Malarial leg" is caused by a poison emanating from the soil. There are two kinds, one due to moist heat, the other to moist cold. It is engendered at any season of the year by prolonged sitting or standing in a damp place, also by suddenly suppressed perspiration,

* 脚氣治法總要, published between the latter half of the 10th and latter part of the 13th century, and is probably the work referred to by Dr. ANDERSON of Tokio as having been republished in Japan. *Vide* his pamphlet on the subject and Guy's Hospital Reports.

as when one is heated by the weather or by spirits, and disrobes when in that condition; and,
according to the patriarchal Emperor, by venereal indulgence when under the influence of
liquor. In the moist heat kind the pulse beats fast; in the moist cold kind it beats slowly.
When the poison rises from the legs to the heart, the mind is affected, the patient mutters,
there are loss of appetite and vomiting, restlessness, difficult respiration and scanty urine. In
the moist warm form of the disease, the legs are painful, and there is fever; in the cold moist
form, the limbs are not painful, and there is no fever. The mouth in both kinds becomes
black, the skin and flesh are painful, particularly on the sides of the chest, and the tendons
become prominent; these symptoms extend gradually to the face and head. Besides moisture
as the exciting cause of the disease, errors in diet are named as predisposing causes. Why
has this disease hitherto escaped detection in China? That is due partly to the fact that the
disease is not a common one, and partly because it belongs to a class of maladies for which
the intervention of foreign physicians is seldom made. Now, however, that attention is called
to the subject, cases are likely soon to be reported. I have heard of one case only—the
subject having but recently engaged my attention. It was that of the mother of a Chinese
officer of the Imperial Maritime Customs. It was an acute attack, and terminated in one week,
fatally. Native physicians pronounced the affection to be malarial leg, and from what is
reported it seems clear that it was a case of the wet form of the malady.

There is reason to believe that it prevails in Tungking, and it is not unlikely that it is
the disease called "mauvais vent" by Abbé RICHARD.*

Epidemics of a very destructive kind prevail among cattle, including the buffalo. The
autumn of 1877 was remarkable for devastation from a murrain in which vast numbers of
domestic animals of every kind perished (the preceding summer was a cholera season). Horned
cattle, including the cow and buffalo, horses, goats, pigs, dogs and poultry, all suffered,—the
bovine race from rinderpest; goats suffered from a foot-and-mouth disease; with regard to the
others my information thus far is defective. The Taotai then ruling was a gentleman of
great benevolence, and rigorously enforced the law which (not, however, to the extent of the
magistrate at Nanking, who about the same time beheaded a Mussulman butcher for the
offence) prohibits the slaughter of cattle, and by way of compensation to farmers whose animals
were superannuated, and from compassion for worn-out cattle, he established an asylum where
the animals were cared for during the balance of life. There were several hundred of these in
sheds situated outside the West Gate, but they all succumbed to the pest immediately after
an infected cow was introduced. The area over which the epidemic prevailed remains to be
ascertained; it affected the whole of this province and portions of Kiangsu and Anhwei.

Two years later, 1879, a murrain of unusual violence prevailed among bullocks and
camels in Mongolia, the transportation of tea between Kalgan and Urga being much impeded
in consequence. A standard work on cow diseases (牛經) gives stercoraceous and mucous

* "Le mauvais vent (Sinicè, morbific vapour?) est une autre espèce qui nous est inconnue. Le mauvais vent ou
l'impression subite d'un air froid, chargé d'exhalations locales, glace tout d'un coup le sang et fait mourir sur le champ
plusieurs personnes; d'autres ne sont qu'estropiées de quelques membres: le plus souvent, la bouche se déforme et tourne
comme dans une attaque de paralysie. Lorsque l'impression est légère on en guérit en se réchauffant. Il y a des remèdes
spécifiques contre ce mal s'ils sont administré à temps."—*Histoire naturelle, civile et politique du Tonquin*, par M. l'Abbé
RICHARD, Chanoine de l'Église royale de Verelai: à Paris, MDCCLXXVIII.

vomiting as pathognomonic of a common epidemic, but it affords no other information that merits transcribing. Pig murrains do not often occur synchronously with cattle plagues. Dr. PORTER SMITH's discovery of trichinæ of pork at Hankow,* and Dr. MANSON's detection of them at Amoy (see last Customs *Medical Reports*), indicate that parasite to be widespread. Further inquiry will probably lead to the discovery of trichiniasis, although, for the reason assigned by Dr. MANSON, the thorough cooking to which pork is subjected in China, the disease probably is of rare occurrence.

Wênchow is an opium producing region and an opium importing one as well. The domestic product is employed largely to adulterate the Indian article,—Patna, not Malwa, opium being thus employed. Native opium, being deficient in alkaloids, produces comparatively transient effect on the system; two or three hours after inhaling the smoker yearns for more whiffs of the pipe. It would be a work of supererogation at this date to comment on the demoralising effects of the use of opium or on its pathological action, but there is scope for remark on medical means of reforming smokers, and on the effects of the habit as it affects reproduction. Nine months ago the Inland Mission established a hospital for ophthalmic and opium patients under the care of A. W. DOUTHWAITE, Esq., who has in that period of time treated above 200 patients, all of whom quitted the institution as cured of the habit, having been under treatment four weeks each on an average. † There is no charge for admission into the institution, patients merely paying for sustenance. The average amount of opium daily

* *Contributions to the Materia-Medica and Natural History of China.*
† Since writing the above, the *First Annual Report of the Wênchow General Hospital and Opium Refuge*, by Mr. DOUTHWAITE, has appeared. I append the statistics as affording useful information on the subject of this paper:—

ANTI-OPIUM HOSPITAL STATISTICS.

| Number of patients admitted | . . . | 213 | Number of patients incurable | . . . . | 2 |
| „ „ cured | . . . | 209 | Expelled for bad conduct | . . . . | 2 |

NUMBER OF YEARS SINCE SMOKING WAS COMMENCED.

9 had smoked 1 year.		4 had smoked 9 years.		1 had smoked 19 years.
10 „ 2 years.		14 „ 10 „		2 „ 20 „
21 „ 3 „		11 „ 12 „		1 „ 21 „
18 „ 4 „		4 „ 14 „		2 „ 23 „
25 „ 5 „		13 „ 15 „		2 „ 24 „
29 „ 6 „		5 „ 16 „		5 „ 25 „
12 „ 7 „		4 „ 17 „		1 „ 29 „
17 „ 8 „		3 „ 18 „		

AGES OF PATIENTS.

Under 20	. . . . . .	3	Over 40 and under 50	. . . .	52
Over 20 and under 30	. . .	64	„ 50 „ 60	. . . .	14
„ 30 „ 40	. . .	79	„ 60 „ 70	. . . .	1

AMOUNT OF OPIUM CONSUMED DAILY BY EACH MAN.

7 consumed 1 mace.		41 consumed 5 mace.		3 consumed 9 mace.
23 „ 2 „		17 „ 6 „		5 „ 10 „
45 „ 3 „		11 „ 7 „		1 „ 12 „
49 „ 4 „		10 „ 8 „		1 „ 15 „

Average, 4½ mace.

4½ mace per day is 1,642 mace, or 10 catties 4 liang=13 lb. 6½ oz. avoirdupois, per annum.

If we consider those who have entered the hospital as fairly representing the opium-smokers of this city, and accept the *lowest* native estimate of the number of smokers—i.e., half the adult males,—then reckon the population at 80,000, we shall find there are at least 10,000 opium-smokers in the city.

smoked by patients treated at Peking by Dr. DUDGEON was 4½ mace, that of Mr. DOUTHWAITE'S.

At the above average of 10 catties 4 liang per annum, 10,000 men would require 102,500 catties of prepared opium for their yearly consumption. Crude opium loses in the process of preparation about one-third in weight; accordingly, 102,500 catties of the extract represents 132,950 catties, or about 1,329 chests of the crude drug.

As only 58 chests of foreign opium paid Customs duty here last year, a great quantity must be smuggled, or brought overland from Ningpo, to supply the market.

QUALITY OF OPIUM SMOKED.

69 smoked Malwa.	25 smoked Patna.	119 smoked native.

The Indian opium contains from 8 to 15 per cent. of morphine. The native drug is only about one-third that strength as it is sold in the shops, but in the Suian district, about 30 miles south of Wênchow, a very superior drug is produced, which those who smoke it declare to be equal to Patna. An opium planter from that district told me that a great quantity is annually sent over the borders to Fukien, where it is sold as Indian opium. It does not become soft when exposed to the air as the Wênchow and Taichau drug does.

	FOREIGN.	NATIVE.
Largest quantity smoked daily	8 mace.	15 mace.
Smallest „ „	1 „	2 „
Largest quantity eaten	1 „	5 „

TIME SPENT IN HOSPITAL.

Longest	40 days.
Shortest	8 „

Average, 21 days.

On leaving the hospital each man takes a supply of tonic medicines, so the average period of treatment is about 30 days.

The following statistics will show the work done during the past 12 months :—

GENERAL HOSPITAL STATISTICS.

Number of out-patients treated during the year	4,030
„ in-patients „ „	45

NATURE OF DISEASES TREATED.

Eye Diseases :—

Purulent ophthalmia	47
Gonorrhœal „	9
Granular „	86
Conjunctivitis	46
Entropion with ulceration of cornea	1,626
Granular lids	205
„ „ with ulceration of cornea	1,030
Superficial ulcers of cornea	190
Deep ulcers of cornea	27
Pterygium	98
Iritis	9
Cyclitis	3
Cataract	2
Night blindness	15
Asthenopia	20

Eye Diseases—cont.

Amblyopia	40
Abscess of orbit	2

General Diseases :—

Syphilis	32
Rheumatism	68
Ulcers and abscesses	146
Ague	57
Bronchitis and asthma	90
Pulmonary consumption	8
Dyspepsia	107
Anæmia	103
Hepatitis	5
Nasal polypi	3
Harelip	1
TOTAL	4,075

OPERATIONS PERFORMED.

For cataract	2
„ pterygium	98
„ entropion	160

For abscess of orbit	2
„ harelip	1
„ nasal polypus	3
TOTAL	266

patients was 3 mace 2 candareens. So extensive is the demand for anti-opium medicines that there are no city walls in the Empire that do not contain the placards of charlatans whose pills, it is vaunted, effect a perfect cure of opium-smoking desire; many of these nostrums are advertised as prepared under foreign auspices, a ruse which facilitates their sale. Opium in some form is always an ingredient of those pills which are most efficacious, and no doubt they effect much good. So long ago as 1844 I adopted a mode of treatment which may be called "thorough," in contradistinction to the above lenitive measures. It consisted in withholding from the first the accustomed narcotic and in combating the fearful consequences. A few hours' deprivation of the drug induces a colliquative diarrhœa, soon followed by seminal emissions, pain in the lumbar region, and an utter prostration. Stimulants, astringents, tonics and nourishing diet served to prop up the miserable patient until a desire was engendered for the new form of excitement, which seemed to bridge over the chasm which separated him from his former life. A taste for alcohol was never acquired by such patients, and there was no difficulty in reducing the dose until it was discontinued altogether. Patients who are cured by the lenitive method are liable to relapses. When tempted, they feel that an easy remedy is within reach, and that there is no danger of a little indulgence proving utterly ruinous, but he who has passed through the "thorough" ordeal is so impressed with its horrors that death by torture could have no greater terrors for him than a repetition of like treatment, and having been emancipated at such a cost he is hardly likely again to become enslaved. Physically and morally speaking, he has taken a new departure, and gradually recovers manhood in every sense; he, however, again becomes liable to attacks of malarial fever and catarrhs,—the narcotic, and a suggestive fact it is, affording him immunity from those disorders. I published an account of my mode of treating opium-smokers * many years ago; it was adopted by the late Dr. OSGOOD of Foochow, who found the new medicine, chloral hydrate, of signal use in meeting the cravings of the patient.

The seminal discharge which speedily follows disuse of opium is noteworthy when considered in connexion with its early use as an aphrodisiac and its employment in bagnios to protract orgasm, and such being the case it is not matter of surprise that its continued action conduces to impotency. To the effects, then, usually attributed to opium-smoking where it is a national habit must be added that of its being to an appreciable extent a check to the growth of population.

The Customs Report on Opium† shows—first, that, allowing 3 mace per day as the average amount of opium consumed by each man, the foreign market supplies only sufficient opium for 1,000,000 of the population; second, that the population of China is about 300,000,000; and third, that the native produce equals at least the amount exported; and therefore that opium-smokers constitute only a third of 1 per cent. of the population. Allowing, as a rule—and the exceptions are extremely rare,—that only the male part of the population smoke opium, and that none under 20 years of age are its victims, we obtain a more accurate view of

* *Chinese Repository*, August 1851.
† *Chinese Imperial Maritime Customs : Special Series : No. 4, Opium.* Published by order of the Inspector General of Customs. Shanghai : Statistical Department of the Inspectorate General, MDCCCLXXXI.

the number of opium-smokers, for the number of men over 20 years of age must be, on the above, about 60,000,000. Therefore we may say that 1 in 60 of the adult male population consumes foreign opium, and the same number consume the native drug; in other words, that about 3½ per cent. of the male population over 20 years of age smoke opium. My own inquiries concerning the amount of opium of native growth in China place it at over four times that of the imported article, which indicates a much larger per-centage of unvirile. This, in view of the fact that population in China is constantly pressing on means of sustenance, may not be thought greatly deplorable, but when it is considered that the progeny of the opium drunkard who has not reached the last stage of decline are indubitably degenerate and inheritors of a propensity to indulge in the emasculating habit, the magnitude of the evil defies the computations of the statistician and eludes the ken of the political economist.*

As the materia medica of China has merited and received attention from foreigners, so their materia alimentaria is worth investigating. Culinary and dietary regulations abound. Particular attention, for example, is called to the importance of selecting edibles for the same meal that are not incompatible; articles which when taken separately are wholesome become noxious when in combination, so much so that such are classed among poisons. The most noted of these is a-mixture of honey and onions. In some provinces they are employed for suicide, and cases are frequently reported of deaths from that cause. The great physician SUN SZEMIAO (early 7th century canonised) is quoted in the *Pêntsao* as stating that raw onions and honey induce purging, and that honey and cooked onions cause death. Doubtless the two combined are so indigestible that, sustained by high medical authorities, they are popularly regarded as poisonous. In like manner honey and Chinese dates (*Zizyphus jujuba*) are interdicted. So also eel and sugar-cane. A death at Shanghai was lately reported from eating crab and persimmons.

In various parts of the Empire and for several years I have sought information on colour-blindness, interrogating painters, dyers and others likely to become acquainted with that visual defect, without finding evidence of its existence. Lately, through the courtesy of Mr. DOUTHWAITE, I obtained the services of his hospital native assistant in subjecting to examination above 1,000 applicants for relief at that institution. The result of the examination, and that which I myself made among the crews of gun-boats,† failed to afford evidence of the existence of Daltonism.‡ The rarity, if not absence, in China of that defect of vision, or rather of the sensorium, and the absence of evidence of its existence except among Europeans and Americans, is suggestive of inquiry if this chromatopseudopsis is not an ethnic characteristic. The examinations instituted in India among candidates for employment on railways were probably restricted to Eurasians, and the cases there discovered may not have been those of natives. Nubians, it has been lately ascertained, are free of the defect.

* The impartial chronicler of opium discussions in China will not overlook the fact that the cultivation of opium in the country is favoured by writers of note. In November last the semi-official *Hsin Pau* had a cleverly-written article defending the culture and use of opium on economic grounds.

† Captain FARROW, of the Customs cruiser *Ling Fêng*, and several commanders of Chinese Imperial gun-boats, kindly allowed me to subject their men to examination.

‡ The irides of those examined were generally dark hazel, the others black—colours prevalent in China.

It having been demonstrated that from 5 to 7 per cent.* of Americans and Europeans are at fault in distinguishing between colours, red and green for example (signal colours), it is presumable that among the hundred or more pilots of the China coast there are several who are thus disqualified from following that vocation, and it would only be in accordance with recent legislation in the West if that most useful class of our fellow-residents were subjected to the usual tests for colour-blindness. At Baltimore recently a pilot who had served 25 years without a collision had his license withdrawn because he was unable to distinguish green from red; which shows that the defect may long exist without mischievous results, and the importance which marine authorities attach to the not too common faculty of discriminating colours aright; at the same time it must be admitted that the Baltimore case seems confirmatory of the opinion of Mr. POLE,† who himself has the defect of "dichromic vision," that there is no more danger of colour-blind engine-drivers or pilots mistaking red for green signals than are those of normal vision, no train or ship collision having thus far been traced to that defect.

Vaccination is making considerable progress in many provinces. Physicians in large cities who make a speciality of infantile diseases often include vaccination in their practice, but the new art is chiefly followed by persons who make it their sole occupation. Unfortunately, the extension of this great improvement cannot be viewed with unmixed satisfaction. It is to be feared that ignorance or dishonesty on the part of vaccinators may delude whole communities by spurious operations, the baneful consequences of which will become apparent when a small-pox epidemic of unusual virulence appears, that disease presenting various phases of violence, from a mild to a terribly malignant form. A reaction may then be looked for which will dispel confidence in the prophylactic,—a danger which will menace society until magistrates interdict the practice of inoculation to all persons not duly qualified and licensed. I am informed by Mr. DOUTHWAITE that at Kinhua vaccination has been taken up by the Buddhist priesthood, their temples having recently become the resort of mothers carrying their infants there for the operation, having implicit confidence in sacerdotal intercession with the gods for success; and as the fraternity surround the act with mystery and imposing ceremonies, they are likely to monopolise the new vocation. In like manner, secular practitioners of vaccination have been induced to resort to various devices to impress parents with the supernatural character of the rite, directing them to make pilgrimages to certain shrines, and the like, during the period of incubation. A native Christian vaccinator who would not thus deceive the people has lost all his practice, and obliged to adopt another calling.

Vaccination will not speedily supersede inoculation, which, since its introduction from Thibet (A.D. 1023-1055), has served to mitigate the violence of small-pox, which was introduced, as I formerly showed, in the 1st century from the then foreign region of Hupeh by the army of the renowned hero MA YÜAN.

* Dr. WILSON found among 1,154 men (about the number examined here), 17.7 per cent. to be colour-blind.

† "Daltonism," by WILLIAM POLE, F.R.S., *Contemporary Review*, May 1880.

Two writers in *Nature*, both having for their theme "Skin-furrows on the Hand," solicit information on the subject from China.* As the subject is considered to have a bearing on medical jurisprudence and ethnology as well, this Report is a suitable vehicle for responding to the demand.

Dr. FAULDS' observations on the finger-tips of the Japanese have an ethnic bearing and relate to the subject of heredity. Mr. HERSCHEL considers the subject as an agent of Government, he having charge for 20 years of registration offices in India, where he employed finger marks as sign manuals, the object being to prevent personation and repudiation. DOOLITTLE, in his *Social Life of the Chinese*, describes the custom. I cannot now refer to native works where the practice of employing digital rugæ as a sign manual is alluded to. I doubt if its employment in the courts is of ancient date. Well-informed natives think that it came into vogue subsequent to the HAN period; if so, it is in Egypt that earliest evidence of the practice is to be found. Just as the Chinese courts now require criminals to sign confessions by impressing thereto the whorls of their thumb-tips—the right thumb in the case of women, the left in the case of men,—so the ancient Egyptians, it is represented, required confessions to be sealed with their thumb-nails,—most likely the tip of the digit, as in China. Great importance is attached in the courts to this digital form of signature, "finger form" (指 模). Without a confession no criminal can be legally executed, and the confession to be valid must be attested by the thumb-print of the prisoner. No direct coercion is employed to secure this; a contumacious culprit may, however, be tortured until he performs the act which is a pre-requisite to his execution. Digital signatures are sometimes required in the army to prevent personation; the general in command at Wênchow enforces it on all his troops. A document thus attested can no more be forged or repudiated than a photograph,—not so easily, for while the period of half a lifetime effects great changes in the physiognomy, the rugæ of the fingers present the same appearance from the cradle to the grave; time writes no wrinkles there. In the army everywhere, when the description of a person is written down, the relative number of volutes and coniferous finger-tips is noted. It is called taking the "whelk striæ," the fusiform being called "rice baskets," and the volutes "peck measures" (螺 紋 箕 斗). A person unable to write, the form of signature which defies personation or repudiation is required in certain domestic cases, as in the sale of children or women. Often when a child is sold the parents affix their finger marks to the bill of sale; when a husband puts away his wife, giving her a bill of divorce, he marks the document with his entire palm; and when a wife is sold, the purchaser requires the seller to stamp the paper with hands and feet, the four organs duly smeared with ink. Professional fortune-tellers in China take into account almost the entire system of the person whose future they attempt to forecast, and of course they include palmistry, but the rugæ of the finger-ends do not receive much attention. Amateur fortune-tellers, however, discourse as glibly on them as phrenologists do of "bumps"—it is so easy. In children the relative number of volute and conical striæ indicate their future; "if there are nine volutes," says a proverb, "to one conical, the boy will attain distinction without toil."

* HENRY FAULDS, Tsukiyi Hospital, Tokio, Japan. W. J. HERSCHEL, Oxford, England.—*Nature*, 28th October and 25th November 1880.

Regarded from an ethnological point of view, I can discover merely that the rugæ of Chinamen's fingers differ from Europeans', but there is so little uniformity observable that they form no basis for distinction, and while the striæ may be noteworthy points in certain medico-legal questions, heredity is not one of them.

It is matter of regret that quinine, the anti-malarial value of which the Chinese fully appreciate, should, owing to its cost, be unobtainable by the masses; it is a national evil and merits attention on the part of the Imperial authorities, who might, there is good reason to believe, do much towards its mitigation. From the result of experiments made by the Dutch in Java and by the English in India in acclimatising cinchona trees, there is sufficient encouragement to attempt their introduction into Yünnan and other southern portions of the Empire. An additional inducement is afforded by the fact that in India cinchona plantations have already become a source of revenue, the trees being found so rich in alkaloids that some plantations have yielded $8,000 per acre. But for the successful acclimatisation of cinchona trees in those countries, the world would soon suffer from a quinine famine, as the cinchona forests of South America are in the course of rapid destruction. At the same time it is extremely desirable that the Imperial Government or the Governor-General of the southern provinces should be moved to introduce eucalyptus trees extensively, the prophylactic of malarial fever, which is so injurious to the best interests of the State. Private enterprise has accomplished something in acclimatising and cultivating eucalyptus, but the aid of Government must be invoked and obtained before that invaluable tree casts its protecting shade over the countless hamlets of fever-haunted regions where lurks the subtle foe of their inmates. The most successful of the attempts that have been made in that direction were with seeds kindly provided by Dr. ABBOTT of the Hobart Town Botanic Garden, to whom I applied for those of trees that flourished in the highest southern latitude and at the highest elevation, as most likely to endure the cold of a Shanghai or Ningpo winter. Although the various species that I experimented with failed in those ports, the plants rarely thriving beyond the third year, yet further south the result has been all that can be desired. It is true that recent observations are unconfirmatory of the anti-miasmatic properties of this exotic in Algeria and California, but if its prophylactic virtues have been exaggerated, there can be no doubt that its extensive culture would be advantageous because of the peculiar value of its wood.* A minister like TSO TSUNGTANG, whose recent work of tree-planting in Kansuh is unequalled by any like feat in history, requires no solicitation to favour such an undertaking as the acclimatisation of useful plants.

Now that the Imperial Government favours the study by its youth of foreign science, it is not premature to lodge a plea in behalf of a scientific pursuit which is practically interdicted; that is, dissection of the human frame. In presenting the subject, it can be shown that neither army nor navy can be effective without a corps of duly qualified surgeons, and that anatomical knowledge is the first thing to be imparted to that branch of the military art, and that such knowledge is to be acquired by dissections alone. By presenting the subject

---

* I prepared an account of the eucalyptus, which was published in Mr. FRYER's Chinese magazine, 格致彙編, in 1879, which induced ex-Minister KUO to apply to me for seeds, which have thus far proved a success in southern Hunan.

discreetly, the prejudices which prevail may soon be overcome. With conservatives like the Chinese, precedent goes very far, and it might not be amiss to remind them how the Emperor HSIAO WU delivered up certain prisoners for a sort of vivisection, from which an inference may be drawn in favour of the delivery for dissection of the bodies of executed criminals. In the year 459 there appeared at the court of that monarch an embassy from the Yüeh-pan (悅般國), a tribe of Huns, whose southern boundary was the volcanic portion of the Tien Shan range. In the train was a magician who professed to be able to sever a man's throat and vessels, and come so near decapitating him that his head would fall back, and though basinfuls of blood flowed, the administration of a drug would arrest the hæmorrhage and cause the wound to heal without a scar! Moved by curiosity, if not by a desire to promote physiological knowledge, His Majesty ordered the experiment to be tried on prisoners. The operation was perfectly successful, and restoration completed in a month. HSIAO WU liberally rewarded the magician, and directed the study of the art. It was remarked that the herb by which the cure was effected was to be found on certain famous hills in China.*

Coming down to a later period, we are told of a Governor ordering the evisceration of 40 criminals and *enceinte* women and children for anatomical purposes, causing examination of the viscera to be made by skilful physicians.† It may be fairly argued that if an Emperor of good repute committed prisoners to what he must have regarded as vivisection, and if a Governor ordered with impunity such cruelties on the living, surely a magistrate may consign the cadavers of the decapitated to anatomists for dissection, a course which, if discreetly done, will occasion no popular ferment, considering how eager the people of this city were the other day to witness the cutting out, by the public executioner, of the heart of a living malefactor: the thousands who witnessed the flagitious act were envied by the rest of the population who were debarred the spectacle. An additional inducement for the utilisation of persons capitally executed is afforded by the fact that it would probably serve as a deterrent to crime, owing to the dread of postmortem mutilation which is generally entertained by all classes of the Chinese. Evidence in support of the utility of postmortem examinations is furnished by the highest medical authority that the Chinese acknowledge, the *Pêntsao*, which narrates the case of a man of rank, who, as well as his slave, suffered from abdominal pains. The slave succumbed to the malady, and the master, opening the body, discovered a red-eyed white turtle, on which he tried the effect of various medicines, none of which killed the animal; by accident, however, it was discovered to be soluble in horse urine, from which he inferred that that article, hitherto unknown as a medicine, would dissolve the tumour that occasioned him so much pain; he tried it and was cured. Since that time equine urine has held a high place in the pharmacopœia for treatment of visceral tumefactions and various other disorders. Its virtues as a medicine might never have become known but for the autopsy in question.

* 太平寰宇記 (A.D. 976–983), book 186. In the Imperial Catalogue this celebrated work on topography is stated to consist of 193 books, which is one less than the actual number. Among my notes from this work, I find the following in relation to the Yüehpan: "Before each of their three daily meals they perform ablutions and gargle." Such an un-Mongolian custom is noteworthy.

† *Mémoires concernant l'Histoire, etc.*, tome viii, p. 261.

7

By adducing facts like these we may gradually reconcile the Chinese to the proposed innovation.

Supplementary Meteorological Note, January 1882.—The year just closed was remarkable for the extraordinary number of typhoons which devastated the China Sea, not less than 20 having been recorded, the last of the series occurring as late as the month of December. Allowing that certain cyclones were counted twice, it must be conceded nevertheless that the season in this respect was unprecedented. It may be remarked also that the fogs which regularly prevail in the latter part of April were denser, more protracted and wider spread than usual. The expression of COLUMBUS with regard to fogs which he encountered off Cape Verd, "that they might be cut with a knife," was peculiarly applicable to those of last spring on this coast and the Yangtze. Besides, the barometrical reading during December was remarkably high, in many places unprecedentedly so. At Wênchow, which is on the isobaric line, 30.02, the aneroid indicated a pressure of 31.20. It differs from the standard barometer of the Shanghai Customs. Coincident with the exceptional season has been, according to the *Sheng Pau*, an unusual number of epidemics in Kiangsu and northern Chêhkiang—autumnal diseases being rife, children chiefly suffering, while about the beginning of December puerperal fever raged in Soochow. Many cases were incurable, and within 10 days several tens of recently delivered women succumbed to the prevailing epidemic.

China, Imperial Maritime Customs, Medical Reports
(1881. 10. 01—1882. 09. 30)

CHINA.

IMPERIAL MARITIME CUSTOMS.

II.—SPECIAL SERIES: No. 2.

MEDICAL REPORTS,

FOR THE HALF-YEAR ENDED 30TH SEPTEMBER 1882.

24th Issue.

PUBLISHED BY ORDER OF

The Inspector General of Customs.

SHANGHAI:
STATISTICAL DEPARTMENT
OF THE
INSPECTORATE GENERAL.
MDCCCLXXXIII.

INSPECTORATE GENERAL OF CUSTOMS,

PEKING, 31st *December* 1870.

SIR,

1.—IT has been suggested to me that it would be well to take advantage of the circumstances in which the Customs Establishment is placed, to procure information with regard to disease amongst foreigners and natives in China; and I have, in consequence, come to the resolution of publishing half-yearly in collected form all that may be obtainable. If carried out to the extent hoped for, the scheme may prove highly useful to the medical profession both in China and at home, and to the public generally. I therefore look with confidence to the co-operation of the Customs Medical Officer at your port, and rely on his assisting me in this matter by framing a half-yearly report containing the result of his observations at.................upon the local peculiarities of disease, and upon diseases rarely or never encountered out of China. The facts brought forward and the opinions expressed will be arranged and published either with or without the name of the physician responsible for them, just as he may desire.

2.—The suggestions of the Customs Medical Officers at the various ports as to the points which it would be well to have especially elucidated, will be of great value in the framing of a form which will save trouble to those members of the medical profession, whether connected with the Customs or not, who will join in carrying out the plan proposed. Meanwhile I would particularly invite attention to—

a.—The general health of....................during the period reported on; the death rate amongst foreigners; and, as far as possible, a classification of the causes of death.

b.—Diseases prevalent at............................

c.—General type of disease; peculiarities and complications encountered; special treatment demanded.

d.—Relation of disease to $\begin{cases} \text{Season.} \\ \text{Alteration in local conditions—such as drainage, &c.} \\ \text{Alteration in climatic conditions.} \end{cases}$

e.—Peculiar diseases; especially leprosy.

f.—Epidemics $\begin{cases} \text{Absence or presence.} \\ \text{Causes.} \\ \text{Course and treatment.} \\ \text{Fatality.} \end{cases}$

Other points, of a general or special kind, will naturally suggest themselves to medical men; what I have above called attention to will serve to fix the general scope of the undertaking. I have committed to Dr. ALEX. JAMIESON, of Shanghai, the charge of arranging the Reports for publication, so that they may be made available in a convenient form.

3.—Considering the number of places at which the Customs Inspectorate has established offices, the thousands of miles north and south and east and west over which these offices are scattered, the varieties of climate, and the peculiar conditions to which, under such different circumstances, life and health are subjected, I believe the Inspectorate, aided by its Medical Officers, can do good service in the general interest in the direction indicated; and, as already stated, I rely with confidence on the support and assistance of the Medical Officer at each port in the furtherance and perfecting of this scheme. You will hand a copy of this Circular to Dr. ...., and request him, in my name, to hand to you in future, for transmission to myself, half-yearly Reports of the kind required, for the half-years ending 31st March and 30th September—that is, for the Winter and Summer seasons.

4.—   *   *   *   *   *

I am, &c.,

(signed)   ROBERT HART,
I. G.

THE COMMISSIONERS OF CUSTOMS,—*Newchwang,*   *Ningpo,*
Tientsin,   *Foochow,*
Chefoo,   *Tamsui,*
Hankow,   *Takow,*
Kiukiang,   *Amoy,*
Chinkiang,   *Swatow,* and
Shanghai,   *Canton.*

SHANGHAI, *1st May 1883*.

SIR,

IN accordance with the directions of your Despatch No. 6 A (Returns Series) of the 24th June 1871, I now forward to the Statistical Department of the Inspectorate General of Customs, the following documents :—

Report on the Health of Newchwang for the eighteen months ended 30th September 1882, pp. 1, 2.

Report on the Health of Chefoo, pp. 3–6 ;

Report on the Health of Wênchow, pp. 18–21 ; each of these referring to the year ended 30th September 1882.

Report on the Health of Ichang, pp. 7–11 ;

Report on the Health of Kiukiang, pp. 12–16 ;

Report on the Health of Ningpo, p. 17 ;

Report on the Health of Amoy, pp. 22–24 ;

Report on the Health of Canton, pp. 25, 26 ;

Report on the Health of Pakhoi, pp. 27–30 ;

Report on the Health of Shanghai, pp. 39–46 ; each of these referring to the half-year ended 30th September 1882.

Notes on an Epidemic Disease observed at Pakhoi in 1882, pp. 31–38.

I have the honour to be,

SIR,

Your obedient Servant,

R. ALEX. JAMIESON.

THE INSPECTOR GENERAL OF CUSTOMS,
PEKING.

The Contributors to this Volume are :—

J. WATSON, M.D., L.R.C.S.Ed. ....,..............................…..... Newchwang.

J. G. BRERETON, L.K.&Q.C.P., L.R.C.S.I. ....…..... Chefoo.

A. HENRY, M.A., L.R.C.P.Ed., L.R.C.S.Ed. .... Ichang.

G. R. UNDERWOOD, M.B., CH.M. .... Kiukiang.

W. A. HENDERSON, L.R.C.P.Ed., L.R.C.S.Ed......................... Ningpo.

D. J. MACGOWAN, M.D. .... Wênchow.

B. S. RINGER, M.R.C.S., L.S.A. .... Amoy.

J. F. WALES, B.A., M.D., CH.M. .... Canton.

J. H. LOWRY, L.R.C.P.Ed., L.R.C.S.Ed. .... Pakhoi.

R. A. JAMIESON, M.A., M.D., M.R.C.S. .... Shanghai.

Dr. D. J. Macgowan's Report on the Health of Wênchow for the Year ended 30th September 1882.

During the past year the few foreigners who reside at Wênchow enjoyed exemption from disease, but the general public health suffered interruption, owing to an exceptionally protracted rainy season, febrile and choleraic maladies prevailing more than usual, the poor being the chief sufferers, who, beside being badly housed, suffered from the enhanced price of rice, which the rains caused by injuring the crop. It is to be feared that the latter half of the year will not prove more favourable in a sanitary point of view. Unfortunately, opportunity for investigation of disease no longer exists at this port, owing to the removal of the Inland Mission Hospital, under Mr. Douthwaite, to Chefoo.

The rains, to which this impairment of the ordinary health of this region is due, commenced earlier, continued longer, and were more copious than usual,—occasioning disastrous floods throughout the catchment of the northern portion of the Nanshan range, causing destruction in the south-western portion of this province, as well as of Southern Kiangsi and Anhwei, and inundations of the Poyang Lake and Lower Yangtze. The occurrence is too recent to ascertain how far these disasters have proved causes of disease.

CHINESE EPIDEMIOLOGICAL NOTES.

Prominence is given to the subject of epidemics in the instructions conveyed in the Circular of the Inspector General inaugurating these Reports, investigations of which call for extensive surveys; a report on the health of any one port may therefore, I assume, include reference to diseases that are found prevailing through the Empire at large.

Information respecting epidemics in the interior is supplied by correspondents of Chinese newspapers; these form the main source of the facts herein submitted: it is therefore meagre, but not an unacceptable contribution to climatal and epidemiological science.

These Chinese medical notices take cognizance, it will be observed, of meteorological and telluric influences as causes of disease, the exceptionally abnormal character of the weather during the summer of 1881, and the following autumn and winter, furnishing apt illustrations. The abnormalities consisted in a series of typhoons, of which there were a score, some of them extending late into the autumn. Then followed an " open winter," which was coincident with a like condition of weather which prevailed over the northern portion of the Europeo-Asiatic continent; at least, the winter was noted in North-eastern Europe as an unprecedentedly mild one. In Northern China, rivers and harbours experienced the ice blockade later, and the thaw occurred earlier, than usual. At the same time, barometric readings, which are always high in China during the winter, indicated a pressure greater than had yet been observed. Only statistical information can determine what effect those abnormal meteorological conditions had on the public health; and in the absence of vital statistics, we may make some use of the consensus of "folk lore." This much is clearly discoverable, that while the atmospheric conditions affected an extensive area, there were no widespread epidemics corresponding to the cyclonic and anti-cyclonic phases that prevailed, those that are reported being local and sporadic.

I append all that has found its way into Chinese newspapers on the public health during the two semi-annual periods under review, divided into the four seasons,—a plan that accords with Chinese usage, which regards certain types of disease as more or less prevalent at certain periods of the year; for example, in spring, (疫) infectious and contagious maladies prevail, as typhus and small-pox; in summer, (痧) spasmodic cholera; in autumn, (痢) diarrhœa and ague; and in winter, (瘟) non-malignant fever.

OCTOBER, NOVEMBER, and DECEMBER 1881.

NANKING (the ancient capital, situated on the right bank of the Yangtze river).—Referring to the early autumn, the reporter notes numerous sunstrokes due to untimely heat. Showers that fell on the 20th September brought down the temperature, but it soon rose again, so that perspiration, even at rest, was excessive, and sleep unobtainable by night,—a state of things which was followed by a virulent form of cholera, from which children suffered most.

In the autumn there was a remarkable mortality among field rats at Nanking. It was first observed on the opposite side of the Yangtze, soon after in the western suburbs of the ancient capital. The animals emerged from holes in dwellings, jumped up, turned round, and fell dead. Baskets and boxes filled with their bodies were cast into the canal. Their colour was darker and their tails were shorter than the common rat. Here was evidently a subsoil poison, which affected the animals precisely in the same way as the malaria of the Yünnan pest (which extended to higher animals and to man). Happily, the subterranean miasm at Nanking did not affect animals that live above ground, nor did subterranean animals communicate the disease in any way.

SOOCHOW (in a lacustrine region, situated south of the Yangtze, on the Grand Canal,—the centre of silk culture; one of the most populous and fertile portions of the globe).—During the preceding summer, owing to alternations of cold winds and excessive heat, agues and bowel complaints raged with violence, children being the chief sufferers. It was given out that the God of Pestilence had descended, and people, discarding doctors and drugs, crowded the temples, entirely neglecting treatment.

The ill-health of summer extended into autumn; diseases prevailed beyond the capacity of doctors to give due attendance on the sick,—the cause of the maladies being untimely cold winds, with inter-missions of extreme heat. Ague and diarrhœa were most prevalent and were very fatal, especially among children over 10 years of age, many of whom died the day they were attacked. In some cases whole households were prostrate at the same time.

YANGCHOW (north of the Yangtze, on the Grand Canal; topographical features like the latter region).—After the summer the heat became more intense, and numerous fatal cases of cholera occurred, but two out of 10 proving curable. At the same time a murrain prevailed among cattle, horses, pigs, and dogs. Similar accounts, except that relative to murrain, came from Ningpo and Hangchow; as Shanghai also suffered, it is probable that disease was unusually rife throughout the coasts of Northern Chêkiang and Kiangsu.

HANKOW, 22nd November.—Since October the weather has been preternaturally warm, summer clothing being in request, and mosquitos abounding; consequent on this unseasonable heat, there has been much sickness, but not of a fatal character. There was much mortality among hens; they were suddenly seized with fits, expiring at once.

JANUARY, FEBRUARY, and MARCH 1882.

HANGCHOW (on the Ch'ient'ang river, at the head of a great estuary, where commences the Grand Canal).—It was reported early in February that the winter weather had been characterised by fluctuations of heat and cold, which caused a large amount of inflammatory disease among children, who fell victims to throat maladies, for which there was no remedy, the disorder proving fatal in a few hours (diphtheria?); and at the time of writing, small-pox existed, children being attacked notwithstanding every precaution was taken to keep them in-doors, and by strict dieting. Besides, inoculated persons, between the age of 40 and 50 years, were confined to bed, their faces being covered with pustules; those cases, though severe, were not fatal, recovering in the course of seven days. Doctors said it was due to suppressed wind in the system, and to unseasonable weather,—sudden alternations of heat and cold,—and belonged to the variolous class of disorders : a "water pox" (varicella?). Its existence augurs well for a healthy spring.

SOOCHOW.—It was thought that as the summer and autumn were unhealthy, winter would bring an improvement, but intractable diseases still prevail, and now puerperal fever exists, not one in 10 recovering; it has been found incurable. Within a few days several tens have succumbed. Another account states that typhoid fever raged to such an extent, particularly among women, as to cause an increase in the price of woven fabrics.

YANGCHOW.—The warmth of last winter indicated, with its snow and rain, a fruitful year, but the cold, or negative principle of nature, being unable to cope with the positive or warm principle, disease became rife, particularly of the throat, among young children, who died a few hours after being attacked,—an utterly inexplicable circumstance.

APRIL, MAY, and JUNE 1882.

NANKING.—A mild winter and paucity of rain caused an unhealthy spring; the ordinary maladies of the season show a disposition to assume a chronic form, being cured with difficulty.

NANCHANG (on the southern shore of Poyang Lake), May.—The very changeable weather during the past season—unseasonable rain and sunshine, heat and cold alternately prevailing, followed by a furious storm, brought a degree of cold that caused extensive sickness, although not of a fatal character, yet it was cured with difficulty. The disorder resembled ague, but ague it was not; one day the patient would be better, and the next day worse,—a somewhat peculiar malady, and one to be guarded against. This region has also suffered from a pig murrain. Those who ate the flesh were attacked with boils.

CANTON, 10th May.—This province has suffered from want of rain, causing a loss of half the crops in some districts. There was much sickness, children being the chief sufferers. A rainfall abated the evil.

JULY, AUGUST, and SEPTEMBER 1882.

YANGCHOW.—In July this city and the adjacent region were revisited by cholera. In the year before, 40,000 fell victims, and now the epidemic is raging with greater violence than at that time. On that occasion the disease came from the north and went south. This year its course has been reversed; it approached from the south, travelled northward; the choleraic wave reached Tientsin and Peking in a mild form. A month later this unfortunate region was visited by three types of disease. The first chiefly affected men; it was caused by cold wind suppressing the summer's heat, inducing fever, which became irregular, some cases experiencing a change between the seventh and tenth days, when the heat gradually subsided, and the patients recovered; others, changing between the third and fifth days, presented petechiæ over the entire body, and succumbed. The second form of the epidemic appeared chiefly in women, who first suffered from chills, followed by fever, which did not subside; it was attended with a dry mouth. Cooling remedies were of no avail. Only two or three out of 10 survived. Thirdly, children suffered from fever, followed by cold, while the whole face broke out into blotches, as in measles; when the eruption came out distinctly the patient took a favourable turn, otherwise the disease changed to a throat-locking malady, and terminated fatally.

CANTON, 1st August.—An epidemic has suddenly appeared in this city which makes its first attack by an excessive thirst and profuse perspiration, afterwards there is a flow of saliva, then the tongue retracts, and the patient dies of suffocation. Doctors direct that in such cases heated lard should be dropped on the tongue, to restore it to position.

HANKOW (on the left bank of the Yangtze, at the embogue of the Han river).—Native doctors report the existence of diarrhœa in the autumn, which when not treated at its commencement becomes intractable. Agues were uncommonly frequent at the same time, and in the cases of the crews of junks that had conveyed rice to Shantung in the spring, it was often fatal. These men returned from their voyage with diarrhœa, the water and food of Shantung not agreeing with them, and hence the ague proved too much for them.

SOOCHOW.—This city also suffered from a virulent form of cholera. It was preceded by agues and diarrhœas; these last assumed a chronic form.

NINGPO.—At the close of summer there was a cattle murrain at Ningpo, in consequence of the heat; it extended to horses, dogs and goats. An epidemic affecting domestic animals generally, such as this, is an unusual occurrence. Cows and buffaloes died after having two or three watery stools, their illness being of a few hours duration. The year 1878 was remarkable for the virulence of this disease, exceeding what living men had before known,—80 per cent. of the cattle perishing. It was not a new disease, but one well known, only appearing at that time with greater intensity. Since then the disease has appeared each autumn.

The mountains to the south of Ningpo, in Fêng-hua and T'ai-chou, appear to be the habitat of a microbe *(Bacillus anthracis?)*, the organism of the splenic disease in cattle, from which that region is seldom free. The equine disease that prevailed simultaneously was probably glanders; ponies at Shanghai suffered from that malady about the same time. Concerning the canine epidemic, information is yet more meagre. The animals were suddenly seized with tremors, and speedily died, somewhat as dogs in China are known to perish when their hearts become clogged with filaria. Ningpo seems to suffer from an undue proportion of rabies; no year passes without the occurrence of several fatal cases of hydrophobia.

NORTHERN FORMOSA.—A detachment of troops from Hunan posted in Northern Formosa all suffered from fever; the type is not reported, only that it was of a fatal character. It has been found that men from the interior of China are less easily acclimatised than those from the adjacent coast. Excessive rains at this period, and the employment of the soldiers as road-makers, contributed to render them more susceptible to disease; and the absence of suitable medical attendance served to increase the disaster.

China, Imperial Maritime Customs, Medical Reports
（1883. 04. 01—1883. 09. 30）

CHINA.

IMPERIAL MARITIME CUSTOMS.

II.—SPECIAL SERIES: No. 2.

MEDICAL REPORTS,

FOR THE HALF-YEAR ENDED 30TH SEPTEMBER 1883.

26th Issue.

PUBLISHED BY ORDER OF

The Inspector General of Customs.

SHANGHAI:
STATISTICAL DEPARTMENT
OF THE
INSPECTORATE GENERAL.

MDCCCLXXXIV.

INSPECTOR GENERAL'S CIRCULAR No. 19 OF 1870.

INSPECTORATE GENERAL OF CUSTOMS,

PEKING, 31st December 1870.

SIR,

1.—IT has been suggested to me that it would be well to take advantage of the circumstances in which the Customs Establishment is placed, to procure information with regard to disease amongst foreigners and natives in China; and I have, in consequence, come to the resolution of publishing half-yearly in collected form all that may be obtainable. If carried out to the extent hoped for, the scheme may prove highly useful to the medical profession both in China and at home, and to the public generally. I therefore look with confidence to the co-operation of the Customs Medical Officer at your port, and rely on his assisting me in this matter by framing a half-yearly report containing the result of his observations at..................upon the local peculiarities of disease, and upon diseases rarely or never encountered out of China. The facts brought forward and the opinions expressed will be arranged and published either with or without the name of the physician responsible for them, just as he may desire.

2.—The suggestions of the Customs Medical Officers at the various ports as to the points which it would be well to have especially elucidated, will be of great value in the framing of a form which will save trouble to those members of the medical profession, whether connected with the Customs or not, who will join in carrying out the plan proposed. Meanwhile I would particularly invite attention to—

a.—The general health of....................during the period reported on; the death rate amongst foreigners; and, as far as possible, a classification of the causes of death.

b.—Diseases prevalent at...........................

c.—General type of disease; peculiarities and complications encountered; special treatment demanded.

d.—Relation of disease to
$\begin{cases} \text{Season.} \\ \text{Alteration in local conditions—such as drainage, etc.} \\ \text{Alteration in climatic conditions.} \end{cases}$

e.—Peculiar diseases; especially leprosy.

f.—Epidemics
$\begin{cases} \text{Absence or presence.} \\ \text{Causes.} \\ \text{Course and treatment.} \\ \text{Fatality.} \end{cases}$

Other points, of a general or special kind, will naturally suggest themselves to medical men; what I have above called attention to will serve to fix the general scope of the undertaking. I have committed to Dr. ALEX. JAMIESON, of Shanghai, the charge of arranging the Reports for publication, so that they may be made available in a convenient form.

3.—Considering the number of places at which the Customs Inspectorate has established offices, the thousands of miles north and south and east and west over which these offices are scattered, the varieties of climate, and the peculiar conditions to which, under such different circumstances, life and health are subjected, I believe the Inspectorate, aided by its Medical Officers, can do good service in the general interest in the direction indicated; and, as already stated, I rely with confidence on the support and assistance of the Medical Officer at each port in the furtherance and perfecting of this scheme. You will hand a copy of this Circular to Dr. ...., and request him, in my name, to hand to you in future, for transmission to myself, half-yearly Reports of the kind required, for the half-years ending 31st March and 30th September—that is, for the Winter and Summer seasons.

4.—   *   *   *   *   *

I am, etc.,

(Signed)   ROBERT HART,
I. G.

THE COMMISSIONERS OF CUSTOMS,—*Newchwang, Ningpo,*
                              Tientsin, Foochow,
                              Chefoo, Tamsui,
                              Hankow, Takow,
                              Kiukiang, Amoy,
                              Chinkiang, Swatow, and
                              Shanghai, Canton.

SHANGHAI, *26th December 1883.*

SIR,

      IN accordance with the directions of your Despatch No. 6 *A* (Returns Series) of the 24th June 1871, I now forward to the Statistical Department of the Inspectorate General of Customs, the following documents:—

    Report on the Health of Shanghai, pp. 1–24;

    Report on the Health of Pakhoi, pp. 35–38;

    Report on the Health of Foochow, pp. 39–43;

    Report on the Health of Ichang, pp. 44–48;

    Report on the Health of Amoy, p. 49;

    Report on the Health of Wênchow, pp. 64–72;

    Report on the Health of Ningpo, p. 73; each of these referring to the half-year ended
        30th September 1883.

    Report on the Health of Kiukiang, pp. 25–30;

    Report on the Health of Chefoo, pp. 31–33; each of these referring to the year ended
        30th September 1883.

    Special articles on—

        The Fevers of Chefoo, p. 34.

        The Operative Treatment of Hepatitis and Hepatic Abscess, pp. 50–63.

    An Appendix giving a translation of a contribution to the history of Syphilis, pp. 74–76.

I have the honour to be,

SIR,

Your obedient Servant,

R. ALEX. JAMIESON.

THE INSPECTOR GENERAL OF CUSTOMS,
    PEKING.

The Contributors to this Volume are:—

R. A. JAMIESON, M.A., M.D., M.R.C.S. .... Shanghai.

G. R. UNDERWOOD, M.B., CH.M. .... Kiukiang.

J. G. BRERETON, L.K.&Q.C.P., L.R.C.S.I. .... Chefoo.

W. L. PRUEN, L.R.C.P.Ed., L.R.C.S.Ed .... „

J. H. LOWRY, L.R.C.P.Ed., L.R.C.S.Ed .... Pakhoi.

T. RENNIE, M.D., CH.M. .... Foochow.

A. HENRY, M.A., L.R.C.P.Ed., L.R.C.S.Ed .... Ichang.

P. MANSON, M.D., CH.M. .... Amoy.

D. J. MACGOWAN, M.D. .... Wênchow.

W. A. HENDERSON, L.R.C.P.Ed., L.R.C.S.Ed. .... Ningpo.

Dr. D. J. Macgowan's Report on the Health of Wĕnchow for the Half-year ended 30th September 1883.

It is remarkable that although this port has repeatedly suffered from Indian cholera since the first invasion of China by that disease, it this season entirely escaped, up to the end of the period under review,* and that although the disease has prevailed elsewhere from Canton to Newchwang and from the seaboard to Ichang or further west. There would be nothing report-worthy but for the occurrence of a case of poisoning from the use of porpoise as food, and for opportunities that have presented of testing the value of musk, so much lauded by the Chinese as a therapeutic agent.

A member of the Customs staff, who for several years suffered from rheumatism, and had become well-nigh saturated in Formosa with potassium iodide, and cinchonised withal for malarial fever, was lately attacked by lumbago, and, after suffering 10 days, made application for treatment. He had been taking his medicine, and had abraded the entire lumbar region by turpentine frictions. For four nights the severity of the pain had prevented sleep. I applied the common Chinese musk plaster (which contains but a pinch of musk), adding to it 4 grains of that drug in a tolerable state of purity. In two hours the patient fell into a quiet sleep; in the morning the pain was barely perceptible, and in three days it wholly disappeared.

About the same time I treated a sprained ankle of a foreign resident in the same manner.

The application was made about 11 hours after the injury. There was extensive tumefaction and intolerable pain, such, in fact, as always attends severe accidents of that kind. Ten hours after the application the pain subsided so far that the patient fell asleep, and in the morning the joint was painful only on pressure. On the fifth day walking was partially resumed, and in a few days more the only trace of the injury was a stiffness of the joint, which continued much longer. The lividity from rupture of vessels lasted five weeks, indicating the severity of the lesion.

Chinese tell of severe cases cured in less time. This case would not have yielded to leeching, embrocation or other modes of treatment in one quarter of that period of cure.

Although musk has been long well known in the West, it seems worth while to translate what Chinese writers have to say about it. There are two sources of supply, the *Moschus moschiferus* (musk-deer), from the western provinces, and the *Viverra civetta*, or civet cat, common in Central China.

The musk-deer is found throughout the mountains of Yünnan, Szechwan and Thibet. It is a timid little animal, and often dies of fright. It feeds on juniper leaves and reptiles; snake bones are found in its stomach. In spring its glandular pouch is greatly swollen and inflamed. The secretion is discharged with the urine. Musk-deer always resort to the same

---

* A fortnight later cholera in a most virulent form appeared, and prevailed for several weeks, but not extensively.

place for urination, covering their urine with earth. In such places deposits of a superior quality are found, amounting sometimes to 15 catties.

A native traveller recently gave the following account of the animal :—

It is in the habit of throwing itself down on the ground in an exhausted state, in order to cool itself and to seek relief from the itching felt round the orifice of its glandular pouch. This emits a very rank odour, and thereby attracts numerous ants, which crawl in and feast upon the highly flavoured secretion. The animal shortly feels relieved by the scratching of the ants, closes the opening by a sort of sphincter, shuts up the ants, and makes off. This operation is repeated day after day, at the expense of the unwitting ants, during the life of the buck (for no musk is obtained from the doe), until a hard, india-rubber-like mass is formed in the distended pouch.

The article, however, which is most prized is that which falls from the musk-deer on the ground, and is gathered in grains that are precious as pearls. This is so pungent that if carried through a garden or woods it prevents fructification. The poisonous effect of fresh musk on vegetation is shown also by the blighted appearance of places which the musk-deer selects for its convenience. For some distance there is an absence of plants, and farther off, leaves exhibit a yellow tinge. Some plants are more susceptible to musk than others, the lichee fruit tree *(Nephelium litchi)* is particularly obnoxious to it. If brought too near the nose it causes inflammation, followed by the appearance of white worms in the nostrils.

It is recorded that a peculiar species, caught by a fisherman, was kept in the imperial garden (A.D. 742-55). Its pouch on being pricked emitted such a strong kind of musk that a single drop in over a gallon and a half of water rendered that fluid so odoriferous that garments sprinkled with it had an ineffaceable perfume. The incised wounds, which were made for obtaining the secretion, were healed by the application of arsenic bisulphide. It is directed that musk which is found in lumps mixed with the blood in the heart of animals that die from fright is not to be employed in medicine; that is, not to be administered internally. Hunters of the musk-deer using its flesh for food never suffer when bitten by the most virulent snakes. Snake-hunters—snakes are pursued because of their attacks on fruit trees—place a bit of musk under the nails of the big toes, which is an unfailing prophylactic.

This valuable substance no sooner leaves the hunter's hand than skilful manipulators adulterate the article for wholesale dealers, who adulterate it for the trade, when it is found to possess about 10 per cent of genuine musk. Fortunate, indeed, are those who obtain the drug having that degree of potency. A genuine musk-bag may be known from the hair internally. False bags are made of the abdominal skin of the musk-deer, and stuffed with the genitals of the civet cat and matters that are undistinguishable.

It is incompatible with alliaceous food; too long carried on the person it induces unusual forms of disease. It expels whatever is noxious in the system, including demoniacal influences; it is an anthelmintic, and cures the bites of venomous serpents; and is fatal to certain plants. Wind that has entered the bones (rheumatism) is expelled by it, but when wind gets between the skin and the flesh, musk, if taken, will drive it into the bones, and the pain is increased. When given for restoration from a swoon, it is to be discontinued as soon as the patient revives. It may be administered with advantage in indigestion from eating fruit. It is to be used when diffusible stimulants, not tonics, are indicated. It is given in fevers of every type, and in tedious parturition. Popularly, it is believed to possess great power as a fœticidal agent, being applied by perpetrators of that heinous crime to the umbilicus, potions of liquor being drunk at the same time. As a calmer of the spirits it is much employed; laid on the pillow it favours pleasant dreams and averts nightmare. It has the effect of ammonia when there is prostration of the vital powers. Externally, it is employed in piles, and is in universal use for plasters, the base of which is composed of wax and resin. They are thick and very adhesive. Druggists who charge their articles with a liberal quantity of the penetrating drug render their plasters highly popular. Shanghai plasters, for this cause mainly, are in general demand.

The analogue of the musk-deer in the secretion of odorous matter is the civet cat, which is found in the central and southern provinces, throughout the Nanshan range. The feline and vulpine appearance of this member of the *Viverridæ* gives it the name in Chinese of "mysterious cat," "fragrant fox," and "supernatural fox," which they describe as hermaphrodite. The pouch and genitals are removed for procuring the secretion, which, to the uninitiated, is palmed off as musk. In a notice of one of these animals obtained from China in 1683, M. POMET, in his history of drugs, states :—

Having kept this creature some days, I perceived that the walls and bars that enclosed it were covered with unctuous moisture, thick and very brown, of a very strong and disagreeable smell, so that during all the time that I kept this animal I took care to gather the civet out of the pouch every other day, and not without some trouble and hazard, because it put the creature to some pain or apprehension of it ; and having done so for months, I had the quantity of an ounce and a half; but it is certain that if the necessary care had been taken, and the beast could be hindered from rubbing itself, I might have got a great deal more.

The Chinese do not keep the animal for obtaining civet, but kill it, cut out the genitals, sprinkle them with liquor, and dry them in the shade.

Besides its use as a medicine, musk is largely consumed in perfumery. The total amount produced is approximatively discoverable from the Imperial Maritime Customs Returns, which for 10 years ending 1882 show exports amounting to 329.38½ piculs, valued at *Hk.Tls* 2,520,364. It will be perceived from the following table that Hankow is the chief mart, that port being nearest (except Ichang) to the source of supply. Tientsin musk is said to be a product of Chihli, but probably Shansi furnishes the greater part.

EXPORT of each PORT for TEN YEARS.

Shanghai	*Piculs*	$43.61\frac{3}{16}$	= *Hk.Tls*	375,527
Canton	,,	$5.87\frac{1}{8}$	,,	26,638
Hankow	,,	$218.30\frac{1}{16}$	,,	1,731,581
Tientsin	,,	$27.46\frac{10}{16}$	,,	191,047
Ichang	,,	$34.13\frac{1}{2}$	,,	195,571
TOTAL	*Piculs*	$329.38\frac{1}{2}$	= *Hk.Tls*	2,520,364

TOTALS for each YEAR.

	QUANTITY.	VALUE.				
	Piculs.	*Hk.Tls.*				
Total 1873	21.23⅓	118,218, averaging about *Hk.Tls.* 56 per catty.				
„ 1874	24.64½	148,239	„		„ 60	„
„ 1875	25.23¾	164,288	„		„ 65	„
„ 1876	25.03¼	209,469	„		„ 84	„
„ 1877	57.53₁₆⁵	479,095	„		„ 83	„
„ 1878	42.85₁₆¹⁵	374,246	„		„ 87	„
„ 1879	37.84½	267,056	„		„ 73	„
„ 1880	41.28	283,016	„		„ 69	„
„ 1881	23.61	202,802	„		„ 86	„
„ 1882	30.11	273,935	„		„ 91	„
Total for 10 years, 1873–82	329.38⅓	2,520,364 { average value for 10 years about } *Hk.Tls.* 76 per catty.				

There are no data for estimating the consumption in China, or the extent to which the foregoing amounts were adulterated.

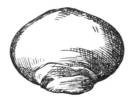

DRIED MUSK-BAG OF THE MOSCHATA (?), YÜNNAN.   (Average size as found in the shops.)

POISONOUS ANIMALS.

Porpoise.—The case of poisoning by eating porpoise (referred to above) did not prove serious, but as death often results from that cause, a summary of Chinese observations on the porpoise may be worth putting on record in these Reports.

The porpoise occupies greater space by far in Chinese ichthyology than any fish. CH'ÊN's *Cyclopædia* quotes 30 authors who refer to it. Few fishes are so prized for their flavour, and none so much condemned for poisonous qualities. Like English, German, French and other maritime people, the Chinese name the animal from its resemblance to a pig,—it is the *ho-t'un,* "river pig." It enters the rivers from the sea early in spring, being most abundant in the Yangtze, which it ascends over 1,000 miles—as far as the rapids allow. On its first appearance it is fat, and less hurtful as food than at a later period. A portion of fat found in the abdomen is so esteemed that it is styled "SI TSZE's milk," that lady being pre-eminent among all comely women for her beauty. One writer attributes the fatness to willow leaf buds, on which the porpoise feeds; but another combats that idea, inasmuch as the fatness is found to exist before the willow begins to sprout. The former observer, it is remarked, lived higher up the Yangtze, where the willow buds and porpoise appear synchronously. Another writer says willow buds are hurtful to fish. Porpoise, it is added, are a terror to fish, none daring to attack them; their appearance in large numbers indicates a blow. A centenarian author who wrote at the close of the twelfth century is quoted to show the risk of indulging in porpoise flesh. He begins by a remark of the renowned poet SU T'UNGPO, that the price of porpoise-eating is death, and then narrates how it nearly happened that he failed to see a full century. He was on a visit to a relative, a literary official at Pangyang, who said that his southern region produced nothing more savoury than porpoise, and then he ordered some to be cooked for a repast. As the two were sitting down to partake of it, they had to rise to receive a guest; at that moment a cat pounced upon the dish, upset it, and, with a dog, ate the dainty contents; but very soon it killed them both, thus plucking death from the watering mouths of guest and host. He adds that in Honan the eating-houses prepare mock porpoise dishes, and that in his opinion, the genuine article being fatal, the imitation should suffice to half kill the eaters. Animals seem to be more obnoxious to the poison than man. One authority says that cats and dogs partaking of it invariably die; and fishermen tell me that carrion birds will not eat porpoise entrails, or if they do, they die speedily. The liver, which is regarded as a great delicacy, is often poisonous; the eyes and the blood, and particularly that part which is found near the back, are always poisonous. All cases of fatal poisoning, however, appear to be due to neglect of certain precautions that require to be observed more minutely after the animals have made their visit to the rivers. In the first place the parts indicated require to be well cut away and the flesh thoroughly washed, and, when cooked, to be well boiled; at Ningpo the boiling is kept up for eight hours by careful people. Further to secure safety the Chinese olive or sugar-cane is boiled with the flesh. A man who happens to be taking as medicine a sort of sage will assuredly be killed if he takes porpoise at the same time. The toxic effects vary according to the portion which is taken. The blood and liver are generally poisonous, the fat causes swelling and numbness of the tongue, eating the eyes produces dimness of vision. On the lower Yangtze the fat is prepared for food by mixing it with liquor dregs and for a time burying it. With regard to the whole " river pig " a proverb says, " Eat it if you wish to discard life." Antidotes to porpoise-poisoning are the cosmetic which women use to give red colour to their lips, or the Chinese olive and camphor soaked together in water.

Notwithstanding that magistrates issue proclamations from time to time cautioning people against the use of porpoise flesh, scarcely a spring passes without fatal cases of poisoning from that cause. The *Shênpao* lately reported 11 deaths that occurred at Yangchow from eating portions of that fish.

Poisonous Fish.—The Ningpo gazetteer describes a fish, popularly called "tiger fish," which by its needle-like tail inflicts poisonous wounds on men and kills fish; men thus wounded suffer excruciating and protracted pain, say the people, who also declare that the spinous tail, if driven into a tree, will kill it. Somewhat similar is the "tiger fish," with hedgehog-like spines, which, piercing men, occasion pain; its bite is poisonous, and so is its flesh. On the coast of Chêkiang and Fukien the "swallow-red fish" is found, which resembles the "ox-tailed fish." It darts with extreme velocity, inflicting painful wounds on mussel divers. Yet worse is the poisonous wound inflicted by a species of ray which has three spines in its tail; the pain is such as to keep the sufferer groaning for successive days and nights.

A sort of sturgeon is found at Soyang which resembles a pig; its colour is yellow. Its stench forbids near approach, and it is very poisonous; notwithstanding, when properly prepared, it is considered fit food for the Emperor, for it constitutes an article of tribute.

A silure, or mud fish, is hurtful, particularly the kind with reddish eyes and no gills. No kind is to be eaten with cow liver, or with wild boar or venison. A small species of shark called "white shark," having a rough skin and hard flesh, is slightly poisonous. Several kinds of eels are represented as hurtful. Some Ningpo people will not eat eels without first testing them. They are placed in a deep water-jar, and if on the approach of a strong light they spring up, they are thrown away as not fit for food. There is a kind of eel that has its head turned upward that is not to be eaten. Eels that have perpendicular caudal fins are to be discarded; also those with white spotted backs, those without gills, the "four-eyed" kind, the kind with black striped bellies, and the kind that weigh 4 or 5 catties. The *Pênts'ao* shows the fallacy of the popular belief that eels spring from dead men's hair, by stating that they have eggs.

The "stone-striped fish" is described as causing vomiting. It resembles the roach, and is a foot long, with tiger-like markings. There are no males among these fish. According to native report, the females copulate with snakes, and have poisonous roes. In the south these fish are hung on trees where wasps' nests are found, by which means birds are attracted that devour the wasps. They swim on the surface of the water, but on the approach of men, dive down.

A curious account is given of a poisonous lacertian. It is amphibious, living in mountain creeks. Its fore-feet are like those of a monkey, its hinder resemble those of a dog; it has a long tail, is 7 or 8 feet long, and has the cry of a child, which is indicated by the mode of writing one of its names. It climbs trees, and in times of drought, fills its mouth with water, and, concealing itself in jungle, covering its body with leaves and grass, expands its jaws; birds, seeing the water therein contained, attempt to slake their thirst in the trap, when they are soon gulped down. The poison that it contains is removed by suspending it from trees, and beating it until it all flows out in the form of a white fluid.

There is a curious tortoise not named in the books, to which Kiangsu people give the names "ash ground tortoise" and "earth duke snake," because of its long tail. It spurts from its mouth a cobweb-like string against a stem of grass, and animals or insects treading on it are bitten, and sure to die from the poison; men also are killed by it. It is supposed to be blind, and for that reason projects its secretion as a feeler. It is found from the fifth to the seventh month. Making every allowance for exaggeration, it would seem to relate to an animal of considerable interest.

Of fishes that are wholesome at ordinary times and hurtful at others, the shad, *shih-yü, i.e.,* periodical fish, is the most remarkable. Its oil is regarded by the Chinese as a remedy in consumption and in cases where cod-liver oil is employed. When the *shih-yü* ascends the Yangtze as far as Szechwan, it becomes poisonous, and is there known as the "pest fish"—a change that is due, doubtless, to exhaustion from its enormous expenditure of strength in overcoming the torrential rapids that impeded its course. According to the gazetteer of the Kienli district, shad can ascend no higher than "White Snail Rapids," at which place they are largely caught; that is, about 1,100 miles from the sea. When they ascend as high as the Little Orphan, they show signs of change, for according to a popular superstition they receive at that islet an imprint on their heads, which is the seal of the Goddess of Mercy of that place; an inflammation probably occasioned by their encountering the current thus far, and an earnest of the deterioration which awaits them by the time a few reach their limits in Szechwan, where they become "pest fish"—about 1,300 miles from the sea. Carp are sometimes poisonous. There is a kind found in creeks that have poisonous brains, and a species that has two tendons on the back where the blood is black; these carp are not to be eaten. In cooking carp the fumes are to be avoided, or within three days dimness of vision will ensue. They are not eatable when epidemics prevail, when there is looseness of the bowels, or constipation, or when mercury is being taken; nor should they be eaten with dogs' flesh. Perch also are sometimes slightly poisonous, even the famous species found at Sungkiang, having "four gills," are at times unwholesome; when it proves so, the juice of reed-roots is to be given. A fish resembling the silure is slightly noxious. One writer says the same of the excellent barbel, "which are best cooked on plantain leaves."

The chelonia furnish poisonous species, as the three-footed, the red-footed, the single-eyed, the non-retractable head and foot, the sunken-eyed, the abdominal marked 卜, the abdominal marked 王, and the abdominal snake-figured kinds; also a mountain species, called "drought terrapin;" none of these are to be eaten. Edible kinds are not to be eaten with spinach nor hen's eggs, ducks or rabbits; pregnant women partaking of them will bring forth short-necked children; consumptive persons troubled with abdominal swellings should not use them for food. These are not fabulous, but misdescribed animals. The kind which does not retract head and feet is destitute of "petticoat" (that is, the leathery border of the carapace); eating this stops the breath. There is a jingling proverb which says the three and the four toed terrapins may be eaten; while the five-toed, which are transformed snakes, and the six-toed, which are transformed scorpions, are fatal poisons. The three-legged terrapin is found in pools on Chünshan, a hill in Ich'êng, Yangchow (Kiangsu), which a myth represents as a transformation of Yü the Great. It is very cold in its nature, and poisonous; fatal to those who partake of it. A man of T'aitsang ordered his wife to cook a three-legged terrapin, which he ate, and went to bed; soon after he was changed to blood and water, his hair alone remaining. Neighbours, suspecting foul play, informed the magistrate, HWANG TINGSHÊN, who could make nothing of the case, but ordered a prisoner who was condemned to death to eat one of those tripedal chelonians; the consequence was that nothing was left of the miserable culprit but bloody water and hair, whereupon the widow was acquitted. The learned author of the *Materia Medica*, who was less credulous than most men of his day, says, on quoting the above case, that it is not reasonable to suppose that this poison should dissolve a man in that fashion, and cites another authority who says that the animal may be eaten with impunity. He then gives the names of certain maladies for which the three-legged terrapin is prescribed. It does not seem to have occurred to the author in reviewing the above medico-legal case, that the accused widow found in the magistrate no unfriendly judge. Three-legged turtles are found in the markets at times, the fourth leg having evidently been bitten off in some contest.* Crustaceans are also sometimes poisonous; 15 kinds of crabs are interdicted as food. The antidotes for crab-poisoning are sweet basil or thyme or reed-root juice, the juice of squash or of garlic, etc. If women eat crabs during pregnancy they will suffer from cross-presentations. Crabs are not to be eaten with persimmons. The flesh of the king crab is sometimes poisonous, and is employed as an anthelmintic. Field and ditch prawns are described as poisonous. Many will be glad to hear that there are no admonitions against oyster-eating, although it is known that they and other shell-fish are sometimes poisonous.

FISH-POISONING.

Allied to the subject of poisonous fishes is that of fish-poisoning. At an early stage of their history, anterior perhaps to the legendary period when it is said the Chinese made the discovery of fire, and ere they had acquired the art of fishing, they found dead fish floating on the surface of streams, and in the course of time observed that the fall of certain seeds into the water was followed by the rise of fish, and then commenced the practice, which has continued to the present day, of catching fish by poisoning them. In Western China, says a writer quoted in the *Cyclopædia*, the waters are perfectly clear, and the people do not use nets in fishing, but in the winter season construct rafts, and from these throw on the water a mixture of wheat and the seeds of a species of polygonum pounded together; which, being eaten by the fish, they are killed and rise to the surface, but in a short time they come to life again. This they call "making the fish drunk." In this part of China, seeds of the *Croton tiglium* are employed very extensively for the same purpose. They are powdered and cast into the water, and being, like the polygonum, extremely acrid, speedily kill the fish and crustaceans that partake of them; these seeds render them colourless and flavourless, but not hurtful. Purchasers are never deceived, as their appearance discloses their mode of death; they are bought by the poor because of their cheapness. Similar modes of poisoning fish prevail on portions of the Grand Canal adjacent to the Yangtze, which sometimes call forth magisterial interdicts as damaging to the public health. As foreigners often travel through those parts, they would do well to bear the fact in mind. One of the district magistrates of Soochow lately issued a proclamation forbidding the sale of the "thunder duke creeper," which miscreants employ for catching fish, terrapins, prawns, crabs and the like, killing them, and injuring men. It is during the fourth month that care is most required, the practice being more common at that time.

METEOROLOGICAL.

I am indebted to Comte D'ARNOUX for an abstract of meteorological observations for the half-year.

---

* While our author holds to the existence of three-legged turtles and terrapins, he gives place to an exposure from another writer of a fraud respecting three-legged toads, a fraud that may be detected by macerating the animal. Belief in the existence of toads with three legs is fostered by legends of one of the genii, who is pictured as bestriding an animal of this description; images of the same are worn also on children's caps as charms.

ABSTRACT of METEOROLOGICAL OBSERVATIONS taken at WÊNCHOW during the Half-year
ended 30th September 1883.

DATE.		Barometer.	THERMOMETER.		Hu-midity, 0-100.	Ne-bulosity, 0-10.	RAINFALL.		REMARKS.
			Diurnal Mean Temperature in Shade.	Extreme Temperature in Shade.			No. of Days.	Total during Month.	
1883.		Inches.	° F.	° F.				Inches.	
April	Max......	30.29	67.8	83	95				Thunderstorms with heavy rain on 14th, 17th and 20th.
	Mean ...	30.01	64.2	...	80.5	6.4	16	5.25	
	Min.......	29.69	60.6	52	50				
	Range ...	0.60	7.2	31	45				
May	Max......	30.14	73.0	82	100				9th, 7.45 P.M.: squall, N.W.; very heavy rain. 15th, 1.45 P.M.: squall, N.N.W.; heavy rain.
	Mean ...	29.93	69.8	...	83.8	8.7	24	6.84	
	Min.......	29.70	66.6	60	46				
	Range ...	0.44	6.4	22	54				
June	Max......	30.03	82.7	96	95				21st, 5.30 A.M.: heavy wind and rain squall from N.W. 25th, 8 P.M.: wind and rain squall from N.W.
	Mean ...	29.89	78.4	...	78.7	6.8	12	5.00	
	Min.......	29.71	74.1	62	46				
	Range ...	0.32	8.6	34	49				
July	Max......	29.96	89.5	94	95				3rd, 4th, 5th, 5 P.M.: heavy wind and rain squall, from N.W. on the 3rd, and from W. on the 4th and 5th.
	Mean ...	29.82	85.4	...	78.9	6.9	12	6.60	
	Min.......	29.63	81.4	75	64				
	Range ...	0.33	7.6	19	31				
August	Max......	30.04	87.0	92	96				5th: typhoon passing to the eastward; strong wind squalls from W.N.W. and N.N.W. 6th, 2 A.M.: very heavy rain. 24th: typhoon passing to the eastward; 1 A.M. to 5 A.M., blowing very hard, N.W. and N.N.W.
	Mean ...	29.79	83.4	...	78	6.1	15	13.51	
	Min.......	29.39	79.9	75	58				
	Range ...	0.65	7.1	17	38				
September	Max......	30.26	83.4	93	100				20th: very heavy rain.
	Mean ...	30.19	79.7	...	77	7	8	2.37	
	Min.......	29.76	75.9	67	59				
	Range ...	0.50	7.5	26	41				

Chinal，Imperial Maritime Customs，Medical Reports
（1883. 10. 01—1884. 03. 31）

CHINA.

IMPERIAL MARITIME CUSTOMS.

II.—SPECIAL SERIES: No. 2.

MEDICAL REPORTS,

FOR THE HALF-YEAR ENDED 31st MARCH 1884.

27th Issue.

PUBLISHED BY ORDER OF

The Inspector General of Customs.

SHANGHAI:
PUBLISHED AT THE STATISTICAL DEPARTMENT OF THE INSPECTORATE GENERAL OF CUSTOMS,
AND SOLD BY
Messrs. KELLY & WALSH, SHANGHAI, YOKOHAMA, AND HONGKONG.

LONDON: P. S. KING & SON, CANADA BUILDING, KING STREET, WESTMINSTER, S.W.

1884.

INSPECTOR GENERAL'S CIRCULAR No. 19 OF 1870.

INSPECTORATE GENERAL OF CUSTOMS,

PEKING, 31st December 1870.

SIR,

1.—IT has been suggested to me that it would be well to take advantage of the circumstances in which the Customs Establishment is placed, to procure information with regard to disease amongst foreigners and natives in China; and I have, in consequence, come to the resolution of publishing half-yearly in collected form all that may be obtainable. If carried out to the extent hoped for, the scheme may prove highly useful to the medical profession both in China and at home, and to the public generally. I therefore look with confidence to the co-operation of the Customs Medical Officer at your port, and rely on his assisting me in this matter by framing a half-yearly report containing the result of his observations at..................upon the local peculiarities of disease, and upon diseases rarely or never encountered out of China. The facts brought forward and the opinions expressed will be arranged and published either with or without the name of the physician responsible for them, just as he may desire.

2.—The suggestions of the Customs Medical Officers at the various ports as to the points which it would be well to have especially elucidated, will be of great value in the framing of a form which will save trouble to those members of the medical profession, whether connected with the Customs or not, who will join in carrying out the plan proposed. Meanwhile I would particularly invite attention to—

a.—The general health of....................during the period reported on; the death rate amongst foreigners; and, as far as possible, a classification of the causes of death.

b.—Diseases prevalent at...........................

c.—General type of disease; peculiarities and complications encountered; special treatment demanded.

d.—Relation of disease to $\begin{cases} \text{Season.} \\ \text{Alteration in local conditions—such as drainage, etc.} \\ \text{Alteration in climatic conditions.} \end{cases}$

e.—Peculiar diseases; especially leprosy.

f.—Epidemics $\begin{cases} \text{Absence or presence.} \\ \text{Causes.} \\ \text{Course and treatment.} \\ \text{Fatality.} \end{cases}$

Other points, of a general or special kind, will naturally suggest themselves to medical men; what I have above called attention to will serve to fix the general scope of the undertaking. I have committed to Dr. ALEX. JAMIESON, of Shanghai, the charge of arranging the Reports for publication, so that they may be made available in a convenient form.

564212

3.—Considering the number of places at which the Customs Inspectorate has established offices, the thousands of miles north and south and east and west over which these offices are scattered, the varieties of climate, and the peculiar conditions to which, under such different circumstances, life and health are subjected, I believe the Inspectorate, aided by its Medical Officers, can do good service in the general interest in the direction indicated; and, as already stated, I rely with confidence on the support and assistance of the Medical Officer at each port in the furtherance and perfecting of this scheme. You will hand a copy of this Circular to Dr. ...., and request him, in my name, to hand to you in future, for transmission to myself, half-yearly Reports of the kind required, for the half-years ending 31st March and 30th September—that is, for the Winter and Summer seasons.

4.—   *   *   *   *   *

I am, etc.,

(Signed)   ROBERT HART,

I. G.

THE COMMISSIONERS OF CUSTOMS,—*Newchwang, Ningpo, Tientsin, Foochow, Chefoo, Tamsui, Hankow, Takow. Kiukiang, Amoy, Chinkiang, Swatow,* and *Shanghai, Canton.*

SHANGHAI, *1st July 1884.*

SIR,

In accordance with the directions of your Despatch No. 6 *A* (Returns Series) of the 24th June 1871, I now forward to the Statistical Department of the Inspectorate General of Customs, the following documents :—

Report on the Health of Ichang, pp. 1, 2 ;

Report on the Health of Kiukiang, pp. 3-6 ;

Report on the Health of Canton, pp. 7, 8 ;

Report on the Health of Wênchow, pp. 9–18 ;

Report on the Health of Amoy, pp. 19–21 ;

Report on the Health of Shanghai, pp. 29–43 ; each of these referring to the half-year ended 31st March 1884.

Report on the Health of Newchwang for the eighteen months ended 31st March 1884, pp. 22–28.

A special article on Distomata Hominis, pp. 44–54.

An Appendix of translations of—

A monograph on Sprue, pp. 55–85 ;

Note on an Affection of the Sympathetic Plexuses of the Intestinal Wall, pp. 86–91.

I have the honour to be,

SIR,

Your obedient Servant,

R. ALEX. JAMIESON

THE INSPECTOR GENERAL OF CUSTOMS,
PEKING.

The Contributors to this Volume are :—

A. HENRY, M.A., L.R.C.P.Ed. .... Ichang.

G. R. UNDERWOOD, M.B., CH.M. .... Kiukiang.

J. F. WALES, B.A., M.D., CH.M. .... Canton.

D. J. MACGOWAN, M.D. .... Wênchow.

B. S. RINGER, M.R.C.S., L.S.A. .... Amoy.

W. MORRISON, M.B., CH.M. .... Newchwang.

WALLACE TAYLOR, M.D. .... Osaka, Japan.

R. A. JAMIESON, M.A., M.D., M.R.C.S. .... Shanghai.

For everything enclosed within square brackets [ ], the compiler is responsible.

Dr. D. J. MACGOWAN'S REPORT ON THE HEALTH OF WÊNCHOW

For the Half-year ended 31st March 1884.

In my last half-yearly Report I remarked that the cholera epidemic then prevailing in so many portions of the Empire had left this port unscathed, but I was obliged to append a footnote admitting its appearance in the middle of October, about the time of its subsidence at Foochow, Ningpo and other places.

During the months preceding, the rainfall was less than usual, while from September to the rise of the disease no rain had fallen. Rice-fields, usually very moist, had become dry, and the water in the canals (no longer flowing, but dammed up) was greatly reduced in quantity, and consequently more charged with excreta. At such times, on the alluvial coast region of Chêkiang and Kiangsu certain telluric and atmospheric conditions tend to develop zymotic disease. In other parts of the country, however, the same disorder occurred under dissimilar conditions, unusual rainfall being followed by cholera, the same as where drinking water had been scarce and polluted.

References to the cholera outbreak of 1883 are to be found in the last issue of these Reports, which I supplement by a summary of what has appeared on the subject in the vernacular press. It extended on the coast from Canton to Newchwang, and from Shanghai to Hsüchow, on the upper part of the middle Yangtze, over 1,500 miles from its mouth; but while visiting all the towns of the central and lower divisions of the Great River, it spared those situated on its affluents.

Dr. Edwards of the Inland Mission at Chêngtu informs me that that city (provincial capital of Szechwan) was exempt.

Accounts of its appearance at Canton, Swatow, Foochow, Ningpo, Shanghai, Newchwang, Hangchow, Soochow, Yangchow, Nanking, Wuch'ang and Ichang were published in the native papers, but the information is not of much value. At Wuch'ang it prevailed in July and August (two months later than at Ichang), and followed a protracted wet season, when that weather was suddenly interrupted by a period of cold.

At Soochow, medicines proving inert, recourse was at last had to snails (with which the shrivelled fingers were tipped), when some recovered, which caused the disorder to be styled " snail-head disease."

It lingered at Yangchow until the end of September. It is stated that the opium smokers of that city suffered from the epidemic more than other classes.

In Soochow it continued until October, 9 cases out of 10 being fatal. At Ningpo the epidemic was denominated the "midnight-moon disease," because of the periods of its commencement and fatal termination. "Not 1 in 10 of the attacked survived."

The history of Indian cholera in China remains to be written. As a contribution I submit the following, which embraces information derived from an *Essay on Leg-contracting Spasms*, published in 1860 by Hsü Tzǔmo of Kiahsing, in which it is stated that the disease made its first appearance in 1821.* He does not say whence it came, but medical tradition at Ningpo refers its origin to the Straits, whence it was conveyed to Fukien by junk. From that province it extended to Canton, and passing thence into Kiangsi, it next advanced into Chêkiang and Kiangsu, presenting the features of an imported epidemic.

Wênchow tradition gives 1820 as the date of its appearance in southern Chêkiang, which, if correct, shows that it had come from Fukien, which is very probable. That year may therefore be accepted as the date of the advent of Indian cholera in China.

It slowly advanced up the Yangtze, a fearful outbreak which is still remembered for its violence occurring at Ch'ungch'ing in 1825. Northward it seems to have travelled less leisurely, but definite information is still wanting from that quarter of the Empire, and from Korea and Japan, where it proved extremely virulent.

Becoming endemic in all parts of the Empire, it has for over 40 years frequently assumed an epidemic character, sometimes extending over the whole of Eastern Asia, at others restricted to a single province or part of a province.

A remarkable and tragical medical delusion characterised the first epidemic. Theory and almost universal practice forbids the employment of the class of "warming medicines" in warm weather, as also the use of cooling ones in cold weather. Cooling remedies alone were resorted to when this form of cholera first appeared, and apparently for a generation later, the result being that "not 1 in 100 patients were cured." The credit of reversing the practice is ascribed to our author. Hsü commences his essay on epidemic cholera by saying that the term "contracting-leg spasm" was formerly unknown, but dates from the summer and autumn of 1821, when it arose suddenly.

The disease is characterised by either vomiting or purging, or both together, accompanied by abdominal pain, which feature is sometimes absent. After several discharges from the stomach and bowels, the feet contract, or the hands and feet, when the pain becomes more severe, and immediately the skin and muscles shrink, the breath is shortened, the voice falters and fails, the eyes sink, there is a craving for cold drinks, the body is covered with icy cold perspiration, the six pulses (three are recognised at each wrist) cease, and death supervenes in half a day. Persons attacked in the morning die at evening, or attacked at night, die in the morning, or, still more rapidly, fall down dead in the street. Persons attending on patients or visiting them catch the disorder and succumb sooner than the patients themselves.

Doctors treated the disease as common cholera, and did not cure 1 in 100. Since the malady has been recognised as originating in the three *yin* (lungs, heart, kidneys), warming remedies have been administered to correct the *yang* (positive or male principle, as contradistinguished from the *yin*, negative or female principle), such as ginseng, ginger, aconite (*A. variegatum*), and cinnamon. Patients have been loath to use those warming medicines, or have employed them too sparingly, and they were not cured. Wealthy people in particular were averse to the change.

Those are to be compassionated who, living in secluded places, are unable to obtain medical attendance, and those in cities who, attacked at midnight, are unable to call a physician until the disease becomes incurable.

* A year earlier has been given by the Rev. W. C. Milne (*Chinese Repository*, "Asiatic Cholera in China") for its first appearance in Chêkiang, owing to his assigning 1820 as the first year of Tao Kuang, according to rule. But that Emperor decreed that the year following his accession should be styled the first of his reign.

Generally the disease is violent in proportion to the heat of the season; as the weather cools, the disorder abates. In winter there are few that die after half a day's illness; although the treatment may be slight, patients gradually recover. In summer and autumn, on the contrary, light attacks rapidly become violent, and if not promptly treated terminate fatally. "On this account," says the author, "I have carefully prepared this essay, selecting prescriptions to avert calamity, with the request that gentlemen will bear them in mind, to be prepared for epidemics."

It is not a little marvellous that such a misapprehension should have long existed touching the proper way of treating the new epidemic, seeing that Chinese systematic works on medicine describe one form of cholera as characterised by all the symptoms that impart to epidemic cholera an extraordinary degree of terror, including contractions, which gave its name to the epidemic from India, and for which warming remedies are prescribed by those old writers. Retraction of the testicles is also named, but suppression of urine is not mentioned in those works, nor by our author, although that symptom has always been mentioned in cases reported as Indian cholera in this country.

In fine, Indian cholera in China differs from the common cholera of the country only in its epidemic character, the former being migratory, the latter stationary. In its marches from region to region it is as irregular here as in its Gangetic home, leaping over certain districts, sometimes to return, and at others not. Instead of moving as though air-borne or conveyed by persons, it rises here and there as if it had been awaiting the concurrence of certain telluric and atmospheric conditions for its development—conditions that exist in one district but are absent in a contiguous locality, and that are wholly absent sometimes for successive years. Its history indicates either that a specific germ was conveyed from abroad or that there suddenly arose successively from south to north a series of conditions which favoured the development of a virulent form of endemic cholera which became epidemic.

The account of the cholera at Soochow makes us acquainted with a Chinese superstition that is familiar to all Western peoples, namely, the belief that owls are harbingers of evil, their discordant hooting prognosticating death. The cholera epidemic in that city was characterised by screams of the "cat-head eagle" (horned owl). Men on hearing its notes rushed out with flambeaux to kill or drive it away. It seems that the owl of those parts appears and disappears at intervals, its visit proving always fatal to somebody.

Concerning the processions that take place to exorcise demons of pestilence, a writer in the *Shênpao* makes sensible remarks: "Epidemics are ordered by Providence; neither gods nor demons have any influence in the matter. Men ignorant of this resort to superstitious practices as if they were insane." He then proceeds to describe the processions, and he might have added another reason against them besides their uselessness. Being usually conducted in hot weather, with great exposure to heat, and involving excessive fatigue, they render the participants more susceptible to morbid influences.

CATTLE DISEASE.

In 1882 northern Chêkiang suffered from an epizootic that extended to horses, goats and dogs—cattle chiefly suffering. Last year cattle suffered extensively from the same cause. A rinderpest is endemic in the mountainous region of T'aichow, whence this last epizootic reached Ningpo as epidemic cholera subsided. I find no account of Foot-and-Mouth disease in China.

A correspondent of the *Shênpao* advised the killing of diseased animals to prevent contagion spreading, and the burial of carcasses, instead of their being cast into canals and rivers. The Huangp'u received so many that the authorities of Sungkiang and Kiahsing were petitioned to interdict it. Interment is objected to because decomposition in the soil is regarded as unhealthy. The same writer recommends *Robinia amara*—a pleasant, bitter root-tonic—to be mixed with the animals' food. Cattle-sheds should be fumigated by burning aromatic pastilles, whose odorous fumes are used for disinfecting the rooms of the dead and of patients suffering from contagious fevers and the like. It would appear from the inertness of their medicines, the uselessness of their writings on cattle maladies, and from the great mortality that attends their epizootic murrains, that the Chinese have no remedy for rinderpest.

PORPOISE POISON.

As a supplement to what I wrote in my last Report on this subject, I would add the following. Five persons died at Anch'ing in April last from eating porpoise. In one family a father and son were the victims; in one vomiting was induced, in the other emetics failed to act; both died. In another family a father, mother and daughter died from the same cause. They suffered much pain, with swelling of the abdomen, skin purple and benumbed, with greenish saliva from the mouth. This is the only report of cases of this kind where symptoms are given. It would seem that porpoise-poisoning is commoner on the Yangtze than on the coast, as if the ascent of the Great River rendered porpoise less fit for food, as it does the shad. It is well known that sailors eat porpoise caught at sea with impunity, and islanders, as the Japanese, rarely suffer from porpoise eating.

NOTES ON CHINESE SYPHILOGRAPHY.

The last issue of these Reports contains a translation of a " Contribution to the History of Syphilis," by Dr. SCHEUBE of Leipzig, in which the author quotes a Japanese work showing that syphilis was known in Japan anterior to A.D. 806. Having had long in hand a treatise on the history and treatment of syphilis in China, I am moved by Dr. SCHEUBE'S article to publish at once so much of my essay as is of present interest.

Unless syphilis had an independent origin in Japan, its genesis must be referred to China, as it was a common disorder in Canton at a period probably anterior to the ninth century, whence it spread to all portions of the Empire.

The earliest Chinese work in which syphilis has been described is the *Dermatology* of TOU HANCH'ING, imperial physician during the Northern Sung, at an uncertain period of the eleventh century. The blocks from which that early book on cutaneous diseases was printed having perished, it was recut by a descendant of the author in the reign of LUNG CH'ING (1567-72) and printed with additions that are not distinguishable from the original treatise. Although ancient, the work is much valued, and is now to be found in almost every medical library. It is in six volumes, containing 13 sections. Soyang in Honan was at that time the metropolis, and the residence of the court physician.

According to our dermatologist, syphilis invaded Central China from Canton, then known only as a fit place for penal servitude, criminals being banished to that province, and officers who were in disgrace sent to govern it, or, in other words, there was little intercourse between the far South and the Great Plain. From Canton it spread over the Empire, the períod assigned being the latter part of the eleventh century of our era. How there happens to be a record of its existence in Japan at the beginning of the ninth century, as shown by Dr. SCHEUBE, at a period so much earlier than the date of its appearance in Central China, is matter for conjecture; possibly it had an independent origin in that country, extending thence to Canton. Most probably the disease was conveyed to Japan by junk from that port, where it is likely that it prevailed for ages before it commenced its northward course. Assuming that syphilis was imported into Europe, its place of export is determined by this record. It may have been by caravan, but presumably it was by ship, Arabians being the carriers of commodities between Canton and the Arabian Gulf in the eighth century, if not anterior to the Hegira.

Not only did syphilis originate in China (perchance one of several spots on the globe entitled to that bad distinction), but the Chinese were the first to employ mercury in its treatment, a mode of cure repudiated by our author, who claims merit for neutralising its poisonous effects on those who had been subjected to a mercurial course. It will be observed, however, that he employed it (unconsciously) in another form. According to his etiology, syphilis owes its origin at Canton to a predisposing climatal diathesis; persons having sexual intercourse while suffering from malarial cachexia developing a poison communicable even by means of ordinary fugitive contact in crowded thoroughfares—a notion that has been long abandoned by practitioners.

It is fit that some of his views should be given in his own words. He begins his chapter on syphilis by saying :—

Venereal ulcers [*Mei-ch'uang*, "tree-strawberry ulcers"] were formerly unknown. An examination of their origin shows that they arose in Canton towards the close of the Wu Wei period and calamitously overspread the land, and now, in the early part of the present cycle, the human frame has deteriorated and the seasons are irregular, and sexual intercourse is rendered very liable to communicate the syphilis poison. Once effected, the morbid action is of more than ordinary violence, penetrating the marrow of the bones and permeating the muscles, flowing into the blood-vessels, and entering the male and female genitals, or abiding in the system or coming to the surface, or attacking the intestines or the orifices (eyes, nostrils, mouth, ears, fundament, urethra). There are some lesions that from beginning to end remain in one place, and there are some that move to other regions; some that leap from one viscus over one adjacent to a more distant one, and some that remain fixed in one organ. The various appearances are numerous, each requiring its special treatment.

Next follows an account of the *tu* or poison in each of the five viscera—liver, kidneys, stomach, lungs and heart.

Liver.—When the poison enters the liver it first affects the urethra,* when the tendons become painful, and next ulcers appear on the ear or neck or axilla, resembling amomum capsules. In severe forms the tendons cannot be moved. Extending from the liver to the stomach, the limbs become tumefied and painful, the legs and skin as if worm-eaten; advancing

---

* [History repeats itself in medical theories just as in political and social theories and combinations of circumstances. HAESER (*Lehrbuch der Geschichte der Medicin und der epidemischen Krankheiten.* Jena, 1882, Bd. iii, S. 259) thus sums up the views of the earliest European writers on syphilis :—"Man dachte sich das syphilitische Gift . . . . . als eine dem kranken Körper in seiner Totalität beiwohnende verborgene Eigenschaft *(totius substantiæ qualitas occulta)*, welche im Körper des Angesteckten vor Allem auf die Leber, den Heerd der Blutbereitung, wirkt, indem sie daselbst eine Veränderung des Blutes, eine Art der *putredo* erzeugt. Durch die von der Leber entspringenden Adern verbreitet sich die Verderbniss zu allen Körpertheilen, am frühesten zu den Genitalien, welche sich vor allen übrigen Organen durch die Weite ihrer *Poren* auszeichnen."] ,

to the heart, ulcers appear on the skin like dark specks, causing both pain and itching. When instead of moving from the liver to other viscera it becomes lodged in that viscus, the large tendons become painful, and after a long time ulcers appear on the neck and knees.

Kidneys.—When syphilis penetrates the kidneys, it begins by producing sores on the genitals, followed by pains in the bones. Ulcers appear within the ears, on the scrotum, on the vertex, on the back between the shoulders, presenting the appearance of rotten persimmon, and are called genital corroding ulcers. When virulent the poison destroys the male and female organs of generation.

Stomach.—When the poison enters the stomach, ulcers appear on the margin of the hairy scalp, round the mouth, and on the arms. When virulent it extends to the kidneys; the bones become painful and their marrow heated, and tumefactions appear over the coccyx, in the popliteal space and soles of the feet. Advancing to the lungs, the skin becomes scabby, resembling purplish-red flowers; the scales falling, leave white spots. Remaining lodged in the stomach, lesions of that organ and of the intestines are caused, and reddish lines appear on the skin.

Lungs.—When the poison enters the lungs, ulcers appear in the armpits, on the chest, and on the cheeks, like blooming flowers, and are vulgarly called "cotton-flower ulcers." When severe, the poison, concentrating in the throat, extending from the lungs to the liver, causes pain in the tendons on certain days of the calendar, or in cloudy weather from 4 to 7 P.M.

Advancing from the liver to the kidneys, eruption of the scrotum is caused, both painful and itching. The poison lurking in the lungs produces reddish-white spots on the skin, and when chronic occasions lesions of chest, arms, and legs.

Heart.—In the heart the poison displays its action in ulcers on the shoulders and chest, the heads being dark purple, exactly like "tree-strawberry ulcers." In severe forms the virus attacks the iris, extending to the lungs, breaking out in the throat, and gradually the septum of the nose becomes as if worm-gnawed and destroyed, attended with great salivation. Moving on to the stomach, it produces "goose-feet scales," benumbing hands and feet. Remaining stationary in the heart, the poison causes the fall of finger-nails. Our author remarks on the mode of communication and the prognosis as follows :—

This disease is not due solely to sexual intercourse, but arises in vitiated constitutions, or it may be caught, either by young or old, in crowded thoroughfares or in latrines, or when chatting with the infected,— the poison in those cases appearing either immediately or long after exposure. The whole body suffers pain. Sometimes it is painless, and incautiously communicated in the marital couch ; in some cases women not themselves suffering transfer the poison to children.

It is a disease of the vessels, and the poison is either superficial or deep, and the medicines act, some slowly, others promptly. Examining the pulse, the symptoms and appearance of the malady indicate whether it is to be vigorously attacked, or the patient fortified (heroic or expectant, according to circumstances), avoiding an error of a hair's breadth. Half a month suffices for the cure of a case in which the poison has not extended beyond the viscus first attacked. In cases where three viscera are affected, a month's treatment is required for cure; when all are affected, 50 days are required for restoration to health ; but only by that mode of treatment which is admitted by the intelligent throughout the land. The disease is as easily cured (by my treatment) as it is easily acquired, and no purplish-red discoloration is left behind ; no pain or inconvenience follows, nor danger of communicating it, nor of impairing progeny, nor of injuring the digestion, nor of harming the constitution. The remedies will continue to be used unchanged through the remote future, they being like the royal way—beneficial, genii-like. There are those who bunglingly rely on sudorifics, laxatives, topical applications, fumigations, lotions, as remedies that quickly afford relief, ignorant of the lurking of the poison in the system, which, later, causes lesions of the intestines and all the above-named affections of the five viscera, which shows their treatment to be inefficacious.

I, on the contrary, am able to name the time of recovery, and am able also to expel the mercurial poison (administered according to the prevailing mode), so that to the end of his days the patient shall not suffer.

The controversy that our author commenced regarding the use of mercury in the treatment of syphilis still continues, but those who, like him, denounce its employment in one form—protochloride,—ignorantly use the bisulphide. In the great work that was compiled by and issued under imperial auspices in 1717, *Golden Mirror of Eminent Medical Authors, compiled by Imperial Authority*, the chapter on syphilis states that while mercury appears to effect a speedy cure, it merely drives the poison into the bones, whence, after a protracted lodgment, it reappears in the forms that we designate secondary and tertiary.

Further information is then conveyed in answer to questions that are supposed to be propounded by a pupil to the author—a most ancient mode of communicating instruction by Chinese writers.

The answer to the first question is interesting :—

If it be asked "How did the venereal malady arise?" I answer that, Canton being marshy and hot, without frost and snow, insects and serpents there do not burrow or become torpid, and garbage accumulating on the ground, in the eleventh month (commencement of winter) its moisture and the mountain malaria, mutually fermenting, induced in the physically vitiated what were called genital corroding ulcers, which, like creeping plants or permeating dyes, infected brothels ; originating in telluric influences, it became epidemic.

If it be asked "Seeing that syphilis arose from telluric causes, how comes it to be called the Canton ulcer?" I answer, the "Canton ulcer" belongs to the small-pox class of disorders, which also was formerly unknown. Small-pox arose in the North ; its infection came thence to the South during the Han period (B.C. 206 to A.D. 220), and was called "Hun pox."

Next follows a record of cases illustrating the author's method of treating primary, secondary and tertiary forms of syphilis, although not recognising such distinctions. I translate the first and second cases.

A student, 18 years of age, living in the country, suffered from loss of hair and eyebrows ; his whole frame was bent and contorted : he had been treated for rheumatism. On examination of patient's pulse I found it sunken, impeded and slow, which indicated that the metal element (lungs) oppressed the wood element (liver), owing to syphilitic poison. I administered the discutient infusion composed of [here follows a prescription containing 10 vegetable ingredients].

Next I gave the compound bezoar and toad-venom pill [composed of bezoar, toad-venom,* musk, olibanum, red sulphide of mercury and bisulphide of arsenic]. This induced a profuse perspiration.

Next I gave the antidotal pill No. 2 [composed of bezoar, amber, silkworms, nitrate of potash, sulphate of iron, salt, alum, burnt hair, etc., with mercury and arsenic as before]. With that antidotal pill I gave at the same time the "gentian-decoction laxative" [composed of gentian, rhubarb and other

---

* No account has yet been given to foreigners of this acrid article. It is obtained from the toad by tying oil-paper over its head and then striking the animal, when it ejects the secretion in considerable quantity. The material is carefully removed from the paper, dried, and formed into thin circular cakes an inch or two in diameter, which, from being milky white at first, turn nearly black. When of good quality it is worth its weight in silver. Inferior kinds are imported from Siam and Japan : the Chinese comes from Szechwan, and is chiefly employed in sternutatory powders.

vegetable simples]. After 10 days' use of those medicines a miliary eruption appeared, which soon desquamated. In something over 20 days the poison had been neutralised ; the hair of the eyebrows and of the head grew again.

The second of the 29 cases given by the imperial dermatologist was that of—

A poet's wife, to whom her husband communicated the Canton ulcer. After taking many medicines they were both cured, as they imagined ; but all their children dying in early infancy, I was consulted. I told them that their children had all died from inherited syphilis.

In such cases children are born without integument, or with various ulcers or tumefactions or scaly eruptions—all congenital. I could find nothing abnormal in the pulse of the father ; his system was in equilibrium. But the disorder lurked in the mother's system in a severe form, to the injury of the uterus. I prescribed the "comforting decoction" [consisting of 10 vegetable ingredients].

Twenty of these decoctions were given, and at the same time pill No. 9 [composed of tiger-bone, terrapin plastron, red sulphide of mercury, bisulphide of arsenic, etc.].

After administering the above I gave the compound flavouring pill [vegetable].

Under this treatment the patient in less than a year bore a son, and two years later a daughter ; the children took small-pox inoculation mildly, and were free of disease.

INTRODUCTION OF SMALL-POX AND INOCULATION INTO CHINA.

Incidental allusion is made by the imperial dermatologist to the first appearance of variola in China, which he assigns to the period of the Han dynasty (B.C. 206 to A.D. 220), and names the hereditary enemies of China, the Huns, as communicating that disease, which was accordingly denominated "Hun pox." More precise is the statement of the *Eastern* [*Korean*] *Precious Mirror of Medical Practice*, which states that the disease first appeared at the close of the Chou and commencement of the Han dynasties (B.C. 256–205). Indubitably, then, it made its first appearance (since history began) in the middle of the third century before the Christian era, whither it came from Mongolia ; but two and a quarter centuries later it entered China from the South, when it was regarded as a new disease. In A.D. 48 the renowned warrior MA YÜAN conducted a campaign against the Wuling aborigines (south-west of Tungting Lake, Hunan), and brought back with him the "captives'-pox," implying that his prisoners conveyed the infection, and according to several high authorities, such as the *Sombre Pearls of Chihshui* (genii remedies from a place of genii) and the *Correct Treatment of Small-pox*, the "captives'-pox" was the origin of small-pox in the Middle Kingdom. It would seem that the epidemic from the steppes had so long disappeared as to have been forgotten at the time when it was conveyed into the country by barbarians from sub-tropical regions.

The earliest medical writer on small-pox was CH'IEN CHUNGYANG, of the Northern Sung—10th century.*

INOCULATION.

Dr. COLLINSON (*Small-pox and Vaccination medically considered*) is quoted as saying "The Chinese practised inoculation from the sixth century." I have been unable to discover an earlier account of its origin than that given in the above-named *Correct Treatment of*

---

* When the Chinese had occasion to devise a character for expressing the new disease, they united two radicals (疒, *ping*, "sickness," and 豆, *tou*, "lentil-bean," and made 痘, *tou),* using "bean" as the phonetic, both being ideographic : "a disease with bean-shaped pustules."

Small-pox, which states that the art was first taught by a nun in the reign of JÊN TSUNG (A.D. 1023–63). That reign was signalised by a famous premier, WANG TAN, a great statesman and scholar. Small-pox had deprived him of all his children, and when in old age a son was born to him he was most solicitous to secure for that child a safe attack of the fell disorder, and summoning a council of physicians whose speciality was infantile diseases, he inquired if they understood the treatment of small-pox. The faculty disclaimed profound knowledge of the malady, but knew something of it. They were dismissed, each with a fee of *Tls.* 10, the minister remarking that what they understood they could accomplish, adding that when the child was attacked they should be sent for to prescribe, and in the event of their success they should be liberally compensated.

An officer at the capital, a native of Szechwan, hearing of the circumstance, obtained an introduction to the minister and gave him the following information. A young woman of Kiangsu vowed to quit the world, and, rejecting marriage, devoted herself to the worship of Buddha, but refused submission to the tonsure, preferring to retain her hair. She wandered to Omei Mountain (sacred to Sakyamuni, contiguous to Thibet), and on its summit lived in a reed hut. The women of all that region became her disciples, fasting, reciting prayers and doing good. Recently she told her followers that she had been inspired to impart instruction in implanting small-pox, which consisted in selecting scabs from cases that had had but few pustules, and these pointed, round, red, and glossy, full of greenish-yellow pus that became thick. The scabs to be used when a month old, or in hot weather those that had fallen only 15 or 20 days might be used, while winter ones should be 40 or 50 days old before using, which may be in spring or autumn. Take 8 grains of the desiccated scabs and 2 grains of *Uvularia grandiflora*; pound the two together in a clean earthen mortar. Select lucky and eschew unlucky days for implanting. Employ for the operation a silver tube curved at the point; blow the prepared matter into the right nostril in the case of a boy, and into the left in girls; six days after there is slight fever, which on the following day increases greatly; in two or three days more an eruption appears, charged with matter, and then scabs. Not one in 10, not one in 100, that does not recover. All the inhabitants of the region adjacent to Omei Mountain adopted the practice, praying her to perform the operation. On hearing this the minister sent for the venerable recluse, who came to the capital and operated successfully. She refused to accept reward, saying "I am a pilgrim, and have no need of silver or silk. If your excellency will on the one hand serve the Emperor loyally, and on the other be an exemplary model to the mandarinate, giving stability to the State and soothing outside regions, thereby preserving the people in peace, that will be a greater recompense for me than gifts of silver or silk." She returned to the sacred mountain, and some years later informed her followers that she was not uterine born, but was an incarnation of the Goddess of Mercy, and had come to preserve the lives of children by implanting small-pox, "which," said she, "I have taught you, that you should impart the art to others." On hearing this announcement the women all worshipped her, lauding her righteousness, asking by what title they should invoke her. She answered, "As Your Ladyship the Celestial Mother," adding, "whenever anyone shall offer incense and prayers to me, invoking my intervention, I will from heaven manifest myself by turning malignant into benignant cases;" whereon she was transformed, that is, she died. Every official temple has a shrine to this "Goddess of Small-pox," and many cities have temples for her exclusive worship. Evidently, inoculation had been taught at Omei Mountain by some Thibetan monk, who had acquired his art in India, where it appears to have been known in high antiquity.

METEOROLOGICAL.

Again I am indebted to Comte d'Arnoux for a half-year's meteorological record.

ABSTRACT of METEOROLOGICAL OBSERVATIONS taken at WÊNCHOW during the Half-year ended 31st March 1884.

DATE.	Barometer.	THERMOMETER.		Hu-midity, 0–100.	Ne-bulosity, 0–10.	RAINFALL.		REMARKS.
		Diurnal Mean Temperature in Shade.	Extreme Temperature in Shade.			No. of Days.	Total during Month.	
1883.	*Inches.*	° F.	° F.				*Inches.*	
October { Max	30.46	77.4	83	91			0.01	
Mean	30.19	72.8	...	65.6	4.8	1		
Min	30.00	68.3	58	32				
Range	0.46	9.1	25	59				
November { Max	30.39	62.1	76	100			7.10	Heavy rain on 6th, 8th, and 21st.
Mean	30.25	60.9	...	79	8.6	19		
Min	30.02	59.7	47	44				
Range	0.37	2.4	29	56				
December { Max	30.64	54.0	63	93			0.87	
Mean	30.36	49.6	...	71.7	4	5		
Min	30.20	45.2	39	37				
Range	0.44	8.8	24	56				
1884.								
January { Max	30.55	53.6	64	100			1.35	
Mean	30.32	50.3	...	79.7	7.7	11		
Min	30.05	47.0	36	40				
Range	0.50	6.6	28	60				
February { Max	30.54	49.2	65	100			5.54	On the 4th, snow on the hills.
Mean	30.30	46.1	...	79.5	6.6	13		
Min	30.00	43.0	34	56				
Range	0.54	6.2	31	44				
March { Max	30.44	58.2	74	100			7.61	Heavy rain on 6th and 16th. 6th: moon halo. 28th: very high tide, 19 feet, being 2 feet higher than ordinary high springs.
Mean	30.12	54.6	...	82.2	7.1	16		
Min	29.80	51.1	41	50				
Range	0.64	7.1	33	50				

China, Imperial Maritime Customs, Medical Reports
(1891. 04. 01—1891. 09. 30)

CHINA.

IMPERIAL MARITIME CUSTOMS.

II.—SPECIAL SERIES: No. 2.

MEDICAL REPORTS,

FOR THE HALF-YEAR ENDED 30TH SEPTEMBER 1891.

42nd Issue.

PUBLISHED BY ORDER OF

The Inspector General of Customs.

SHANGHAI:
PUBLISHED AT THE STATISTICAL DEPARTMENT OF THE INSPECTORATE GENERAL OF CUSTOMS,
AND SOLD BY
KELLY & WALSH, LIMITED: SHANGHAI, HONGKONG, YOKOHAMA, AND SINGAPORE.
LONDON: P. S. KING & SON, CANADA BUILDING, KING STREET, WESTMINSTER, S.W.

1894.

[*Price* $1.]

INSPECTOR GENERAL'S CIRCULAR No. 19 of 1870.

INSPECTORATE GENERAL OF CUSTOMS,

PEKING, 31st December 1870.

SIR,

1.—IT has been suggested to me that it would be well to take advantage of the circumstances in which the Customs Establishment is placed, to procure information with regard to disease amongst foreigners and natives in China; and I have, in consequence, come to the resolution of publishing half-yearly in collected form all that may be obtainable. If carried out to the extent hoped for, the scheme may prove highly useful to the medical profession both in China and at home, and to the public generally. I therefore look with confidence to the co-operation of the Customs Medical Officer at your port, and rely on his assisting me in this matter by framing a half-yearly report containing the result of his observations at.................upon the local peculiarities of disease, and upon diseases rarely or never encountered out of China. The facts brought forward and the opinions expressed will be arranged and published either with or without the name of the physician responsible for them, just as he may desire.

2.—The suggestions of the Customs Medical Officers at the various ports as to the points which it would be well to have especially elucidated, will be of great value in the framing of a form which will save trouble to those members of the medical profession, whether connected with the Customs or not, who will join in carrying out the plan proposed. Meanwhile I would particularly invite attention to—

a.—The general health of.................during the period reported on; the death rate amongst foreigners; and, as far as possible, a classification of the causes of death.

b.—Diseases prevalent at..........................

c.—General type of disease; peculiarities and complications encountered; special treatment demanded.

d.—Relation of disease to { Season.
Alteration in local conditions—such as drainage, etc.
Alteration in climatic conditions.

e.—Peculiar diseases; especially leprosy.

f.—Epidemics { Absence or presence.
Causes.
Course and treatment.
Fatality.

Other points, of a general or special kind, will naturally suggest themselves to medical men; what I have above called attention to will serve to fix the general scope of the undertaking. I have committed to Dr. ALEX. JAMIESON, of Shanghai, the charge of arranging the Reports for publication, so that they may be made available in a convenient form.

3.—Considering the number of places at which the Customs Inspectorate has established offices, the thousands of miles north and south and east and west over which these offices are scattered, the varieties of climate, and the peculiar conditions to which, under such different circumstances, life and health are subjected, I believe the Inspectorate, aided by its Medical Officers, can do good service in the general interest in the direction indicated; and, as already stated, I rely with confidence on the support and assistance of the Medical Officer at each port in the furtherance and perfecting of this scheme. You will hand a copy of this Circular to Dr. ...., and request him, in my name, to hand to you in future, for transmission to myself, half-yearly Reports of the kind required, for the half-years ending 31st March and 30th September—that is, for the Winter and Summer seasons.

4.—   *   *   *   *   *

I am, etc.,

(Signed)   ROBERT HART,

I. G.

THE COMMISSIONERS OF CUSTOMS,—*Newchwang,   Ningpo,*
Tientsin,   Foochow,
Chefoo,   Tamsui,
Hankow,   Tainan,
Kiukiang,   Amoy,
Chinkiang,   Swatow, and
Shanghai,   Canton.

SHANGHAI, 15th July 1894.

SIR,

In accordance with the directions of your Despatch No. 6 *A* (Returns Series) of the 24th June 1871, I now forward to the Statistical Department of the Inspectorate General of Customs, the following documents :—

Report on the Health of Wuhu for the two and a half years ended 30th September 1891, pp. 21-26.

Report on the Health of Seoul (Corea) for the year ended 30th June 1891, pp. 7-9.

Report on the Health of Swatow for the year ended 30th September 1891, pp. 4-6.

Report on the Health of Chemulpo (Corea) for the half-year ended 30th April 1891, p. 10.

Report on the Health of Kiukiang, pp. 1-3;

Report on the Health of Ichang, pp. 11, 12;

Report on the Health of Pakhoi, pp. 17, 18;

Report on the Health of Wenchow, pp. 19, 20;

Report on the Health of Shanghai, pp. 43-47; each of these referring to the half-year ended 30th September 1891.

Medical Report on Chungking, pp. 13-16.

Abdominal Hysterectomy in Japan, pp. 27-33.

The Influenza Epidemics in Foochow, 34-36.

On Mr. J. T. ROE's Theory that Influenza is Endemic in China, pp. 37-42.

I have the honour to be,

SIR,

Your obedient Servant,

R. ALEX. JAMIESON.

THE INSPECTOR GENERAL OF CUSTOMS,
PEKING.

The Contributors to this Volume are :—

GEORGE R. UNDERWOOD, M.B., C.M., L.R.C.S.Ed. .... Kiukiang.

HENRY LAYNG, M.R.C.S., L.R.C.P. .... Swatow.

J. WILES, M.R.C.S., L.S.A. .... Seoul, Corea.

E. B. LANDIS, M.D. .... Chemulpo, Corea.

E. A. ALDRIDGE, L.M.&L.R.C.P.I., M.R.C.S. .... Ichang.

JAMES H. McCARTNEY, M.D. .... Chungking.

A. SHARP DEANE, L.R.C.P.I., L.R.C.S.I. .... Pakhoi.

J. H. LOWRY, L.R.C.P.Ed., L.R.C.S.Ed. .... Wenchow.

ROBERT H. COX, L.R.C.P.I., L.R.C.S.I. .... Wuhu.

WALLACE TAYLOR, M.D. .... Osaka, Japan.

T. B. ADAM, M.D., C.M. .... Foochow.

JAMES CANTLIE, M.A., M.B., F.R.C.S. .... Hongkong.

R. ALEX. JAMIESON, M.A., M.D., M.R.C.P. .... Shanghai.

For everything enclosed within square brackets [   ], the compiler is responsible.

DR. J. H. LOWRY'S REPORT ON THE HEALTH OF WENCHOW

For the Half-year ended 30th September 1891.

FOREIGN POPULATION, WENCHOW AND DISTRICT.

Male adults	12
Female adults	6
Male children	2
Female children	2
TOTAL	22

The general health of foreigners resident at this port was only fairly good during the past six months. Every member of the Customs staff has been under treatment. The new out-door staff quarters, on Conquest Island, will, it is hoped, prove a benefit. So far, both members of the staff who live in them have suffered from malarial fever; but it is possible that the poison entered their systems during the time they lived in the former unhealthy quarters. Time will show whether the new buildings are more healthy.

The season was exceedingly wet, rain having fallen almost continuously from April to September. A glance at the meteorological table shows how large the rainfall has been.

One birth and one death occurred during the period under review.

The death was due to acute dysentery, the subject being a missionary lady brought in from an outlying district. Her case was a severe one, and she died on the second day after arrival.

On 8th September another missionary lady met with a severe accident; she fell from the city wall to the street below, a distance of from 20 to 30 feet, and received a compound fracture of the arm.

During July, when H.B.M.S. *Redpole* was stationed here, the sailors suffered much from diarrhœa and fever; they seldom went ashore, yet they had fever of a malarial type. The ship was lying in mid-river. The diarrhœa was lessened by Surgeon BRADLEY putting a veto on fruit being brought on board.

There was said to be a great deal of sickness in August and September among the native community in the city; no cases, however, came under my notice. But from what I heard, the sickness and increased mortality was due either to cholera or choleraic diarrhœa, probably the latter. I am unable to obtain any reliable details as to the mortality; so it is useless to speculate. It is not surprising that there is sickness in the city, for a privy atmosphere pervades the place. Privies and latrines are numerous in every street, and, I understand, are very profitable mercantile speculations. The city has changed a good deal since

Dr. W. W. MYERS wrote on the "Sanitary Condition of Wenchow." * No doubt the increased population has much to do with the change. The streets are no cleaner than I have observed in other Chinese cities and are very unsavoury, and, as I have already said, a privy atmosphere pervades the place, and must be deleterious to the public health. The pleasant sea breezes which Dr. MYERS speaks of do not seem now to reach us, and the poor "cathedral city," as he calls it, suffers in consequence.

The diseases observed and treated during the past six months have been :—

Remittent fever.	Dysentery.
Intermittent fever.	Bronchial catarrh.
Congestion of liver and biliary derangement.	Bubo, result of strain.
Diarrhœa.	Herpes round folds of axilla.
Eczema.	Hæmorrhoids.
Neuralgia.	Compound fracture of arm.
Cardiac palpitation.	Incised wound of hand.
Aural catarrh.	Vermes.
Hernia.	Cancer of womb.
Nerve prostration and debility.	Varnish or lacquer poisoning.

Two cases of varnish-poisoning came under my notice. They reminded me much of erysipelas. Recovery was slow, and treatment seemed useless, as I believe other observers have found it.

I append an abstract from the Customs meteorological observations taken at this port (latitude, 28° 1′ 30″ N. ; longitude, 120° 38′ 28″ 50″ E.).

METEOROLOGICAL TABLE, April to September 1891.

MONTH.	Highest Reading of Barometer.	Highest Day Reading of Thermometer.	RAINFALL.		REMARKS.
			No. of Days.	Quantity.	
	Inches	° F.		Inches	
April..........................	30.400	79	18	6.61	
May...........................	30.346	90	19	7.40	
June..........................	30.056	89	16	7.77	Several severe thunder-storms occurred, but the port has not been visited by any typhoons.
July..........................	30.026	90	17	9.56	
August	30.550	93	16	15.33	
September	30.450	94	12	8.91	

NOTE.—"An 'inch of rain' means a gallon of water spread over a surface of nearly 2 square feet, or 3,630 cubic feet = 100 tons upon an acre."— *Whitaker's Almanack*, 1891, p. 53.

* Customs *Medical Reports*, xv.

China, Imperial Maritime Customs, Medical Reports
（1891. 10. 01—1892. 09. 30）

CHINA.

IMPERIAL MARITIME CUSTOMS.

II.—SPECIAL SERIES: No. 2.

MEDICAL REPORTS,

FOR THE YEAR ENDED 30TH SEPTEMBER 1892.

43rd and 44th Issues.

PUBLISHED BY ORDER OF

The Inspector General of Customs.

SHANGHAI:

PUBLISHED AT THE STATISTICAL DEPARTMENT OF THE INSPECTORATE GENERAL OF CUSTOMS,
AND SOLD BY
KELLY & WALSH, LIMITED: SHANGHAI, HONGKONG, YOKOHAMA, AND SINGAPORE.
LONDON: P. S. KING & SON, 12 AND 14, KING STREET, WESTMINSTER, S.W.

1895.

[*Price* $1.]

INSPECTOR GENERAL'S CIRCULAR No. 19 OF 1870.

INSPECTORATE GENERAL OF CUSTOMS,

PEKING, 31st *December* 1870.

SIR,

1.—IT has been suggested to me that it would be well to take advantage of the circumstances in which the Customs Establishment is placed, to procure information with regard to disease amongst foreigners and natives in China; and I have, in consequence, come to the resolution of publishing half-yearly in collected form all that may be obtainable. If carried out to the extent hoped for, the scheme may prove highly useful to the medical profession both in China and at home, and to the public generally. I therefore look with confidence to the co-operation of the Customs Medical Officer at your port, and rely on his assisting me in this matter by framing a half-yearly report containing the result of his observations at..................upon the local peculiarities of disease, and upon diseases rarely or never encountered out of China. The facts brought forward and the opinions expressed will be arranged and published either with or without the name of the physician responsible for them, just as he may desire.

2.—The suggestions of the Customs Medical Officers at the various ports as to the points which it would be well to have especially elucidated, will be of great value in the framing of a form which will save trouble to those members of the medical profession, whether connected with the Customs or not, who will join in carrying out the plan proposed. Meanwhile I would particularly invite attention to—

a.—The general health of....................during the period reported on; the death rate amongst foreigners; and, as far as possible, a classification of the causes of death.

b.—Diseases prevalent at...........................

c.—General type of disease; peculiarities and complications encountered; special treatment demanded.

d.—Relation of disease to $\begin{cases} \text{Season.} \\ \text{Alteration in local conditions—such as drainage, etc.} \\ \text{Alteration in climatic conditions.} \end{cases}$

e.—Peculiar diseases; especially leprosy.

f.—Epidemics $\begin{cases} \text{Absence or presence.} \\ \text{Causes.} \\ \text{Course and treatment.} \\ \text{Fatality.} \end{cases}$

Other points, of a general or special kind, will naturally suggest themselves to medical men; what I have above called attention to will serve to fix the general scope of the undertaking. I have committed to Dr. ALEX. JAMIESON, of Shanghai, the charge of arranging the Reports for publication, so that they may be made available in a convenient form.

3.—Considering the number of places at which the Customs Inspectorate has established offices, the thousands of miles north and south and east and west over which these offices are scattered, the varieties of climate, and the peculiar conditions to which, under such different circumstances, life and health are subjected, I believe the Inspectorate, aided by its Medical Officers, can do good service in the general interest in the direction indicated; and, as already stated, I rely with confidence on the support and assistance of the Medical Officer at each port in the furtherance and perfecting of this scheme. You will hand a copy of this Circular to Dr. ...., and request him, in my name, to hand to you in future, for transmission to myself, half-yearly Reports of the kind required, for the half-years ending 31st March and 30th September—that is, for the Winter and Summer seasons.

4.—   *   *   *   *   *

I am, etc.,

(Signed)   ROBERT HART,
·I. G.

THE COMMISSIONERS OF CUSTOMS,—*Newchwang*,   *Ningpo*,
                              Tientsin,   *Foochow*,
                              Chefoo,   *Tamsui*,
                              Hankow,   *Tainan*,
                              Kiukiang,   *Amoy*,
                              Chinkiang,   *Swatow*, and
                              Shanghai,   *Canton*.

SHANGHAI, 1st *May* 1895.

SIR,

In accordance with the directions of your Despatch No. 6 *A* (Returns Series) of the 24th June 1871, I now forward to the Statistical Department of the Inspectorate General of Customs, the following documents :—

Report on the Health of Hoihow (Kiungchow) for the fifteen months ended 31st December 1891, pp. 1, 2.

Report on the Health of Tamsui for the two years ended 30th September 1892, pp. 20–24.

Report on the Health of Chinkiang for the year ended 31st March 1892, pp. 10–12.

Report on the Health of Swatow, pp. 13–15 ;

Report on the Health of Shanghai, pp. 27–31 ; each of these referring to the year ended 30th September 1892.

Report on the Health of Wenchow, pp. 3, 4 ;

Report on the Health of Pakhoi, pp. 5–8 ;

Report on the Health of Ichang, p. 9 ; each of these referring to the half-year ended 31st March 1892.

Report on the Health of Chefoo, pp. 16, 17 ;

Report on the Health of Ichang, pp. 18, 19 ;

Report on the Health of Wenchow, pp. 25, 26 ; each of these referring to the half-year ended 30th September 1892.

I have the honour to be,

SIR,

Your obedient Servant,

R. ALEX. JAMIESON.

THE INSPECTOR GENERAL OF CUSTOMS,
    PEKING.

The Contributors to this Volume are :—

WILLIAM KIRK, M.D., M.CH. .... Hoihow (Kiungchow)

J. H. LOWRY, L.R.C.P.Ed., L.R.C.S.Ed. .... Wenchow.

A. SHARP DEANE, L.R.C.P.I., L.R.C.S.I. .... Pakhoi.

E. A. ALDRIDGE, L.M.&L.R.C.P.I., M.R.C.S. .... Ichang.

J. A. LYNCH, M.D., M.CH. .... Chinkiang.

HENRY LAYNG, M.R.C.S., L.R.C.P. .... Swatow.

E. W. VON TUNZELMANN, M.B., M.R.C.S. .... Chefoo.

ALEXANDER RENNIE, M.B., C.M. .... Tamsui.

R. ALEX. JAMIESON, M.A., M.D., M.R.C.P. .... Shanghai.

Dr. J. H. LOWRY'S REPORT ON THE HEALTH OF WENCHOW

For the Half-year ended 31st March 1892.

THE health of foreigners resident here has been generally good during the past six months; there have been few cases of sickness attributable to climatic causes. The winter was fairly mild—certainly up to Christmas we had no serious cold weather. During February and March a thin coating of snow was noticed on the hills. The rainfall has not been so great as in the previous six months. Bronchial catarrh has been very prevalent among both foreigners and natives during the past two months, but, so far, no cases of influenza have been observed. There was no serious epidemic among the native community; chicken-pox had its sway for a time, and two foreign children were attacked.

ACCIDENTS.

"Lawn Tennis Leg."—An ardent tennis player, while playing a quiet game, received suddenly an accident to the calf of his leg, and exclaimed at once to his opponent, "You struck me." He hopped to a seat and was subsequently taken home in a chair, and I saw him shortly after. There was considerable pain in the middle of the calf, and there was a boggy feeling over the painful part. The sufferer was totally unable to put his foot to the ground. I came to the conclusion that some fibres of a muscle, probably the plantaris, had been ruptured. With rest, bandaging, etc., and the subsequent wearing of an elastic stocking, the patient was able to walk with a stick after three weeks. This case is precisely similar to the one reported by Dr. POWELL, of Ottawa, in the *Lancet* of 7th July 1883, and in vol. ii of the *Lancet*, same year, other like cases are reported. In all, the receiver of the injury at once exclaimed, "Someone struck me."

Fracture of Skull.—A Chinese boy, æt. 8 years, fell from the city wall, a distance of 30 feet, and sustained a compound fracture of the right parietal bone about the eminence, besides receiving incised wounds on the right brow and temple. He made a slow but good recovery.

Dislocation of the Wrist.—A Customs coolie, while stepping into a sampan from the jetty, slipped and fell, dislocating his left wrist. I saw him immediately after and reduced the dislocation with ease.

Incised Wounds of Face.—A blind Chinese, æt. 70, while struggling with a thief in the night, fell or was thrown down a narrow stair, receiving severe injuries to the face. There was a large, gaping wound on the chin, and the left half of the upper lip was almost torn off; there were also small incised wounds on the left cheek and brow. By careful suturing, the wounds did well, and very little deformity was left.

Eversion of Finger-nail.—A Chinese actor was bitten on the finger by one of his fellows during a quarrel. A very unhealthy inflammation followed, which necessitated the removal of the nail.

Compound Fracture of the Elbow-joint.—The missionary lady, mentioned in my last Report, who fell from the city wall and received the above injury went up to Shanghai. The surgeons under whose care she was removed a quantity of dead bone. Later—five months after the injury—it was found necessary to amputate the arm at the shoulder-joint, and she subsequently died.

The following medical and surgical cases (foreign and native) have been treated during the period under review :—

Amenorrhœa.	Dyspepsia.
Asthma.	Eversion of finger-nail.
Bronchial catarrh.	Fracture of skull.
Carcinoma of womb.*	Gonorrhœa.
Carbuncle.	Incised wounds of face.
Chicken-pox.	"Lawn tennis leg."
Congestion of liver.	Pharyngitis.
Congestion of lungs.	Phthisis.
Diarrhœa.	Remittent fever.
Dislocation of wrist-joint.	

* Case of old standing, which proved fatal in October, after much suffering.

I append an abstract from the Customs meteorological observations taken at Wenchow (latitude, 28° 1′ 30″ N.; longitude, 120° 38′ 28½″ E.).

METEOROLOGICAL TABLE, October 1891 to March 1892.

MONTH.	BAROMETER.		THERMOMETER.		RAINFALL.	
	Highest.	Lowest.	Highest.	Lowest.	No. of Days.	Quantity.
1891.	*Inches*	*Inches*	° *F.*	° *F.*		*Inches*
October	30.32	29.80	81	65	18	6.18
November	30.65	29.93	76	47	4	2.21
December	30.57	29.90	67	40	12	2.64
1892.						
January	30.60	29.90	65	38	5	0.42
February	30.50	29.75	63	38	19	5.35
March	30.40	29.75	61	38	22	8.02

Dr. J. H. LOWRY'S REPORT ON THE HEALTH OF WENCHOW

For the Half-year ended 30th September 1892.

THERE has been a good deal of sickness among foreigners during the period under review, though the heat has not been so great as during the corresponding period of last year, nor have we had so much rain. A glance at the meteorological table shows a total rainfall of 28 inches, against 55 inches in 1891, and 73 days on which rain fell, against 98.

There has been one birth (still-born), one miscarriage and one death.

Whooping-cough was very prevalent during the months of July and August, and five foreign children were attacked; one child, æt. 4, suffered severely, the cough being very persistent, lasting over three months.

Treatment was very unsatisfactory. Antipyrin—so much praised—was tried and found useless, though pushed. Bromide of ammonium gave better results, but had to be pushed almost to bromism.

There was no epidemic of cholera in the city

The following cases were treated during the six months just ended :—

Cerebral congestion.
Chronic constipation.
Diarrhœa, simple and tropical.
Dislocation of shoulder-joint (reduced).
Dysentery, acute.
Gunshot accident (shots extracted).
Hepatic congestion.

Leucorrhœa.
Lumbago.
Remittent fever.
Removal of impacted fruit-stone from rectum.
(?) Shell-fish poisoning or irritation.
Whooping-cough.
Worms.

(?) Shell-fish Poisoning or Irritation.—Two missionary gentlemen, residing in the same house, took tiffin with a neighbour at noon on 2nd June. At 8 P.M. I was summoned to see them and found both in great agony, and they had been so since 5.30, when vomiting and purging commenced, accompanied by violent colic. So severe were the symptoms that it was late in the night before I could leave my patients. In the morning I found both better, but exhausted, their abdomens tender, slight rise of temperature, bad taste in mouth. I was at a loss to know what had caused such violent gastric and abdominal disturbance, for the tiffin was simple enough. At the request of the gentleman at whose house the meal had been taken, I inspected his kitchen and cooking utensils. I found everything scrupulously clean, no copper utensils had been used and no tinned foods had been eaten. Shrimp curry was the only item on the menu that might have caused trouble. My patients had sat next each other, and were consequently helped to curry in succession; and it seemed possible that some of the shrimps were not fresh and that it fell to their lot to get them, the second man helping himself with the spoon his neighbour had just laid down. The party was a large one, and it is hardly likely that enough shrimps could have been purchased, at

this season, from the same basket ; so they were probably mixed.   Four others, including the host, partook of the same dish, and suffered no evil consequences.   No meal or drink was partaken of between the tiffin and the onset of the symptoms.

Malignant Tropical Diarrhœa.—This case ended fatally.   The patient was first taken ill on 30th August, and died 15th September; total number of days ill, including the one on which she died, 17. The case resembled most what Sir JOSEPH FAYRER describes in his *Tropical Diseases*, page 129.   Never through the sickness did the case take on either a dysenteric or enteric form.   On the 13th day a miscarriage took place and a four-month fœtus was painlessly expelled.   The patient was much worn out prior to her own illness by having had to nurse her children through prolonged whooping-cough.

I append an abstract from the Customs meteorological observations taken at Wenchow (latitude, 28° 1′ 30″ N.; longitude, 120° 38′ 28½″ E.)

METEOROLOGICAL TABLE, April to September 1892.

MONTH.	BAROMETER.		THERMOMETER.		RAINFALL.	
	Maximum.	Minimum.	Maximum.	Minimum.	No. of Days on which Rain fell.	Quantity.
	Inches	*Inches*	° F.	° F.		*Inches*
April	30.170	29.850	73	55	13	4.61
May	29.990	29.600	80	64	14	5.87
June	29.944	29.820	80	73	19	7.71
July	30.030	29.600	92	75	7	1.67
August..................	29.980	29.700	91	75	6	3.37
September...............	30.170	29.570	90	63	14	5.19

China, Imperial Maritime Customs, Medical Reports
(1892. 10. 01—1893. 09. 30)

CHINA.

IMPERIAL MARITIME CUSTOMS.

II.—SPECIAL SERIES: No. 2.

MEDICAL REPORTS,

FOR THE YEAR ENDED 30TH SEPTEMBER 1893.

45th and 46th Issues.

PUBLISHED BY ORDER OF

The Inspector General of Customs.

SHANGHAI:

PUBLISHED AT THE STATISTICAL DEPARTMENT OF THE INSPECTORATE GENERAL OF CUSTOMS,
AND SOLD BY
KELLY & WALSH, LIMITED: SHANGHAI, HONGKONG, YOKOHAMA, AND SINGAPORE.
LONDON: P. S. KING & SON, 12 AND 14, KING STREET, WESTMINSTER, S.W.

1895.

[*Price* $1.]

INSPECTOR GENERAL'S CIRCULAR No. 19 OF 1870.

INSPECTORATE GENERAL OF CUSTOMS,

PEKING, 31st December 1870.

SIR,

1.—IT has been suggested to me that it would be well to take advantage of the circumstances in which the Customs Establishment is placed, to procure information with regard to disease amongst foreigners and natives in China; and I have, in consequence, come to the resolution of publishing half-yearly in collected form all that may be obtainable. If carried out to the extent hoped for, the scheme may prove highly useful to the medical profession both in China and at home, and to the public generally. I therefore look with confidence to the co-operation of the Customs Medical Officer at your port, and rely on his assisting me in this matter by framing a half-yearly report containing the result of his observations at.................upon the local peculiarities of disease, and upon diseases rarely or never encountered out of China. The facts brought forward and the opinions expressed will be arranged and published either with or without the name of the physician responsible for them, just as he may desire.

2.—The suggestions of the Customs Medical Officers at the various ports as to the points which it would be well to have especially elucidated, will be of great value in the framing of a form which will save trouble to those members of the medical profession, whether connected with the Customs or not, who will join in carrying out the plan proposed. Meanwhile I would particularly invite attention to—

a.—The general health of....................during the period reported on; the death rate amongst foreigners; and, as far as possible, a classification of the causes of death.

b.—Diseases prevalent at...........................

c.—General type of disease; peculiarities and complications encountered; special treatment demanded.

d.—Relation of disease to { Season. / Alteration in local conditions—such as drainage, etc. / Alteration in climatic conditions.

e.—Peculiar diseases; especially leprosy.

f.—Epidemics { Absence or presence. / Causes. / Course and treatment. / Fatality.

Other points, of a general or special kind, will naturally suggest themselves to medical men; what I have above called attention to will serve to fix the general scope of the undertaking. I have committed to Dr. ALEX. JAMIESON, of Shanghai, the charge of arranging the Reports for publication, so that they may be made available in a convenient form.

3.—Considering the number of places at which the Customs Inspectorate has established offices, the thousands of miles north and south and east and west over which these offices are scattered, the varieties of climate, and the peculiar conditions to which, under such different circumstances, life and health are subjected, I believe the Inspectorate, aided by its Medical Officers, can do good service in the general interest in the direction indicated; and, as already stated, I rely with confidence on the support and assistance of the Medical Officer at each port in the furtherance and perfecting of this scheme. You will hand a copy of this Circular to Dr. ...., and request him, in my name, to hand to you in future, for transmission to myself, half-yearly Reports of the kind required, for the half-years ending 31st March and 30th September—that is, for the Winter and Summer seasons.

4.—   *   *   *   *   *

I am, etc.,

(Signed)   ROBERT HART,
I. G.

THE COMMISSIONERS OF CUSTOMS,—*Newchwang,   Ningpo,*
Tientsin,   Foochow,
Chefoo,   Tamsui,
Hankow,   Tainan,
Kiukiang,   Amoy,
Chinkiang,   Swatow, and
Shanghai,   Canton.

SHANGHAI, 15*th May* 1895.

SIR,

  IN accordance with the directions of your Despatch No. 6 *A* (Returns Series) of the 24th June 1871, I now forward to the Statistical Department of the Inspectorate General of Customs, the following documents :—

  Report on the Health of Chungking, pp. 2, 3 ;

  Report on the Health of Pakhoi, pp. 8–11 ; each of these referring to the year ended 31st March 1893.

  Report on the Health of Tientsin, p. 1 ;

  Report on the Health of Wenchow, p. 21 ; each of these referring to the half-year ended 31st March 1893.

  Report on the Health of Wuhu for the eighteen months ended 31st March 1893, pp. 4–7.

  Report on the Health of Chefoo, pp. 22, 23 ;

  Report on the Health of Shanghai, pp. 34–38 ; each of these referring to the year ended 30th September 1893.

  Report on the Health of Ichang, pp. 24, 25 ;

  Report on the Health of Kiukiang, pp. 26–28 ;

  Report on the Health of Wuhu, pp. 29, 30 ;

  Report on the Health of Wenchow, p. 31 ;

  Report on the Health of Foochow, pp. 32, 33 ; each of these referring to the half-year ended 30th September 1893.

  Notes on Diseases in North Formosa, pp. 12–20.

I have the honour to be,

SIR,

Your obedient Servant,

R. ALEX. JAMIESON.

THE INSPECTOR GENERAL OF CUSTOMS,
  PEKING.

The Contributors to this Volume are :—

A. IRWIN, F.R.C.S.I. .... Tientsin.

JAMES H. McCARTNEY, M.D. .... Chungking.

ROBERT H. COX, L.R.C.P.I., L.R.C.S.I. .... Wuhu.

A. SHARP DEANE, L.R.C.P.I., L.R.C.S.I. .... Pakhoi.

ALEXANDER RENNIE, M.B., C.M. .... Tamsui.

J. H. LOWRY, L.R.C.P.Ed., L.R.C.S.Ed. .... Wenchow.

E. W. VON TUNZELMANN, M.B., M.R.C.S. .... Chefoo.

E. A. ALDRIDGE, L.M.&L.R.C.P.I., M.R.C.S, ... Ichang.

GEORGE R. UNDERWOOD, M.B., C.M., L.R.C.S,Ed. .... Kiukiang.

T. RENNIE, M.D., CH.M. .... Foochow.

R. ALEX. JAMIESON, M.A., M.D., M.R.C.P. .... Shanghai.

Dr. J. H. LOWRY'S REPORT ON THE HEALTH OF WENCHOW

For the Half-year ended 31st March 1893.

In spite of the very severe winter, there has not been a great deal of sickness among the foreign residents of this port. Not for over 20 years has the district experienced such cold weather. The Chinese suffered severely, and I believe there were many cases of frostbite, though only two came under my notice.

There has been one death, from enteric fever.

The following cases have been under treatment:—

Amputation of fingers.	Frostbites.
Bronchial catarrh.	Palmar abscess.
Cardiac failure.	Pleuritis.
Chronic dysentery.	Pulmonary congestion.
Enteric fever.	Stabbing wounds of face and back.

Enteric Fever.—The patient was a chief petty officer of H.B.M.S. *Linnet*. He was landed from the ship on the 26th January, having been ill since the 10th January, and he died on the 2nd February. No postmortem was made, but from the collapse at the end it was clear that perforation had taken place.

Appended is an abstract from the Customs meteorological observations taken at Wenchow (latitude, 28° 1′ 30″ N.; longitude, 120° 38′ 28¼″ E.).

Meteorological Table, October 1892 to March 1893.

Month.	Barometer.		Thermometer.		Rainfall.	
	Maximum.	Minimum.	Maximum.	Minimum.	No. of Days on which Rain fell.	Quantity.
1892.	*Inches*	*Inches*	° F.	° F.		*Inches*
October	30.336	29.890	80	60	2	2.05
November	30.486	29.670	76	42	15	2.60
December	30.500	30.030	63	36	5	1.70
1893.						
January	30.500	29.950	63	25	5	1.67
February	30.490	30.028	59	33	14	5.06
March	30.500	29.820	70	40	18	4.01

Remarks.—15th and 16th January: snow, 1 inch. 12th and 14th February: snow, 2 inches.

Dr. J. H. LOWRY'S REPORT ON THE HEALTH OF WENCHOW

For the Half-year ended 30th September 1893.

THE health of foreigners was good during the past six months, though the summer has been a trying one, owing to the damp heat which prevailed. During September there was much sickness among the natives, chiefly diarrhœa and fevers.

The following cases have been under treatment:—

Burns of hands.	Incised wound of scrotum.
Diarrhœa.	Remittent fever.
Hepatic congestion.	Uric acid calculus.
Gout.	Worms.

Incised Wound of Scrotum.—In May a somewhat unusual case came under my care. A native was brought to my house in a chair, suffering from a wound in the scrotum, and he had evidently lost much blood, as his clothes were saturated. His story was that while hanging up some clothes he fell from the wall and was hurt. Subsequent inquiries changed the tale. The patient, after having drunk a fair amount of samshu, repaired to one of the brothels of the city, and there received from one of the inmates the wound he showed. After cleansing the parts thoroughly, I found a clean incised wound, measuring 1¼ inch. Five sutures were required to bring the edges together. Fortunately there was no injury to testicle or penis. Under iodoform dressings the wound healed kindly.

I append an abstract from the Customs meteorological observations taken at Wenchow (latitude, 28° 1′ 30″ N.; longitude, 120° 38′ 28½″ E.).

METEOROLOGICAL TABLE, April to September 1893.

MONTH.	BAROMETER.		THERMOMETER.		RAINFALL.	
	Maximum.	Minimum.	Maximum.	Minimum.	No. of Days on which Rain fell.	Quantity.
	Inches	*Inches*	° F.	° F.		*Inches*
April	30.340	29.650	74	50	18	3.53
May	30.200	29.740	81	60	13	3.32
June	30.054	29.730	87	60	17	8.40
July	29.940	29.568	91	74	11	6.05
August	30.036	29.670	90	75	15	6.17
September	30.140	29.394	93	75	19	11.11

China, Imperial Maritime Customs, Medical Reports
(1893. 10. 01—1894. 09. 30)

CHINA.

IMPERIAL MARITIME CUSTOMS.

II.—SPECIAL SERIES: No. 2.

MEDICAL REPORTS,

FOR THE YEAR ENDED 30TH SEPTEMBER 1894.

47th and 48th Issues.

PUBLISHED BY ORDER OF

The Inspector General of Customs.

SHANGHAI:

PUBLISHED AT THE STATISTICAL DEPARTMENT OF THE INSPECTORATE GENERAL OF CUSTOMS,

AND SOLD BY

KELLY & WALSH, LIMITED: SHANGHAI, HONGKONG, YOKOHAMA, AND SINGAPORE.

LONDON: P. S. KING & SON, 12 AND 14, KING STREET, WESTMINSTER, S.W.

1895.

[*Price* $1.]

INSPECTOR GENERAL'S CIRCULAR No. 19 OF 1870.

INSPECTORATE GENERAL OF CUSTOMS,

PEKING, 31st December 1870.

SIR,

1.—IT has been suggested to me that it would be well to take advantage of the circumstances in which the Customs Establishment is placed, to procure information with regard to disease amongst foreigners and natives in China; and I have, in consequence, come to the resolution of publishing half-yearly in collected form all that may be obtainable. If carried out to the extent hoped for, the scheme may prove highly useful to the medical profession both in China and at home, and to the public generally. I therefore look with confidence to the co-operation of the Customs Medical Officer at your port, and rely on his assisting me in this matter by framing a half-yearly report containing the result of his observations at................upon the local peculiarities of disease, and upon diseases rarely or never encountered out of China. The facts brought forward and the opinions expressed will be arranged and published either with or without the name of the physician responsible for them, just as he may desire.

2.—The suggestions of the Customs Medical Officers at the various ports as to the points which it would be well to have especially elucidated, will be of great value in the framing of a form which will save trouble to those members of the medical profession, whether connected with the Customs or not, who will join in carrying out the plan proposed. Meanwhile I would particularly invite attention to—

a.—The general health of....................during the period reported on; the death rate amongst foreigners; and, as far as possible, a classification of the causes of death.

b.—Diseases prevalent at..........................

c.—General type of disease; peculiarities and complications encountered; special treatment demanded.

d.—Relation of disease to { Season. Alteration in local conditions—such as drainage, etc. Alteration in climatic conditions.

e.—Peculiar diseases; especially leprosy.

f.—Epidemics { Absence or presence. Causes. Course and treatment. Fatality.

Other points, of a general or special kind, will naturally suggest themselves to medical men; what I have above called attention to will serve to fix the general scope of the undertaking.

3.—Considering the number of places at which the Customs Inspectorate has established offices, the thousands of miles north and south and east and west over which these offices are scattered, the varieties of climate, and the peculiar conditions to which, under such different circumstances, life and health are subjected, I believe the Inspectorate, aided by its Medical Officers, can do good service in the general interest in the direction indicated; and, as already stated, I rely with confidence on the support and assistance of the Medical Officer at each port in the furtherance and perfecting of this scheme. You will hand a copy of this Circular to Dr. ...., and request him, in my name, to hand to you in future, for transmission to myself, half-yearly Reports of the kind required, for the half-years ending 31st March and 30th September—that is, for the Winter and Summer seasons.

4.—   *   *   *   *   *

I am, etc.,

(Signed)   ROBERT HART,
I. G.

THE COMMISSIONERS OF CUSTOMS,—*Newchwang*, *Ningpo*,
Tientsin, *Foochow*,
Chefoo, *Tamsui*,
Hankow, *Tainan*,
Kiukiang, *Amoy*,
Chinkiang, *Swatow*, and
Shanghai, *Canton*.

TABLE OF CONTENTS.

The Contributors to this Volume are :—

C. C. DE BURGH DALY, M.B., B.CH. .... Newchwang.

JAMES H. McCARTNEY, M.D. .... Chungking.

E. A. ALDRIDGE, L.M.&L.R.C.P.I., M.R.C.S. .... Ichang.

ROBERT H. COX, L.R.C.P.I., L.R.C.S.I. .... Wuhu.

JOHN FRANCIS MOLYNEUX, M.R.C.S., L.R.C.P.Ed. .... Ningpo.

J. H. LOWRY, L.R.C.P.Ed., L.R.C.S.Ed. .... Wenchow.

ALEXANDER RENNIE, M.A., M.B., C.M. .... Canton.

A. SHARP DEANE, L.R.C.P.I., L.R.C.S.I. .... Pakhoi.

E. B. LANDIS, M.D. .... Chemulpo (Jenchuan), Corea.

J. F. WALES, B.A., M.D., CH.M. .... Canton.

J. L. MICHOUD, M.D. .... Mengtsz.

E. H. BALDOCK, M.R.C.S., L.R.C.P. .... Seoul (Corea).

R. ALEX. JAMIESON, M.A., M.D., M.R.C.P. .... Shanghai.

Dr. J. H. LOWRY'S REPORT ON THE HEALTH OF WENCHOW

For the Half-year ended 31st March 1894.

THE general health of the foreign community in this port and district, now numbering 29, has been very good during the past six months. The winter was very mild compared with that of last year, the only cold weather experienced being towards the end of December and first part of January. From October to early in February a very serious drought lasted, and caused much misery among the natives. Enteric fever was said to be rife—a statement hardly to be doubted, seeing that the poorer classes were in desperation for water and took it from where they could get it, even when it was little better than cesspool water.

Owing to the prevalence of small-pox in Shanghai, I vaccinated a number of adults and children. Late in January Dr. ALFRED HOGG, of Aberdeen, arrived here to establish a hospital and dispensary in connexion with the United Methodist Free Church Mission; his services will be greatly appreciated by the native community, and there is a large field for surgical work.

I give a list of the more serious cases that came under my treatment:—

Amenorrhœa.

Blood-poisoning.

Bronchitis.

Diarrhœa.

Influenza.

Remittent fever.

Sprain of shoulder, result of heavy fall.

Tonsillitis, acute, with abscess.

Appended is an abstract from the Customs meteorological observations taken at this port (latitude, 28° 1′ 30″ N.; longitude, 120° 38′ 28½″ E.).

METEOROLOGICAL TABLE, October 1893 to March 1894.

MONTH.	Highest Reading of Barometer.	THERMOMETER.		RAINFALL.	
		Highest by Day.	Highest by Night.	No. of Days on which Rain fell.	Quantity.
1893.	*Inches*	° F.	° F.		*Inches*
October	30.400	75	58	9	4.60
November	30.430	65	48	...	...
December	30.490	66	37	3	0.28
1894.					
January	30.400	57	35	13	3.09
February	30.500	64	38	9	1.20
March	30.500	68	42	17	6.62

Dr. J. H. Lowry's Report on the Health of Wenchow

For the Half-year ended 30th September 1894.

Foreign Population, Wenchow and District.

Male adults	15
Female adults	11
Male children	1
Female children	2
Total	29

The summer has been trying, and there was a good deal of sickness among foreigners. As a slight indication of the amount of sickness, I made 110 visits at the houses of the sick during the months of July, August and September. Among the natives there has been the usual diarrhœa, choleraic diarrhœa, dysentery, and a great deal of fever of a malarial type.

From April to September Dr. Hogg treated, at the dispensary of the United Methodist Free Church Mission, 3,424 medical and surgical cases. Of these, 2,117 were new cases. No record was kept of patients treated up country and on non-dispensary days and hours. During the building of the new British Consulate several cases of accident occurred among the workmen, and they were promptly looked after by Dr. Hogg.

The diseases that I have observed and treated during the past six months have been :—

Choleraic diarrhœa.
Congestion of liver and biliary derangement.
Conjunctivitis.
Constipation.
Diarrhœa, simple and tropical.
Entozoa, intestinal.
Gout.
Hæmaturia.

Hæmorrhoids.
Incised wound of thumb, with sprained arm (result of heavy fall on Customs Jetty).
Remittent fever.
Rheumatic gout.
Sprue or psilosis.
Uterine vomiting (pregnancy).

I append an abstract from the Customs meteorological observations taken at this port.

Meteorological Table, April to September 1894.

Month.	Highest Reading of Barometer.	Highest Day Reading of Thermometer.	Rainfall		Remarks.
			No. of Days.	Quantity.	
	Inches	° *F.*		*Inches*	
April	30.100	75	18	7.20	
May	30.200	78	21	9.05	
June	30.000	86	16	11.05	Typhoon on the 29th June; lowest barometer 28.950.
July	29.980	89	4	0.39	
August	29.984	94	8	4.67	Typhoon on the 3rd August; lowest barometer 29.250.
September	30.130	89	10	3.34	

China, Imperial Maritime Customs, Medical Reports
(1894. 10. 01—1895. 09. 30)

CHINA.

IMPERIAL MARITIME CUSTOMS.

II.—SPECIAL SERIES: No. 2.

MEDICAL REPORTS,

FOR THE YEAR ENDED 30TH SEPTEMBER 1895.

49th and 50th Issues.

PUBLISHED BY ORDER OF

The Inspector General of Customs.

SHANGHAI:
PUBLISHED AT THE STATISTICAL DEPARTMENT OF THE INSPECTORATE GENERAL OF CUSTOMS,
AND SOLD BY
KELLY & WALSH, LIMITED: SHANGHAI, HONGKONG, YOKOHAMA, AND SINGAPORE.
LONDON: P. S. KING & SON, 12 AND 14, KING STREET, WESTMINSTER, S.W.

Price $1.]

1896.

INSPECTOR GENERAL'S CIRCULAR No. 19 OF 1870.

INSPECTORATE GENERAL OF CUSTOMS,

PEKING, 31st December 1870.

SIR,

1.—It has been suggested to me that it would be well to take advantage of the circumstances in which the Customs Establishment is placed, to procure information with regard to disease amongst foreigners and natives in China; and I have, in consequence, come to the resolution of publishing half-yearly in collected form all that may be obtainable. If carried out to the extent hoped for, the scheme may prove highly useful to the medical profession both in China and at home, and to the public generally. I therefore look with confidence to the co-operation of the Customs Medical Officer at your port, and rely on his assisting me in this matter by framing a half-yearly report containing the result of his observations at..................upon the local peculiarities of disease, and upon diseases rarely or never encountered out of China. The facts brought forward and the opinions expressed will be arranged and published either with or without the name of the physician responsible for them, just as he may desire.

2.—The suggestions of the Customs Medical Officers at the various ports as to the points which it would be well to have especially elucidated, will be of great value in the framing of a form which will save trouble to those members of the medical profession, whether connected with the Customs or not, who will join in carrying out the plan proposed. Meanwhile I would particularly invite attention to—

a.—The general health of.....................during the period reported on; the death rate amongst foreigners; and, as far as possible, a classification of the causes of death.

b.—Diseases prevalent at...........................

c.—General type of disease; peculiarities and complications encountered; special treatment demanded.

d.—Relation of disease to $\left\{\begin{array}{l}\text{Season.}\\ \text{Alteration in local conditions—such as drainage, etc.}\\ \text{Alteration in climatic conditions.}\end{array}\right.$

e.—Peculiar diseases; especially leprosy.

f.—Epidemics $\left\{\begin{array}{l}\text{Absence or presence.}\\ \text{Causes.}\\ \text{Course and treatment.}\\ \text{Fatality.}\end{array}\right.$

Other points, of a general or special kind, will naturally suggest themselves to medical men; what I have above called attention to will serve to fix the general scope of the undertaking.

* * * * *

3.—Considering the number of places at which the Customs Inspectorate has established offices, the thousands of miles north and south and east and west over which these offices are scattered, the varieties of climate, and the peculiar conditions to which, under such different circumstances, life and health are subjected, I believe the Inspectorate, aided by its Medical Officers, can do good service in the general interest in the direction indicated; and, as already stated, I rely with confidence on the support and assistance of the Medical Officer at each port in the furtherance and perfecting of this scheme. You will hand a copy of this Circular to Dr. ...., and request him, in my name, to hand to you in future, for transmission to myself, half-yearly Reports of the kind required, for the half-years ending 31st March and 30th September—that is, for the Winter and Summer seasons.

4.—   *   *   *   *   *

I am, etc.,

(Signed)   ROBERT HART,

_I. G._

THE COMMISSIONERS OF CUSTOMS,—_Newchwang,_   _Shanghai,_
Tientsin,   _Ningpo,_
Chefoo,   _Foochow,_
Hankow,   _Amoy,_
Kiukiang,   _Swatow,_ and
Chinkiang,   _Canton._

TABLE OF CONTENTS.

The Contributors to this Volume are :—

C. C. DE BURGH DALY, M.B., B.CH. .... Newchwang.

E. W. VON TUNZELMANN, M.B., M.R.C.S. .... Chefoo.

JAMES H. McCARTNEY, M.D. .... Chungking.

E. RUEL JELLISON, M.D. .... Wuhu.

J. A. LYNCH, M.D., M.CH. .... Chinkiang.

JOHN FRANCIS MOLYNEUX, M.R.C.S., L.R.C.P.Ed. .... Ningpo.

J. H. LOWRY, L.R.C.P.Ed., L.R.C.S.Ed. .... Wenchow.

ALFRED HOGG, M.A., M.B., C.M. ....   ,,

T. RENNIE, M.D., CH.M. .... Foochow.

G. S. .... Lappa.

LEOPOLD G. HILL, M.R.C.S., L.R.C.P. .... Pakhoi.

J. J. DELAY, M.D. .... Lungchow.

J. L. MICHOUD, M.D. .... Mengtsz.

Dr. J. H. Lowry's Report on the Health of Wenchow

For the Half-year ended 31st March 1895.

The health of foreigners during the past half-year has been fairly good. One birth (still-born) and one death have to be recorded. From December to March a severe epidemic of small-pox prevailed in the city and suburbs; the mortality is said to have been very high, chiefly among children, but towards the end of the epidemic adults of both sexes were attacked. It is impossible, as I have found at other ports, to get any reliable information as to the death rate. During the outbreak of bubonic plague at Pakhoi in 1882 I found by inquiring at the coffin shops I was able to make a fair estimate, but here, in a much larger city, this means is not reliable. I have inquired at the Magistrate's yamên, and though that office keeps no official record, it estimates that 4,000 persons died from small-pox. I think, however, from other sources I am justified in stating that about 2,000 died, including adults and children. Strange to say, during December and January an epidemic of measles was also prevalent.

One European, a priest of the Lazarist Mission, contracted small-pox while ministering to some of his folk suffering from the disease. His case ran a simple course and was of the discrete variety. There were no complications and there was no subsequent disfigurement.

In November a case of bubonic plague was discovered by Dr. Hogg on board a steamer that entered from Amoy. The man was not landed, and died after the ship left the port.

The European death above referred to was the result of sprue or psilosis, the subject being a lady who had long suffered from the disease. She contracted it in 1890 at Canton, went to England from there in the same year and was under the care of Dr. Thin, of London, until the autumn of 1893, when she returned to China and placed herself under the treatment of Mr. Peter Sys, of Shanghai. In July 1894 she came under my care, but in spite of every form of treatment the disease made steady headway, and she died in February of this year.

Sprue or psilosis is one of the most formidable tropical diseases we have to deal with. Many of the cases, if taken in time, i.e., sent to Europe and put on strict diet (milk), do well and recover; but again we have them like the case so recently under my observation, where, in spite of change of climate, diet, hygiene, and drugs, the disease makes steady progress to the end.

Dr. Thin's researches on the disease are and have been very valuable. Sir Joseph Fayrer, in his recent article on "Tropical Diarrhœa" in Davidson's *Hygiene and Diseases of Warm Climates* (1893), classifies sprue under this heading, and Dr. Begg, of Hankow, claims that it should be the same *—not a distinct disease. All, I think, agree that there is some special organism at work in the intestinal tract, how brought about we are not positive. Dr. Begg's lines of treatment are, I think, right, but so far we have not enough proof that santonin is the drug. My patient was twice put under the treatment suggested by Dr. Begg, dose and *régime* being followed out exactly. It is true, however, that that treatment was only tried late in the disease, when atrophy had set in and intestinal digestion had long since

* Customs *Medical Reports*, xxxiv.

ceased. The extreme emaciation and night sweats of my patient reminded me much of phthisis, but in the sprue case there was the absence of cough and sputa—replaced by the frequent bowel purging and sore tongue.

A case of puerperal eclampsia occurred in a European, and, though not due in any way to climatic causes, is worthy of mention.

X., a multipara whose confinement was due in three weeks, was suddenly seized on the night of 5th November with eclampsia; unconsciousness followed. Under chloroform the convulsions ceased towards morning, but on the night of the 6th recurred. On the 7th she was free from them, but was still comatose, and during the evening of the same day she was painlessly delivered, without assistance, of a still-born child. Consciousness slowly returned after the birth of the child, there was no recurrence of the convulsions, and the patient made a slow but good recovery. There was no history of kidney trouble, though during September swelled legs and feet had been noticed, which I at the time put down to uterine pressure. As there was nothing to indicate that the eclampsia was due to uræmic poisoning, it was treated on the lines that the disease was a purely functional affection or acute peripheral epilepsy, the administration of chloroform being supplemented by chloral and bromide in moderate doses.

It is hoped that the pathology of this disease will soon be cleared up, considering the high mortality. SPIEGELBERG says that out of every three or four women attacked one dies. I am deeply indebted to Dr. HOGG, of this port, for valuable assistance in the above case.

Measles occurred in a European child, æt. 3. The rash was more profuse and extensive than is usually observed in the European variety, and a flea-bitten appearance of the skin was noticed in some regions. The highest temperature was 103°.2, and there was no fall on the appearance of the eruption. The fever assumed a remittent type all through. The rash did not finally disappear until the 10th day. Itching and tingling were intense from the first—preventing sleep.

The diseases that I have observed and treated during the past six months have been :—

Conjunctivitis.
Ecchymosis of conjunctiva.
Hæmoptysis.
Hæmorrhoids.
Lymphadenitis.
Puerperal eclampsia.

Remittent fever.
Ruteola.
Sprue or psilosis.
Tonsillitis.
Variola.

I append an abstract from the Customs meteorological observations taken at this port.

METEOROLOGICAL TABLE, October 1894 to March 1895.

MONTH.	Highest Reading of Barometer.	Highest Day Reading of Thermometer.	RAINFALL.		REMARKS.
			No. of Days.	Quantity.	
1894.	*Inches.*	° *F.*		*Inches.*	
October	30.270	84	8	3.40	
November	30.400	73	9	0.80	
December	30.540	66	8	0.64	
1895.					
January	30.450	65	13	0.91	Hail and snow, 12th January; 1 inch of snow, 14th January.
February	30.450	66	11	3.49	
March	30.480	75	14	4.21	Thunder, lightning, rain, hail, and snow, 17th March.

Dr. ALFRED HOGG'S REPORT ON THE HEALTH OF WENCHOW

For the Half-year ended 30th September 1895.

Owing to the departure of Dr. J. H. Lowry for Europe, he has left to me, his successor, the completion of the health report for the past six months. The health of the foreigners during that period has not been good, and much sickness prevailed among the natives.

Although the average temperature during the summer was not specially high, yet the period of hot weather was long and sustained, with few intermissions; and as for a large part of that time the atmosphere was humid, close, and oppressive, the hot season was felt by the foreign residents to be particularly trying and enervating. Heavy rains alternated with periods of dry weather, during which the canals and wells got very dry or low, and as the natives largely resort to canal water when well water is scarce, infectious disease had abundant opportunity to spread, and great mortality from cholera resulted.

In the foreign community one birth and two deaths have to be recorded. Of the latter, one was that of a lady who had been resident in the port for about four years. She died at sea, while being removed to Shanghai, from cardiac failure following on heat apoplexy.

The other death was that of a missionary's infant son, who suffered from dyspepsia and was brought to the city by the father for medical consultation. The child was improving under treatment when he was suddenly seized with severe diarrhœa, abdominal pain, and collapse, and died in 20 hours. The fact that four or five Chinese in the same compound showed identical symptoms, with a fatal termination in most of the cases, made it plain that the cause was Asiatic cholera. How the child became infected could not be traced.

Among foreigners, the cases that came up for treatment comprised :—

Diarrhœa.	Anæmia.
Remittent fever.	Fatty degeneration of heart.
Rheumatic gout.	Acute congestion of the liver.
Bronchial catarrh.	Acute and chronic tonsillitis and pharyngitis.
Gout.	Cholera.
Conjunctivitis.	Otitis.

A considerable number of serious cases among Chinese were also treated.

One was a case of dysentery in a cook in foreign employ. The disease started during his master's absence from the city, and was allowed to progress for a day or two before medical aid was sought. Notwithstanding treatment by ipecacuanha in large doses, the case terminated fatally.

Another man came with a bullet lying in his left temple, the result of a skirmish with pirates three months previously. The bullet had struck him on the forehead and nearly penetrated to the brain, then travelled round, and lodged close to the ear. It was extracted, and rather profuse hæmorrhage from a branch of the temporal followed, ligature of the vessel being managed with difficulty, owing to the soft, friable nature of the adjoining tissues. The wound healed well.

A severe bullet wound in the forearm, a large burn on the arm and forearm from a gunpowder explosion, and a huge scalp wound were conspicuous among a large number of minor and major ailments treated at the dispensary of the Methodist Free Church Mission.

I append an abstract from the Customs meteorological observations taken at this port.

METEOROLOGICAL TABLE, April to September 1895.

MONTH.	Highest Reading of Barometer.	Highest Reading of Thermometer.	RAINFALL		REMARKS.
			No. of Days.	Quantity.	
	Inches.	° *F.*		*Inches.*	
April	30.040	79	17	4·54	3rd, 4th, 7th, and 29th thunder and lightning.
May	30.300	81	24	8.25	19 days fog.
June....................	30.050	92	7	2.40	10 days fog.
July	29.990	92	16	6.40	6 days thunder and lightning.
August	29.974	93	9	8.47	9 days thunder and lightning.
September................	30.180	90	13	5.13	8 days fog. Heavy gale of wind on the 5th; lowest reading of barometer at 3 P.M., 29.368.

China, Imperial Maritime Customs, Medical Reports
(1895. 10. 01—1896. 03. 31)

CHINA.

IMPERIAL MARITIME CUSTOMS.

II.—SPECIAL SERIES: No. 2.

MEDICAL REPORTS,

FOR THE HALF-YEAR ENDED 31st MARCH 1896.

51st Issue.

PUBLISHED BY ORDER OF

The Inspector General of Customs.

SHANGHAI:
PUBLISHED AT THE STATISTICAL DEPARTMENT OF THE INSPECTORATE GENERAL OF CUSTOMS,
AND SOLD BY
KELLY & WALSH, LIMITED: SHANGHAI, HONGKONG, YOKOHAMA, AND SINGAPORE.
LONDON: P. S. KING & SON, 12 AND 14, KING STREET, WESTMINSTER, S.W.
1897.

[*Price* $1.]

INSPECTOR GENERAL'S CIRCULAR No. 19 OF 1870.

INSPECTORATE GENERAL OF CUSTOMS,

PEKING, 31st December 1870.

SIR,

1.—IT has been suggested to me that it would be well to take advantage of the circumstances in which the Customs Establishment is placed, to procure information with regard to disease amongst foreigners and natives in China; and I have, in consequence, come to the resolution of publishing half-yearly in collected form all that may be obtainable. If carried out to the extent hoped for, the scheme may prove highly useful to the medical profession both in China and at home, and to the public generally. I therefore look with confidence to the co-operation of the Customs Medical Officer at your port, and rely on his assisting me in this matter by framing a half-yearly report containing the result of his observations at..................upon the local peculiarities of disease, and upon diseases rarely or never encountered out of China. The facts brought forward and the opinions expressed will be arranged and published either with or without the name of the physician responsible for them, just as he may desire.

2.—The suggestions of the Customs Medical Officers at the various ports as to the points which it would be well to have especially elucidated, will be of great value in the framing of a form which will save trouble to those members of the medical profession, whether connected with the Customs or not, who will join in carrying out the plan proposed. Meanwhile I would particularly invite attention to—

a.—The general health of....................during the period reported on; the death rate amongst foreigners; and, as far as possible, a classification of the causes of death.

b.—Diseases prevalent at...........................

c.—General type of disease; peculiarities and complications encountered; special treatment demanded.

d.—Relation of disease to $\begin{cases} \text{Season.} \\ \text{Alteration in local conditions—such as drainage, etc.} \\ \text{Alteration in climatic conditions.} \end{cases}$

e.—Peculiar diseases; especially leprosy.

f.—Epidemics $\begin{cases} \text{Absence or presence.} \\ \text{Causes.} \\ \text{Course and treatment.} \\ \text{Fatality.} \end{cases}$

Other points, of a general or special kind, will naturally suggest themselves to medical men; what I have above called attention to will serve to fix the general scope of the undertaking.

* * * * *

3.—Considering the number of places at which the Customs Inspectorate has established offices, the thousands of miles north and south and east and west over which these offices are scattered, the varieties of climate, and the peculiar conditions to which, under such different circumstances, life and health are subjected, I believe the Inspectorate, aided by its Medical Officers, can do good service in the general interest in the direction indicated; and, as already stated, I rely with confidence on the support and assistance of the Medical Officer at each port in the furtherance and perfecting of this scheme. You will hand a copy of this Circular to Dr. ...., and request him, in my name, to hand to you in future, for transmission to myself, half-yearly Reports of the kind required, for the half-years ending 31st March and 30th September—that is, for the Winter and Summer seasons.

4.—   *   *   *   *   *

I am, etc.,

(Signed)   ROBERT HART,

I. G.

THE COMMISSIONERS OF CUSTOMS,—*Newchwang,   Shanghai,*
Tientsin,   Ningpo,
Chefoo,   Foochow,
Hankow,   Amoy,
Kiukiang,   Swatow, and
Chinkiang,   Canton.

TABLE OF CONTENTS.

The Contributors to this Volume are :—

J. J. MATIGNON, M.D... Peking.

C. C. DE BURGH DALY, M.B., B.CH. .... Newchwang.

JAMES H. McCARTNEY, M.D.. Chungking.

JOHN D. THOMSON, M.B., C.M. .... Hankow.

GEORGE R. UNDERWOOD, M.B., C.M., L.R.C.S.Ed. .... Kiukiang.

E. H. HART, M.D. .... Wuhu.

ALFRED HOGG, M.A., M.B., C.M. .... Wenchow.

HENRY LAYNG, M.R.C.S., L.R.C.P. .... Swatow.

H. M. McCANDLISS, M.D. .... Hoihow (Kiungchow).

Dr. ALFRED HOGG'S REPORT ON THE HEALTH OF WENCHOW

For the Half-year ended 31st March 1896.

DURING the period under review the health of the foreign community has been very good, except in October.

In the summer there was a severe outbreak of cholera in and around the city, which lasted till the end of October; but the advent of cooler weather, and some heavy showers to replenish the stagnant canals and wells, resulted in the disappearance of this scourge, but not until four foreigners and a large number of natives had fallen victims to it.

The infection somehow gained entrance into one of the mission compounds here, and manifested its presence by carrying off a European infant and three Chinese schoolgirls.

Immediately afterwards one of the missionaries in the compound was attacked. The symptoms were at first amenable to treatment, and great hopes were entertained of his recovery; but the shock to the system was too severe, and he succumbed in four days.

His wife was also seized, on the second day of his illness, and, in spite of prompt attention, died in 40 hours.

Another colleague took ill on Sunday morning, collapsed in a few hours, and expired within 24 hours.

In connexion with these cases I have to record my grateful thanks to Dr. J. H. LOWRY, of the Customs here, who had fortunately been detained by the non-arrival of the steamer, and also to Dr. PENNY, of H.B.M.S. *Firebrand*, which was then in port. Both these gentlemen rendered valuable assistance in the work of nursing and attending the patients.

Among other cases in the foreign community I attended the following:—

Bronchial catarrh.	Dyspepsia.
Malarial fever.	Tonsillitis.
Insomnia.	Prolapsus ani.

One lady had a severe attack of intermittent fever, with pulmonary complications, and, owing to delay in seeking advice and treatment, the case for a time assumed a somewhat serious aspect, but ended satisfactorily.

A large number of Chinese have been seen and prescribed for at the Free Methodist Dispensary. Pulmonary diseases, especially phthisis, seem to be largely prevalent among them.

I append an abstract from the Customs meteorological observations of the port, for which I am indebted to Mr. W. G. HARLING.

METEOROLOGICAL TABLE, October 1895 to March 1896.

Month.	Barometer.		Thermometer.		Rainfall.	
	Highest.	Lowest.	Maximum.	Minimum.	No. of Days.	Quantity.
1895.	*Inches.*	*Inches.*	° *F.*	° *F.*		*Inches.*
October	30.300	29.900	82	59	12	2.08
November........................	30.600	30.040	78	48	3	1.64
December........................	30.524	30.000	68	38	7	1.31
1896.						
January........................	30.500	29.912	65	37	9	3.33
February........................	30.500	29.980	66	35	13	3.74
March	30.460	29.830	64	35	6	1.40

China, Imperial Maritime Customs, Medical Reports
(1896. 04. 01—1896. 09. 30)

CHINA.

IMPERIAL MARITIME CUSTOMS.

II.—SPECIAL SERIES: No. 2.

MEDICAL REPORTS,

FOR THE HALF-YEAR ENDED 30TH SEPTEMBER 1896.

52nd Issue.

PUBLISHED BY ORDER OF

The Inspector General of Customs.

SHANGHAI:
PUBLISHED AT THE STATISTICAL DEPARTMENT OF THE INSPECTORATE GENERAL OF CUSTOMS,
AND SOLD BY
KELLY & WALSH, LIMITED: SHANGHAI, HONGKONG, YOKOHAMA, AND SINGAPORE.
LONDON: P. S. KING & SON, 12 AND 14, KING STREET, WESTMINSTER, S.W.

[Price $1.]   1898.

INSPECTOR GENERAL'S CIRCULAR No. 19 OF 1870.

INSPECTORATE GENERAL OF CUSTOMS,

PEKING, 31st December 1870.

SIR,

1.—IT has been suggested to me that it would be well to take advantage of the circumstances in which the Customs Establishment is placed, to procure information with regard to disease amongst foreigners and natives in China; and I have, in consequence, come to the resolution of publishing half-yearly in collected form all that may be obtainable. If carried out to the extent hoped for, the scheme may prove highly useful to the medical profession both in China and at home, and to the public generally. I therefore look with confidence to the co-operation of the Customs Medical Officer at your port, and rely on his assisting me in this matter by framing a half-yearly report containing the result of his observations at..................upon the local peculiarities of disease, and upon diseases rarely or never encountered out of China. The facts brought forward and the opinions expressed will be arranged and published either with or without the name of the physician responsible for them, just as he may desire.

2.—The suggestions of the Customs Medical Officers at the various ports as to the points which it would be well to have especially elucidated, will be of great value in the framing of a form which will save trouble to those members of the medical profession, whether connected with the Customs or not, who will join in carrying out the plan proposed. Meanwhile I would particularly invite attention to—

a.—The general health of....................during the period reported on; the death rate amongst foreigners; and, as far as possible, a classification of the causes of death.

b.—Diseases prevalent at............:.............

c.—General type of disease; peculiarities and complications encountered; special treatment demanded.

d.—Relation of disease to
{ Season.
{ Alteration in local conditions—such as drainage, etc.
{ Alteration in climatic conditions.

e.—Peculiar diseases; especially leprosy.

f.—Epidemics
{ Absence or presence.
{ Causes.
{ Course and treatment.
{ Fatality.

Other points, of a general or special kind, will naturally suggest themselves to medical men; what I have above called attention to will serve to fix the general scope of the undertaking.

3.—Considering the number of places at which the Customs Inspectorate has established offices, the thousands of miles north and south and east and west over which these offices are scattered, the varieties of climate, and the peculiar conditions to which, under such different circumstances, life and health are subjected, I believe the Inspectorate, aided by its Medical Officers, can do good service in the general interest in the direction indicated; and, as already stated, I rely with confidence on the support and assistance of the Medical Officer at each port in the furtherance and perfecting of this scheme. You will hand a copy of this Circular to Dr. ...., and request him, in my name, to hand to you in future, for transmission to myself, half-yearly Reports of the kind required, for the half-years ending 31st March and 30th September—that is, for the Winter and Summer seasons.

4.—   *   *   *   *   *

I am, etc.,

(Signed)   ROBERT HART,

I. G.

THE COMMISSIONERS OF CUSTOMS,—*Newchwang, Shanghai,*
Tientsin, Ningpo,
Chefoo, Foochow,
Hankow, Amoy,
Kiukiang, Swatow, and
Chinkiang, Canton.

TABLE OF CONTENTS.

The Contributors to this Volume are :—

C. C. DE BURGH DALY, M.B., B.CH. .... Newchwang.

E. W. VON TUNZELMANN, M.B., M.R.C.S. .... Chefoo.

JAMES H. McCARTNEY, M.D. .... Chungking.

JOHN D. THOMSON, M.B., C.M. .... Hankow.

E. H. HART, M.D. .... Wuhu.

ALFRED HOGG, M.A., M.B., C.M. .... Wenchow.

J. J. DELAY, M.D. .... Lungchow.

Dr. ALFRED HOGG'S REPORT ON THE HEALTH OF WENCHOW

For the Half-year ended 30th September 1896.

THE health of the foreign community, as well as of the Chinese, has been fairly good during this half-year, and there have been very few cases of any serious import. The weather for a large part of the time was rainy, and the summer was cooler than for several years past. Fortunately, too, the city has not been visited by cholera this summer, and as yet no case of it has come under my notice, though attacks of diarrhœa have been common, as usual.

There have been no deaths; but one birth occurred—a male, large and well developed. There was excess of liquor amnii, which, coupled with the large size of the infant, induced severe postpartum hæmorrhage, owing to uterine inertia and retained placenta. This was controlled, however, by injections of hot water, and ergot internally, and the mother rallied quickly afterwards.

An elderly member of the Customs staff suffered severely from a hot burst in June, showing symptoms of heat apoplexy, and had to be ordered away to a cooler spot during the summer months.

While the s.s. *Poochi* was in port the captain and officers, along with the steward and table "boys" and two members of the Customs staff who had been dining on board, were all variously seized with fever, or diarrhœa, or both. It was a week before two of them recovered. The cause was strongly suspected to be due to some ice-cream which had been partaken of on the previous day.

Among the cases treated have been :—

Malarial fever.	Rupture of cornea.
Diarrhœa.	Incipient typhoid.
Gastritis.	Stomatitis.
Conjunctivitis.	Laryngitis and pharyngitis.
Interstitial keratitis.	Asthma (spasmodic).

There have also been large numbers of Chinese treated at the dispensary of the Methodist Mission.

For the meteorological table I am indebted to Mr. BENSON, Harbour Master.

METEOROLOGICAL TABLE, April to September 1896.

MONTH.	BAROMETER.		THERMOMETER.		RAINFALL.	
	Maximum.	Minimum.	Maximum.	Minimum.	No. of Days.	Quantity.
	Inches.	*Inches.*	° *F.*	° *F.*		*Inches.*
April	30.280	29.640	78	51	15	5.04
May	30.266	29.650	88	60	17	3.74
June	30.080	29.594	93	66	15	12.47
July	29.986	29.460	93	73	13	12.93
August	30.064	29.700	94	77	8	4.34
September	30.200	29.830	93	72	12	1.77

China, Imperial Maritime Customs, Medical Reports
（1896. 10. 01—1897. 09. 30）

CHINA.

IMPERIAL MARITIME CUSTOMS.

II.—SPECIAL SERIES: No. 2.

MEDICAL REPORTS,

FOR THE HALF-YEAR ENDED 30TH SEPTEMBER 1897.

54th Issue.

PUBLISHED BY ORDER OF

The Inspector General of Customs.

SHANGHAI:
PUBLISHED AT THE STATISTICAL DEPARTMENT OF THE INSPECTORATE GENERAL OF CUSTOMS,
AND SOLD BY
KELLY & WALSH, LIMITED: SHANGHAI, HONGKONG, YOKOHAMA, AND SINGAPORE.
LONDON: P. S. KING & SON, 12 AND 14, KING STREET, WESTMINSTER, S.W.
1898.

[*Price* $1.]

INSPECTOR GENERAL'S CIRCULAR No. 19 of 1870.

INSPECTORATE GENERAL OF CUSTOMS,

PEKING, 31st December 1870.

SIR,

1.—IT has been suggested to me that it would be well to take advantage of the circumstances in which the Customs Establishment is placed, to procure information with regard to disease amongst foreigners and natives in China; and I have, in consequence, come to the resolution of publishing half-yearly in collected form all that may be obtainable. If carried out to the extent hoped for, the scheme may prove highly useful to the medical profession both in China and at home, and to the public generally. I therefore look with confidence to the co-opera- tion of the Customs Medical Officer at your port, and rely on his assisting me in this matter by framing a half-yearly Report containing the result of his observations at.................upon the local peculiarities of disease, and upon diseases rarely or never encountered out of China. The facts brought forward and the opinions expressed will be arranged and published either with or without the name of the physician responsible for them, just as he may desire.

2.—The suggestions of the Customs Medical Officers at the various ports as to the points which it would be well to have especially elucidated, will be of great value in the framing of a form which will save trouble to those members of the medical profession, whether connected with the Customs or not, who will join in carrying out the plan proposed. Meanwhile I would particularly invite attention to—

a.—The general health of....................during the period reported on; the death rate amongst foreigners; and, as far as possible, a classification of the causes of death.

b.—Diseases prevalent at...........................

c.—General type of disease; peculiarities and complications encountered; special treatment demanded.

d.—Relation of disease to { Season. Alteration in local conditions—such as drainage, etc. Alteration in climatic conditions.

e.—Peculiar diseases; especially leprosy.

f.—Epidemics { Absence or presence. Causes. Course and treatment. Fatality.

Other points, of a general or special kind, will naturally suggest themselves to medical men; what I have above called attention to will serve to fix the general scope of the undertaking.

* * * * *

3.—Considering the number of places at which the Customs Inspectorate has established offices, the thousands of miles north and south and east and west over which these offices are scattered, the varieties of climate, and the peculiar conditions to which, under such different circumstances, life and health are subjected, I believe the Inspectorate, aided by its Medical Officers, can do good service in the general interest in the direction indicated; and, as already stated, I rely with confidence on the support and assistance of the Medical Officer at each port in the furtherance and perfecting of this scheme. You will hand a copy of this Circular to Dr. ...., and request him, in my name, to hand to you in future, for transmission to myself, half-yearly Reports of the kind required, for the half-years ending 31st March and 30th September—that is, for the Winter and Summer seasons.

4.—   *   *   *   *   *

I am, etc.,

(Signed)   ROBERT HART,
I. G.

THE COMMISSIONERS OF CUSTOMS,—*Newchwang,* *Shanghai,*
Tientsin, *Ningpo,*
Chefoo, *Foochow,*
Hankow, *Amoy,*
Kiukiang, *Swatow,* and
Chinkiang, *Canton.*

TABLE OF CONTENTS.

The Contributors to this Volume are :—

J.-J. MATIGNON, M.D. .... Peking.

C. C. DE BURGH DALY, M.B., B.CH. .... Newchwang.

H. R. ROBERTSON, M.D. .... Tientsin.

JAMES H. MCCARTNEY, M.D. .... Chungking.

EDGERTON H. HART, M.D. .... Wuhu.

J. A. LYNCH, M.D., M.CH. .... Chinkiang.

ALFRED HOGG, M.A., M.B., C.M. .... Wenchow.

Dr. ALFRED HOGG'S REPORT ON THE HEALTH
OF WENCHOW

For the Year ended 30th September 1897.

THE former six months, up to March, were not characterised by much illness among the foreign residents, so that there was hardly sufficient material for a detailed Report. The last six months, however, up to the end of September, have not the same good record to show, and very few of the residents have escaped suffering from some ailment or other, diarrhœa during the autumn having been the prevailing complaint.

The earlier part of the year was very wet, and remained comparatively cool to the end of June. Even afterwards the heat was not excessive, and the maximum daily temperature was seldom above 90° F., but the excess of moisture in the air and the frequent advent of rain during the afternoon made the summer a very trying one, and the health of the community suffered in proportion. During the autumn sudden changes of temperature were not uncommon, the difference between the maximum and minimum occasionally being more than 10°.

During the period under review one birth and two deaths have occurred in the community. In the former case, a primipara, labour commenced and terminated in a little over two hours, and was quite normal. Both of the cases that terminated fatally occurred in the autumn, in September. One, a female child of 14 months, had slight diarrhœa for a day or two, which was treated by the parents. On the 3rd day, as the symptoms persisted and the child was much weaker, they called in medical aid. The same evening the child, which had previously refused food, took a hearty meal, and about two hours after had a severe attack of colic with hyperexia, the temperature rising to 108° F. In spite of treatment collapse followed, and by morning the child succumbed. Two other children in the same family had diarrhœa subsequently, but recovered. About three weeks after the mother was attacked by dysentery with profuse diarrhœa and considerable tenesmus. Ipecacuanha in 30-grain doses, along with 15 minims of nepenthe, was prescribed every eight hours, along with occasional enemas of opium and irrigation of colon by nitrate of silver (weak solution). Though the ipecacuanha and enemas were badly borne by the patient, an improvement took place up to the 5th day, when symptoms of collapse appeared, and a few hours afterwards the patient was delivered of a six months' fœtus. No external hæmorrhage occurred, but the diarrhœa still persisted and was accompanied by severe sickness, which greatly exhausted the patient. Signs of heart failure appeared. Stimulants and peptonised food were administered freely, with some effect, and intravenous injection of saline solution with only transient improvement, and the patient died of heart failure on the 7th day.

Several of the residents had attacks of diarrhœa, but in two of them it was very persistent and recurred time after time. In one case, after repeated trials of aromatic powder of chalk with opium, bismuth, salol, and catechu, recourse was had to peptonising the food, which resulted in cure. The other case was associated with hepatitis and gastric catarrh, and was treated by mineral acids, astringents, and bismuth.

Among the other cases treated were:—

Muscular rheumatism.
Acute diarrhœa.
Chronic diarrhœa.
Nervous irritability and prostration.
Urticaria.
Myalgia and neuralgia.
Insomnia.
Injury to shoulder and ankle.
Rheumatic arthritis.
    „   iritis.

Dyspepsia.
Otorrhœa.
Boils.
Anæmia.
Malaria.
Pruritus.
Constipation.
Hæmorrhoids.
Small-pox.

The case of small-pox occurred on board the steamer in port, and the patient was treated in Shanghai at the General Hospital, and recovered.

METEOROLOGICAL TABLE, October 1896 to September 1897.

MONTH.	BAROMETER.		THERMOMETER.		RAINFALL.	
	Highest.	Lowest.	Maximum.	Minimum.	No. of Days.	Quantity.
1896.	*Inches.*	*Inches.*	° *F.*	° *F.*		*Inches.*
October	30.390	30.000	88	63	12	8.63
November	30.440	29.882	75	55	5	1.85
December	30.720	30.134	66	29	4	0.97
1897.						
January	30.652	30.000	66	30	12	5.05
February	30.706	30.104	54	28	20	6.65
March	30.520	29.970	69	38	22	6.42
April	30.330	29.900	77	45	16	7.66
May	30.244	29.600	81	57	20	8.20
June	30.100	29.750	89	62	23	16.55
July	30.082	29.710	95	67	8	0.70
August	30.100	29.500	92	75	14	5.19
September	30.270	29.820	89	63	16	5.88

I am indebted to the courtesy of the Harbour Master for the above summary of the meteorological conditions that prevailed during the period reported on.

China, Imperial Maritime Customs, Medical Reports
(1897. 10. 01—1898. 09. 30)

CHINA.

IMPERIAL MARITIME CUSTOMS.

II.—SPECIAL SERIES: No. 2.

MEDICAL REPORTS,

FOR THE HALF-YEAR ENDED 30TH SEPTEMBER 1898.

56th Issue.

PUBLISHED BY ORDER OF

𝕿𝖍𝖊 𝕴𝖓𝖘𝖕𝖊𝖈𝖙𝖔𝖗 𝕲𝖊𝖓𝖊𝖗𝖆𝖑 𝖔𝖋 𝕮𝖚𝖘𝖙𝖔𝖒𝖘.

SHANGHAI:

PUBLISHED AT THE STATISTICAL DEPARTMENT OF THE INSPECTORATE GENERAL OF CUSTOMS,
AND SOLD BY
KELLY & WALSH, LIMITED: SHANGHAI, HONGKONG, YOKOHAMA, AND SINGAPORE.
LONDON: P. S. KING & SON, 2 AND 4, GREAT SMITH STREET, WESTMINSTER, S.W.

1899.

[Price $1.]

INSPECTOR GENERAL'S CIRCULAR No. 19 of 1870.

INSPECTORATE GENERAL OF CUSTOMS,

PEKING, 31st *December* 1870.

SIR,

1.—IT has been suggested to me that it would be well to take advantage of the circumstances in which the Customs Establishment is placed, to procure information with regard to disease amongst foreigners and natives in China; and I have, in consequence, come to the resolution of publishing half-yearly in collected form all that may be obtainable. If carried out to the extent hoped for, the scheme may prove highly useful to the medical profession both in China and at home, and to the public generally. I therefore look with confidence to the co-operation of the Customs Medical Officer at your port, and rely on his assisting me in this matter by framing a half-yearly Report containing the result of his observations at..................upon the local peculiarities of disease, and upon diseases rarely or never encountered out of China. The facts brought forward and the opinions expressed will be arranged and published either with or without the name of the physician responsible for them, just as he may desire.

2.—The suggestions of the Customs Medical Officers at the various ports as to the points which it would be well to have especially elucidated, will be of great value in the framing of a form which will save trouble to those members of the medical profession, whether connected with the Customs or not, who will join in carrying out the plan proposed. Meanwhile I would particularly invite attention to—

a.—The general health of....................during the period reported on; the death rate amongst foreigners; and, as far as possible, a classification of the causes of death.

b.—Diseases prevalent at............................

c.—General type of disease; peculiarities and complications encountered; special treatment demanded.

d.—Relation of disease to $\begin{cases} \text{Season.} \\ \text{Alteration in local conditions—such as drainage, etc.} \\ \text{Alteration in climatic conditions.} \end{cases}$

e.—Peculiar diseases; especially leprosy.

f.—Epidemics $\begin{cases} \text{Absence or presence.} \\ \text{Causes.} \\ \text{Course and treatment.} \\ \text{Fatality.} \end{cases}$

Other points, of a general or special kind, will naturally suggest themselves to medical men; what I have above called attention to will serve to fix the general scope of the undertaking.

3.—Considering the number of places at which the Customs Inspectorate has established offices, the thousands of miles north and south and east and west over which these offices are scattered, the varieties of climate, and the peculiar conditions to which, under such different circumstances, life and health are subjected, I believe the Inspectorate, aided by its Medical Officers, can do good service in the general interest in the direction indicated; and, as already stated, I rely with confidence on the support and assistance of the Medical Officer at each port in the furtherance and perfecting of this scheme. You will hand a copy of this Circular to Dr. ...., and request him, in my name, to hand to you in future, for transmission to myself, half-yearly Reports of the kind required, for the half-years ending 31st March and 30th September—that is, for the Winter and Summer seasons.

4.—   *   *   *   *   *

I am, etc.,

(Signed)   ROBERT HART,
I. G.

The Commissioners of Customs,—*Newchwang,   Shanghai,*
Tientsin,   Ningpo,
Chefoo,   Foochow,
Hankow,   Amoy,
Kiukiang,   Swatow, and
Chinkiang,   Canton.

TABLE OF CONTENTS.

The Contributors to this Volume are:—

D. RANKINE, M.A., M.B.C.M. .... Ichang.

F. T. D. CLINDENING, M.R.C.S.E., L.R.C.P.L. .... Kiukaing.

J. A. LYNCH, M.D., M.CH. .... Chinkiang.

HERBERT J. HICKIN, M.B. .... Ningpo.

ALFRED HOGG, M.A., M.B., C.M. .... Wenchow.

RODERICK J. J. MACDONALD, M.D. .... Wuchow.

Dr. ALFRED HOGG'S REPORT ON THE HEALTH OF WENCHOW

For the Year ended 30th September 1898.

DURING the period under review the health of the foreign community has been, on the whole, very good, with the exception of the end of 1897. There have been fewer cases of illness, and these of a less serious nature.

This summer has been a cool one compared with others, and as we were without the usual heavy rains of May and June, there was very little of the close damp weather so prevalent during these months.

The most distressing event in one's practice was the death of a lady very much esteemed in the community, the result of confinement following on dysenteric diarrhœa.

Medical advice was sought for, about the end of October, for symptoms pointing to proctites and internal hæmorrhoids consequent on pregnancy. Irregular diarrhœa and occasional touches of hæmorrhage persisted in spite of various remedies, gradually increasing in severity till finally they assumed somewhat of a dysenteric character, greatly reducing the patient, so that grave fears were entertained for the result. These were, unhappily, justified by the end of November, when, on the 26th, the patient was prematurely confined and delivered of a male child, who survived for 30 hours. The patient rallied somewhat after the ordeal, but the diarrhœa still continued, and she succumbed on the 29th.

There was one other birth, a healthy male child, the subject being a primipara who came in from an out-station to be confined. The labour was normal and tedious, and necessitated chloroform.

Among the cases treated in the ordinary course of work were as below :—

Amenorrhœa.	Iritis.
Ascarides.	Laryngitis.
Atonic dyspepsia.	Lupus exedens.
Boils.	Malarial fever.
Constipation.	Measles.
Diarrhœa.	Otorrhœa.
Dysmenorrhœa.	Ovaritis.
Enteritis.	Pregnancy.
Febricula.	Psoriasis.
Fracture of clavicle.	Renal colic.
Gout.	Rheumatism.
Hepatic dyspepsia.	Sprain of ankle.
Incised wound of palm.	Syncope.
Internal hæmorrhoids.	

During the temporary absence of the writer from the port there occurred a rice riot, but none of the foreigners were molested.

Dr. KIRK, who was in the port for a short time, rendered much assistance in the medical work, and his presence was much appreciated at operations in the hospital.

A large amount of practice amongst the Chinese has been carried on at the Methodist Free Church Hospital and dispensary, involving much minor surgery.

I am indebted to the kindness of the Harbour Master, Mr. KINDBLAD, for the meteorological report appended.

METEOROLOGICAL TABLE, October 1897 to September 1898.

MONTH.	BAROMETER.		THERMOMETER.		RAINFALL.	
	Maximum.	Minimum.	Maximum.	Minimum.	No. of Days.	Quantity.
1897.	*Inches.*	*Inches.*	° *F.*	° *F.*		*Inches.*
October...........................	30.384	30.052	82	54	18	5.64
November..........................	30.544	30.100	82	40	5	1.88
December..........................	30.654	30.150	67	33	7	1.26
1898.						
January...........................	30.734	30.130	65	33	9	1.02
February..........................	30.420	29.760	69	36	14	5.01
March.............................	30.460	29.980	75	36	13	3.01
April.............................	30.380	29.700	78	46	16	7.45
May...............................	30.410	29.680	87	56	19	6.89
June..............................	30.050	29.640	90	60	15	7.99
July..............................	30.070	29.800	92	72	5	5.15
August............................	29.980	29.525	93	71	19	15.22
September.........................	30.130	29.800	92	69	11	4.96

China，Imperial Maritime Customs，Medical Reports
（1898. 10. 01—1899. 09. 30）

CHINA.

IMPERIAL MARITIME CUSTOMS.

II.—SPECIAL SERIES: No. 2.

MEDICAL REPORTS,

FOR THE HALF-YEAR ENDED 30TH SEPTEMBER 1899.

58th Issue.

PUBLISHED BY ORDER OF

The Inspector General of Customs.

SHANGHAI:

PUBLISHED AT THE STATISTICAL DEPARTMENT OF THE INSPECTORATE GENERAL OF CUSTOMS,

AND SOLD BY

KELLY & WALSH, LIMITED: SHANGHAI, HONGKONG, YOKOHAMA, AND SINGAPORE.

LONDON: P. S. KING & SON, 2 AND 4, GREAT SMITH STREET, WESTMINSTER, S.W.

[Price $1.]   1900.

INSPECTOR GENERAL'S CIRCULAR No. 19 OF 1870.

INSPECTORATE GENERAL OF CUSTOMS,

PEKING, 31st December 1870.

SIR,

1.—IT has been suggested to me that it would be well to take advantage of the circumstances in which the Customs Establishment is placed, to procure information with regard to disease amongst foreigners and natives in China; and I have, in consequence, come to the resolution of publishing half-yearly in collected form all that may be obtainable. If carried out to the extent hoped for, the scheme may prove highly useful to the medical profession both in China and at home, and to the public generally. I therefore look with confidence to the co-operation of the Customs Medical Officer at your port, and rely on his assisting me in this matter by framing a half-yearly Report containing the result of his observations at.................upon the local peculiarities of disease, and upon diseases rarely or never encountered out of China. The facts brought forward and the opinions expressed will be arranged and published either with or without the name of the physician responsible for them, just as he may desire.

2.—The suggestions of the Customs Medical Officers at the various ports as to the points which it would be well to have especially elucidated, will be of great value in the framing of a form which will save trouble to those members of the medical profession, whether connected with the Customs or not, who will join in carrying out the plan proposed. Meanwhile I would particularly invite attention to—

a.—The general health of....................during the period reported on; the death rate amongst foreigners; and, as far as possible, a classification of the causes of death.

b.—Diseases prevalent at...........................

c.—General type of disease; peculiarities and complications encountered; special treatment demanded.

d.—Relation of disease to ⎰ Season.
  ⎱ Alteration in local conditions—such as drainage, etc.
  ⎰ Alteration in climatic conditions.

e.—Peculiar diseases; especially leprosy.

f.—Epidemics ⎰ Absence or presence.
  ⎱ Causes.
  ⎰ Course and treatment.
  ⎱ Fatality.

Other points, of a general or special kind, will naturally suggest themselves to medical men; what I have above called attention to will serve to fix the general scope of the undertaking.

3.—Considering the number of places at which the Customs Inspectorate has established offices, the thousands of miles north and south and east and west over which these offices are scattered, the varieties of climate, and the peculiar conditions to which, under such different circumstances, life and health are subjected, I believe the Inspectorate, aided by its Medical Officers, can do good service in the general interest in the direction indicated; and, as already stated, I rely with confidence on the support and assistance of the Medical Officer at each port in the furtherance and perfecting of this scheme. You will hand a copy of this Circular to Dr. ……………, and request him, in my name, to hand to you in future, for transmission to myself, half-yearly Reports of the kind required, for the half-years ending 31st March and 30th September—that is, for the Winter and Summer seasons.

4.—   *   *   *   *   *

I am, etc.,

(Signed) ROBERT HART,

Inspector General.

To

THE COMMISSIONERS OF CUSTOMS.

TABLE OF CONTENTS.

The Contributors to this Volume are :—

J.-J. Matignon, M.D. .... Peking.

C. C. de Burgh Daly, M.B., B.Ch. .... Newchwang.

H. Rennie Robertson, M.D. .... Tientsin.

John Francis Molyneux, M.R.C.S., L.R.C.P.Ed. .... Chefoo.

Herbert J. Hickin, M.B. .... Ningpo.

Alfred Hogg, M.A., M.B., C.M. .... Wenchow.

Henry Layng, M.R.C.S., L.R.C.P. .... Swatow.

Roderick J. J. Macdonald, M.D. .... Wuchow.

J. H. Lowry, L.R.C.P.Ed., L.R.C.S.Ed. ⎫
H. M. McCandliss, M.D.   ⎬ .... Hoihow and Kiungchow.

A. Sharp Deane, F.R.C.S. .... Pakhoi.

E. Reygondaud, M.D. .... Mengtsz.

Laurent Gaide, M.D. .... Szemao.

DR. ALFRED HOGG'S REPORT ON THE HEALTH OF WENCHOW

For the Year ended 30th September 1899.

THE health of the foreign community here during the period under review has been, on the whole, very good, and consequently affords little material to report about. Judging by the description of other ports, Wenchow may, I think, be considered as one of the healthiest and cleanest, though rather damp and depressing at certain seasons. Indeed, the chief complaint about it is on the ground of ennui.

The streets are for the most part raised in the middle by a causeway of bricks set on edge, or else paved with large, long blocks of granite, and, as a rule, drain into a canal running alongside each street, communicating with the river by outlets at certain places. Consequently, a heavy rain scours the streets and drains off into the river at low water.

The water supply is good, though the wells are often contaminated, giving rise at times to epidemics of cholera or typhoid. Malarial fever is common, but not of a severe type.

During the winter months several of the community suffered from colds and catarrhs, through exposure to changes of temperature, but none of the cases were of a serious nature. One or two residents had occasional attacks of fever, from getting a chill, but the malaria was not originally contracted here.

The summer heat this year commenced early, and was very trying at first; but in August, after getting a share of two typhoons, there was a considerable amelioration of heat.

Two old China residents had to be invalided home, one from heart disease and dropsy, the other from general debility.

Among the cases treated were—

Bronchial catarrh.	Acute gastritis.
Rheumatism.	Dysmenorrhœa.
Neuralgia.	Pregnancy.
Malaria.	Syncope.
Podagra.	Rupture of soleus.
Chronic urticaria.	Sprain of gluteus and quadratus
Dyspepsia.	lumborum.
Diarrhœa.	

The writer had also the misfortune to sustain a fracture of the clavicle, between the conoid and trapezoid ligaments, but it united very well without deformity.

For the accompanying meteorological report I have to thank the Harbour Master, Mr. MÜLLER.

METEOROLOGICAL TABLE, October 1898 to September 1899.

MONTH.	BAROMETER.		THERMOMETER.		RAINFALL.	
	Maximum.	Minimum.	Maximum.	Minimum.	No. of Days.	Quantity.
1898.	*Inches.*	*Inches.*	° F.	° F.		*Inches.*
October	30.330	29.880	85	56	8	8.20
November	30.580	29.930	75	40	8	5.35
December	30.500	30.130	65	34	2	0.36
1899.						
January	30.500	30.100	66	34	7	1.56
February	30.500	29.900	64	35	11	3.76
March	30.500	30.000	70	40	10	1.39
April	30.350	29.800	76	41	13	4.25
May	30.300	29.850	83	57	19	10.45
June	30.170	29.700	87	64	10	3.98
July	29.975	29.490	93	72	9	2.10
August	30.030	29.650	96	72	16	10.70
September	30.200	29.850	88	64	11	5.90

China, Imperial Maritime Customs, Medical Reports
(1901. 10. 01—1902. 09. 30)

CHINA.

IMPERIAL MARITIME CUSTOMS.

II.—SPECIAL SERIES: No. 2.

MEDICAL REPORTS,

FOR THE YEAR ENDED 30TH SEPTEMBER 1902.

63rd and 64th Issues.

PUBLISHED BY ORDER OF

The Inspector General of Customs.

SHANGHAI:
PUBLISHED AT THE STATISTICAL DEPARTMENT OF THE INSPECTORATE GENERAL OF CUSTOMS,
AND SOLD BY
KELLY & WALSH, LIMITED: SHANGHAI, HONGKONG, YOKOHAMA, AND SINGAPORE.
LONDON: P. S. KING & SON, 2 AND 4, GREAT SMITH STREET, WESTMINSTER, S.W.

ice $2.]

1903.

INSPECTOR GENERAL'S CIRCULAR No. 19 OF 1870.

INSPECTORATE GENERAL OF CUSTOMS,

PEKING, 31st *December* 1870.

SIR,

1.—It has been suggested to me that it would be well to take advantage of the circumstances in which the Customs Establishment is placed, to procure information with regard to disease amongst foreigners and natives in China; and I have, in consequence, come to the resolution of publishing half-yearly in collected form all that may be obtainable. If carried out to the extent hoped for, the scheme may prove highly useful to the medical profession both in China and at home, and to the public generally. I therefore look with confidence to the co-operation of the Customs Medical Officer at your port, and rely on his assisting me in this matter by framing a half-yearly Report containing the result of his observations at.................upon the local peculiarities of disease, and upon diseases rarely or never encountered out of China. The facts brought forward and the opinions expressed will be arranged and published either with or without the name of the physician responsible for them, just as he may desire.

2.—The suggestions of the Customs Medical Officers at the various ports as to the points which it would be well to have especially elucidated, will be of great value in the framing of a form which will save trouble to those members of the medical profession, whether connected with the Customs or not, who will join in carrying out the plan proposed. Meanwhile I would particularly invite attention to—

a.—The general health of....................during the period reported on; the death rate amongst foreigners; and, as far as possible, a classification of the causes of death.

b.—Diseases prevalent at...........................

c.—General type of disease; peculiarities and complications encountered; special treatment demanded.

d.—Relation of disease to { Season. Alteration in local conditions—such as drainage, etc. Alteration in climatic conditions.

e.—Peculiar diseases; especially leprosy.

f.—Epidemics: { Absence or presence. Causes. Course and treatment. Fatality.

Other points, of a general or special kind, will naturally suggest themselves to medical men; what I have above called attention to will serve to fix the general scope of the undertaking.

3.—Considering the number of places at which the Customs Inspectorate has established offices, the thousands of miles north and south and east and west over which these offices are scattered, the varieties of climate, and the peculiar conditions to which, under such different circumstances, life and health are subjected, I believe the Inspectorate, aided by its Medical Officers, can do good service in the general interest in the direction indicated; and, as already stated, I rely with confidence on the support and assistance of the Medical Officer at each port in the furtherance and perfecting of this scheme. You will hand a copy of this Circular to Dr. ...., and request him, in my name, to hand to you in future, for transmission to myself, half-yearly Reports of the kind required, for the half-years ending 31st March and 30th September—that is, for the Winter and Summer seasons.

4.—   *   *   *   *   *

I am, etc.,

(Signed)   ROBERT HART,
Inspector General.

To

THE COMMISSIONERS OF CUSTOMS.

TABLE OF CONTENTS.

The Contributors to this Volume are:—

H. Rennie Robertson, B.A., M.D., B.CH. .... Tientsin.

Otto Gulowsen, M.D. .... Chefoo.

J. A. Thomson, B.SC., M.B., CH.B. (Aberd.) .... Hankow.

David Brown, M.B., B.CH. .... Wuhu.

W. E. Macklin, M.D. .... Nanking.

J. A. Lynch, M.D., M.CH. .... Chinkiang.

J. B. Fearn, M.D. .... Soochow.

W. E. Plummer, M.D. .... Wenchow.

B. Stewart Ringer, M.D., M.R.C.S., L.S.A. .... Canton.

Sidney L. Lasell, M.D. .... Hoihow and Kiungchow.

J. H. Lowry, L.R.C.P.Ed., L.R.C.S.Ed. .... Pakhoi.

Georges Barbézieux, M.D. .... Mengtsz.

G. A. Sautarel, M.D. .... Szemao.

Dr. W. E. PLUMMER'S REPORT ON THE HEALTH OF WENCHOW

For the Half-year ended 31st March 1902.

SINCE my arrival at this port, in the latter part of October last year, I have paid 63 professional visits to European members of the Customs staff; but, with one exception, there have been no serious cases of illness. The one patient who has been seriously ill suffered from a severe attack of malaria, but as he had had two similar attacks when in Canton, on which account he was transferred here last year, I think there is no doubt that the disease was not acquired in Wenchow.

The other members of the European community, mostly missionaries, have enjoyed good health during this period.

There has been one birth.

In the Mission Hospital I have treated a number of bullet wounds. Those brought in soon after the injury recovered, among these being a young man who was shot through the left lung. A man whose femur had been smashed by a pirate's bullet was brought up a week after the fight, having been detained by his captors. He was in a very serious condition, and as we could not promise to cure him, his friends preferred to take him home. Another man who was stabbed by pirates is at present under treatment, and although his condition is serious, it is hoped he will pull round.

Among the general cases which have been treated are the following :—

1.—A sarcoma, as big as a large cocoa-nut, was removed from the back of a girl aged 12. For three days after the operation the pulse was 150 and the temperature 101° F. On the third day both these symptoms subsided ; the pulse and temperature became normal, and the wound was perfectly healed in a fortnight. No cause was discovered for the abnormal pulse.

2.—A semi-chronic abscess of undiscovered origin. The patient, a young farmer, aged 32, first noticed swelling of the left buttock and thigh three months before admission ; this swelling was accompanied by pain and hardening of the tissues. The symptoms have gradually increased. On admission the upper half of the left thigh behind was swollen, the swelling being most prominent on the posterior and inner aspect, just below the gluteal fold. At this point the skin had a dusky red colour, and on careful palpation, fluctuation was obtained. All round, for about 6 inches, and especially down the thigh, the tissues were indurated and gave much the same impression to the fingers as conveyed when examining a patient with elephantiasis. An incision was made over the most prominent part of the swelling and a little watery pus evacuated. During the following six weeks the discharge, at first copious, gradually diminished, and at the same time the induration and swelling subsided. I have been unable to find any literature out here giving a detailed account of the clinical course of a filarial abscess. I have wondered if that disease might be the cause of this patient's trouble.

3.—There has been quite an epidemic of ophthalmia among the Chinese clinically indistinguishable from the gonorrhœal ophthalmia seen in England. Many of the victims do not come up for treatment until the disease has been in progress for two or three months and the sight is lost. When seen early these cases have been rapidly cured by painting with silver nitrate.

This winter has been remarkably fine and exceptionally dry, practically no rain having fallen for four months on end. The canals have been in a filthy condition for three months and the wells dry, so that all drinking water has had to be brought from a distance; yet I have not heard of there being an unusual amount of sickness amongst the natives.

There are three things which as a new-comer have impressed me :—

(1.) When chloroform is administered to the Chinese they almost invariably go under without making a sound or movement, and when emerging from the effects of the anæsthetic there is no sickness, and food can be taken almost at once and retained. This is very different from the 24 hours misery which usually follows the inhalation of chloroform in England.

(2.) Most of the cases of malarial fever which I have seen have not been ushered in by the rigor described in the text-books, and the fever is usually continued and not intermittent; this is, I am told, a very common experience here. The fever subsides under full doses of quinine in one to three days.

(3.) The number of patients who are troubled with worms has surprised me. In almost every case that I have come across where there has been stomach trouble, pain, colic wind, or other symptoms of indigestion, a dose of santonin has been followed by the expulsion of worms. A woman, aged 58, began to be troubled with fits, apparently hysterical in character; she also suffered from indigestion. After a dose of santonin worms were expelled, and the fits have not returned.

The following meteorological observations have been kindly supplied by Mr. J. H. NIGHTINGALE, the Harbour Master :—

METEOROLOGICAL TABLE, 1901.

MONTH.	THERMOMETER.			BAROMETER.		RAINFALL.	
	Highest.	Lowest.	Mean.	Highest.	Lowest.	Days on which Rain fell.	Quantity.
	° F.	° F.	° F.	Inches.	Inches.		Inches.
January	66	39	52.5	30.400	29.970	17	3.60
February	61	27	44.0	30.590	30.090	1	0.12
March	68	36	52.0	30.525	29.900	15	2.85
April	74	45	59.5	30.375	29.680	19	9.81
May	83	57	70.0	30.300	29.750	20	7.24
June	85	64	74.5	30.010	29.650	17	8.20
July	92	69	80.5	29.954	29.700	14	7.22
August	89	74	81.5	29.990	29.210	19	14.57
September	88	67	77.5	30.220	29.220	6	3.82
October	81	60	70.5	30.400	29.900	10	6.10
November	74	44	59.0	30.490	30.100	3	0.06
December	68	34	51.0	30.557	30.015	9	1.63

Dr. W. E. PLUMMER'S REPORT ON THE HEALTH OF WENCHOW

For the Half-year ended 30th September 1902.

CHOLERA began in this city about the middle of July, but the disease was reported to be in the P'ing-yang-hsien two or three months earlier. It rapidly spread, and at the end of a fortnight cases were occurring all over the city. The mortality was highest at the end of July; during August and the first half of September the deaths became fewer daily. This summer there has been an unusual absence of rain, so that everything was dry and water scarce. On the 15th September a heavy shower of rain fell during the night and partly refilled the canals. This downpour was coincident with a sudden increase in the number of deaths from cholera; the epidemic seemed to have taken a new lease of life, and during this relapse the mortality was greater than during the first attack. At the time of writing—19th October—the disease is again dying down.

Those best able to judge estimate that the deaths from cholera in the city amounted to 5,000 or 6,000, while in the whole prefecture at least 30,000 are said to have died.

e first attack of cholera was subsiding, a very severe form of malarial fever spread over th ole district. The inhabitants of the hills, who have enjoyed relative immunity from cholera, suffered as much as the dwellers in the plains. The mortality directly resulting from this disease has been considerable.

During this period foreigners have enjoyed immunity from cholera; but the general health has been below the average, fever, diarrhœa, or debility having affected most of the community.

China, Imperial Maritime Customs, Medical Reports
(1903. 04. 01—1903. 09. 30)

CHINA.

IMPERIAL MARITIME CUSTOMS.

II.—SPECIAL SERIES: No. 2.

MEDICAL REPORTS,

FOR THE YEAR ENDED 31st MARCH 1904.

66th and 67th Issues.

PUBLISHED BY ORDER OF

The Inspector General of Customs.

SHANGHAI:

PUBLISHED AT THE STATISTICAL DEPARTMENT OF THE INSPECTORATE GENERAL OF CUSTOMS;

AND SOLD BY

KELLY & WALSH, LIMITED: SHANGHAI, HONGKONG, YOKOHAMA, AND SINGAPORE;

MAX NOESSLER: BREMEN, SHANGHAI, AND YOKOHAMA.

LONDON: P. S. KING & SON, 2 AND 4, GREAT SMITH STREET, WESTMINSTER, S.W.

[Price $1.50]

1905.

INSPECTOR GENERAL'S CIRCULAR No. 19 of 1870.

INSPECTORATE GENERAL OF CUSTOMS,
PEKING, 31st *December* 1870.

SIR,

1.—IT has been suggested to me that it would be well to take advantage of the circumstances in which the Customs Establishment is placed, to procure information with regard to disease amongst foreigners and natives in China; and I have, in consequence, come to the resolution of publishing half-yearly in collected form all that may be obtainable. If carried out to the extent hoped for, the scheme may prove highly useful to the medical profession both in China and at home, and to the public generally. I therefore look with confidence to the co-operation of the Customs Medical Officer at your port, and rely on his assisting me in this matter by framing a half-yearly Report containing the result of his observations at.................upon the local peculiarities of disease, and upon diseases rarely or never encountered out of China. The facts brought forward and the opinions expressed will be arranged and published either with or without the name of the physician responsible for them, just as he may desire.

2.—The suggestions of the Customs Medical Officers at the various ports as to the points which it would be well to have especially elucidated, will be of great value in the framing of a form which will save trouble to those members of the medical profession, whether connected with the Customs or not, who will join in carrying out the plan proposed. Meanwhile I would particularly invite attention to—

a.—The general health of....................during the period reported on; the death rate amongst foreigners; and, as far as possible, a classification of the causes of death.

b.—Diseases prevalent at...........................

c.—General type of disease; peculiarities and complications encountered; special treatment demanded.

d.—Relation of disease to { Season. Alteration in local conditions—such as drainage, etc. Alteration in climatic conditions.

e.—Peculiar diseases; especially leprosy.

f.—Epidemics: { Absence or presence. Causes. Course and treatment. Fatality.

Other points, of a general or special kind, will naturally suggest themselves to medical men; what I have above called attention to will serve to fix the general scope of the undertaking.

3.—Considering the number of places at which the Customs Inspectorate has established offices, the thousands of miles north and south and east and west over which these offices are scattered, the varieties of climate, and the peculiar conditions to which, under such different circumstances, life and health are subjected, I believe the Inspectorate, aided by its Medical Officers, can do good service in the general interest in the direction indicated; and, as already stated, I rely with confidence on the support and assistance of the Medical Officer at each port in the furtherance and perfecting of this scheme. You will hand a copy of this Circular to Dr. ...., and request him, in my name, to hand to you in future, for transmission to myself, half-yearly Reports of the kind required, for the half-years ending 31st March and 30th September—that is, for the Winter and Summer seasons.

4.— * * * * *

I am, etc.,

(Signed) ROBERT HART,
Inspector General.

To

THE COMMISSIONERS OF CUSTOMS.

TABLE OF CONTENTS.

The Contributors to this Volume are:—

J. H. McCartney, m.d. .... Chungking.

A. Sharp Deane, f.r.c.s. .... Wuhu.

J. S. Grant, m.d. .... Ningpo.

W. E. Plummer, m.d. .... Wenchow.

H. M. McCandliss, m.d. .... Hoihow.

E. C. Davenport, m.b. .... Canton.

J. H. Lowry, l.r.c.p.ed., l.r.c.s.ed. .... Pakhoi.

Georges Barbézieux, m.d. .... Mengtsz.

Ram Lall Sircar, m.d. .... Tengyueh.

Dr. W. E. PLUMMER'S REPORT ON THE HEALTH OF WENCHOW

For the Half-year ended 30th September 1903.

THIS year Wenchow has been free from cholera, notwithstanding our frequent communication with Shanghai.

In March this district was visited by an epidemic of cerebro-spinal meningitis. Only two cases came under my personal observation, as nearly all the sufferers were country people. In the P'ing-yang-hsien the mortality was considerable, and there were many deaths after only one or two days illness. The symptoms of the cases observed followed the description of the disease given in "OSLER'S Medicine" (second edition) very closely.

During April and May malarial fever in a very severe form was prevalent and caused many deaths.

Dysentery has been epidemic here during the last three months, viz., July, August, and September. All the cases that have come under my notice in adults have yielded to ipecacuanha in a most gratifying manner, but in one case, a baby, this drug did not succeed in controlling the disease.

Cases of dengue have been brought into this port from Ningpo, and one or two Wenchow men have developed the disease, but there has been no epidemic such as at present obtains in Ningpo and Shanghai. The only foreigner who suffered is one who brought the disease with him and developed symptoms the day after arrival. Wenchow escaped this disease in exactly the same way last year.

This year the Methodist Mission has acquired a bungalow on one of the hills, at a height of 1,200 feet above the sea, distant an hour and a half's journey from the city. The ladies and children who have resided there during the hot months have the unusual experience of having passed the summer at Wenchow without becoming pale and anæmic.

Plague has not yet been seen in Wenchow, although we are in frequent communication with Foochow by junks. The oldest residents are not aware that this disease has ever appeared here.

After an experience of two years I have not met a case of leprosy, nor have I seen a case of undoubted typhoid fever, although from 200 to 300 patients have come under my observation every week at the mission hospital. Syphilis is exceedingly prevalent; gonorrhœa, gonorrhœal rheumatism, and gonorrhœal ophthalmia patients are seen almost every day. Cancer has not come as frequently under my observation here as in England; sarcoma, however, appears to be quite as much in evidence here as there.

China， Imperial Maritime Customs， Medical Reports
（1910. 04. 01—1910. 09. 30）

CHINA.

IMPERIAL MARITIME CUSTOMS.

II.—SPECIAL SERIES: No. 2.

MEDICAL REPORTS,

FOR THE HALF-YEAR ENDED 30TH SEPTEMBER 1904

TO

THE HALF-YEAR ENDED 30TH SEPTEMBER 1910.

SIXTY-EIGHTH TO EIGHTIETH ISSUES.

Published by Order of the Inspector General of Customs.

SHANGHAI:
PUBLISHED AT THE STATISTICAL DEPARTMENT OF THE INSPECTORATE GENERAL OF CUSTOMS;
AND SOLD BY
KELLY & WALSH, LIMITED: SHANGHAI, HONGKONG, YOKOHAMA, AND SINGAPORE.
MAX NOSSLER: BREMEN AND SHANGHAI.
TIENTSIN PRESS, LIMITED: TIENTSIN.
NEW YORK: G. E. STECHERT & CO., 151-155, WEST 25TH STREET.
LONDON: P. S. KING & SON, 2 AND 4, GREAT SMITH STREET, WESTMINSTER, S.W.

[Price $2.]   1911.

TABLE OF CONTENTS.

The Contributors to this Volume are :—

T. L. BRANDER, M.D. .... Newchwang

J. H. McCARTNEY, M.D. .... Chungking.

C. W. FREEMAN, M.D. .... ,,

GEO. F. STOOKE, L.R.C.P. .... Ichang.

ANDREW GRAHAM, M.D. .... ,,

H. G. BARRIE, M.D., C.M. .... Changsha.

FRANK A. KELLER, M.D. .... ,,

E. H. HUME, M.D. .... ,,

A. C. LAMBERT, M.D. .... Kiukiang.

M. URBÁNEK, M.D. .... Chinkiang.

CHARLES FISHER MILLS, M.D. .... Ningpo.

E. WILMOT SMERDON, M.D. .... Wenchow.

J. A. McDONALD, M.D. .... Kongmoon.

PHILIP REES, M.D. .... Wuchow.

H. M. McCANDLISS, M.D. .... Hoihow.

S. ABBATUCCI, M.D. .... Pakhoi.

R. ASCORNET, M.D. .... ,,

— POUTHION, M.D. .... ,,

G. BARBÉZIEUX, M.D. .... Mengtsz.

RAM LALL SIRCAR, M.D. .... Tengyueh.

WIHAL CHAND, M.D. .... ,,

N. CHAND, M.D. .... ,,

REPORT ON THE HEALTH OF WENCHOW FOR THE HALF-YEAR ENDED 30TH SEPTEMBER, 1910.

By Dr. E. WILMOT SMERDON.

For the half-year ending 30th September the general health of the port has been very good. The foreign community, small at any time, was further reduced at the beginning of this period by some leaving for home on furlough, and during the hotter part of July to September the great majority went away to bungalows or other resorts. To this is largely due the prevailing absence of any serious illness; but the lack in no way gives an indication of the extremely irksome and depressing climatic condition, which, combined with the want of any social excitement, causes a feeling of malaise and continuous headaches and petty ailments almost to be the normal state of many.

Bowel trouble of a peculiarly chronic and recurrent type is the most frequent cause for any prolonged care. Starting with a tendency to constipation it leads on to a low colitis, with traces of blood and mucus, and only slight fever, but with tenesmus and much abdominal tenderness. Resembling occult chronic dysentery, there are, however, no amoebae found on miscroscopical examination.

The Chinese have been markedly exempt from an epidemic of any magnitude, Plague and cholera being unknown, and dysentery has not been so rife. This is attributable in a large degree to the unusually heavy and continuous rainfall last quarter.

In the Methodist Hospital of 120 beds the diseases most frequently met with are on the medical side, pulmonary tuberculosis (very common), conjunctival complaints, and chronic dysentery (occasionally sprue). Corresponding with these, and in some measure due to them or similar causes, we have surgically to deal with necrosis of long bones (especially femur) and cervical glands, entropion (very common), and fistula in ano.

Santonin is a routine course, varied by thymol. Quinine is the one drug that all prize, even the up-country yokel of most conservative tastes taking it as a panacea, for malarial infection is the rule. Venereal diseases are only too common and the number of primary infections by the pharynx in innocent individuals is quite pitiful. Fifty per cent

WENCHOW.

of our practice comprises ulcers of the legs and face.   Thiersch-grafting for the huge ulcers on the legs of rice cultivators gives a very fair result after return to work.

Appended is a meteorological table, kindly prepared and furnished to me by Capt. A. Walker, the Harbour Master, to whom I am indebted for the trouble taken.

METEOROLOGICAL SUMMARY.

Port of Wenchow, April to September, 1910, inclusive.

MONTH.		Average Max. Temp.	Average Min. Temp.	Rainfall.
April ...	..	64.4° F.	54° F.	4.02 ins. on 16 days.
May ...	...	75.9	63.5	7.95 ins. on 18 days.
June ...	...	87.4	74.2	6.43 ins. on 11 days.
July ...	...	92.6	78.1	12.07 ins. on 13 days.
August	...	89.7	77.2	14.58 ins. on 17 days.
September	...	84.23	72.73	7.61 ins. on 9 days.

Giving an average mean temperature of 75° with rain every other day.

China, Imperial Maritime Customs, Medical Reports
(1913. 10. 01—1914. 03. 31)

THE

China Medical Journal

VOLUME XXX

1916

SHANGHAI:

PRINTED BY THE PRESBYTERIAN MISSION PRESS

1916

CUSTOMS REPORT,—HEALTH OF WENCHOW

During the half-year ending March 31, 1914, Wenchow has been free from any great epidemics. The last case of Cholera was reported about the middle of October, 1913. At Christmas time small-pox was in the city; but few patients sought foreign aid.

Among the foreigners, there has been one case of sprue, in a young lady who had been resident in this district for some five years. The disease was not far advanced, and she has returned to England. A son has been born to a British member of the Customs Staff.

The Methodist Mission Hospital has been busy. About half the cases admitted as in-patients have been uninteresting ulcers, and diseases of the eye. The former are lesions of syphilitic, traumatic and septic origin; and among the latter are glaucoma in all its stages, iritis and cataract.

The more interesting cases includes gun-shot wounds; many of the victims are Fukienese men, and the wounds are inflicted by pirates who attack their junks at sea.

Ascites is common,—renal, cardiac and other cases due to some form of portal obstruction, with or without enlargement of the liver or spleen; such cases usually hurry out of Hospital as soon as they are relieved of the excessive fluid, and a diagnosis is not made. One woman, aged about 50, with ascites, was admitted weighing 125 catties, and left ten days later weighing 45 catties !

There have been several cases of granulomata. These occur for the most part on the lower half of the body, in young adult males. They do not conform to any of the familiar types of this class; and do not respond to anti-syphilitic treatment. They are limited to the skin and subcutaneous tissue, and are characterised by extreme chronicity. A history of ten or fifteen years in a man of 25 is common. They are often limited to one thigh, or one buttock. The tumours are at first isolated, about the size of a cherry stone, palpable but not visible, and seem to be lying in the subcutaneous tissues. Gradually they become visible, and the skin over them becomes smooth; the tumour is now the size of a hazel-nut and blue. Satellites appear and an area as large as the palm of the hand is involved. The skin assumes a deep suffused red colour and ulceration sets in. Ultimately the area is as large as the extended hand, with fungating ulcers the size of golf balls. There is no evidence of any spontaneous healing. Removal of the whole affected area, with skin-grafting where necessary, gives very good immediate results.

There has been one instructive case of quinine poisoning. A young man was admitted at about noon, with a temperature of 104⁸. The malarial parasite was demonstrated in the blood. By 9.00 a.m. the next day he had had three doses of grs. x. of quinine sulphate in solution; and at 10.00 a.m., two hours before the rigor was expected, he had a further dose of grs. xii. All that day he appeared to be perfectly well, but in the evening he complained of slight darkness of vision. A tabloid of quinine bisulphate grs. v. was given in the evening; and this was the last dose of quinine. On the following day he complained of complete blindness. After seven days he could count fingers with difficulty; and then he left Hospital, and took to Chinese treatment. After four months he can see in day-light and by electric light, but must be led about in a room lighted by oil lamps. There has been no return of the malaria. The dispenser denied the possibility of an error in the dose.

W. B. G. ANGUS.

CUSTOM HOUSE, WENCHOW, April 20, 1914.

China, Imperial Maritime Customs, Medical Reports
(1914. 06—1915. 09)

THE

China Medical Journal

VOLUME XXX

1916

SHANGHAI:
PRINTED BY THE PRESBYTERIAN MISSION PRESS
1916

CUSTOMS MEDICAL REPORT: HEALTH OF WENCHOW, CHEKIANG.

By E. T. A. STEDEFORD, M.B., B. Ch.

June-September, 1914. During this period the health among the foreign residents has been good. There has been one case of amoebic dysentery (June) and one case of typhoid fever complicated with cholecystitis (August). Death rate *nil*.

Among the native population syphilis and tuberculosis are extremely common. Syphilitic patients practically always come to hospital in the tertiary stage. Tuberculosis of bones and joints is very prevalent and the Chinese are learning the value of operation in these cases, sometimes presenting themselves with the request to have the diseased bone removed.

Trachoma attacks a large proportion of the population and is responsible for most of the cases of blindness. It is rarely possible to get Chinese to submit to treatment long enough to effect a cure.

Leprosy does not seem to be very common. I have only seen the anæsthetic variety here.

During the short time I have been here I have been struck with the great frequency among tumours of the innocent variety—mainly fibroids.

Cholera, which often visits the city in the latter part of the summer, has not appeared yet. There have been no epidemics.

October, 1914-March, 1915. The health of the foreign community has been excellent.

A very large part of the work among Chinese has been surgical. Tumours, tuberculosis of bones, joints, and glands, eye operations, especially for entropion, fistulæ, sinuses, and piles account for the greater percentage of these cases.

There is a form of ascites prevalent here in men, and more rarely in women, from the country districts, which is not accompanied by enlargement of the liver or spleen. The liver is sometimes reduced in size but not always. In about one-third of the cases a history of diarrhœa occurring near the beginning of the trouble can be obtained. Schistosomum ova have only been found in the fæces of a few cases. The disease may be fatal in a few months, or may last over a year. I have not observed a case that lasted more than eighteen months.

Two cases of ankylostomiasis were seen. There was one case of anæsthetic leprosy, a boy aged nineteen years. According to the evidence of a neighbour, the boy's father, who died when the boy was three years old, had paralysed and anæsthetic hands and an ulcer on the sole of the foot. The boy had anæsthetic patches involving the 4th and 5th fingers and the neighbouring area of the palm of each hand, and a patch on the left buttock. There was commencing *main-en-griffe* of the left hand and paralysis of the left orbicular muscle. The ulnar, external peroneal, and great auricular nerves were thickened. The knee-jerks were exaggerated and the jaw-jerk was present.

The following is a peculiar case, the only one of its kind seen, in which no diagnosis was made. Boy, aged 18. On the right leg there was a line of ulcers extending from the base of the second toe across the dorsum of the foot to the front of the internal malleolus, thence up the leg to the middle of the thigh exactly along the course of the internal saphenous vein. The ulcers had raised bases and varied in size from a few millimeters to 1½ centimeters in diameter ; in some places they were almost contiguous, in others they were separated by an interval of 2 or 3 centimeters. Above the middle of the thigh, on a continuation of the same line, there were two small reddish nodules apparently about to break down. The patient said the trouble had begun five months before with small, hard, painful nodules at the base of the second toe ; in about a fortnight these nodules had ulcerated. Similar swellings breaking down into ulcers had arisen progressively up the leg. There was no anæsthesia or paralysis. Treatment with mercury and arsenic and with local applications of caustics, had no curative effect. The patient did not stay long enough for potassium iodide to be tried

Rheumatic fever is a curiosity here ; one case, the only one during the year, was treated.

Towards the end of March epidemics of measles and smallpox broke out. As the Chinese do not bring these cases to the hospital, I have no first-hand acquaintance with these epidemics except in the case of a mission boarding school which was invaded by measles, and there all the cases ran the common course and no complications followed. From hearsay the smallpox epidemic does not appear to have been severe.

April-September, 1915. There has been a fair amount of sickness among the small foreign community here during these months.

A case of diphtheria occurred in April which quickly cleared up under antitoxin treatment. Round-worms and abscess of the arm in a child of sixteen months caused great constitutional disturbance and wasting.

A case of acute otitis media subsided without suppuration.

In September there was a case of fever, of which the cause is not clear, with two relapses, and apyrexial intervals of eleven and twelve days. When I was called to see the patient, a middle-aged man, he was suffering from fever and severe abdominal pain. He thought the fever had been present also on the two preceding evenings. The pain soon subsided, but the fever lasted for two days more, rising to over 103° F. at night and coming down to 99.°5 or 100° in the morning. During the fever the pulse was rapid (110-130) but regular ; after the disappearance of the fever the patient became collapsed, the pulse remaining rapid (110-120) and becoming bigeminal. It slowed down and became regular in two days and patient improved greatly. The next attack of fever occurred eleven days after its first disappearance. The previous day the patient had walked about ¼ mile and exerted himself more than since getting up. This attack lasted three days and was accompanied by irregular pulse. The fever and irregularity disappeared together. The second relapse took place in another twelve days. It was less severe and unaccompanied by any irregularity of the heart. It lasted three days.

During the summer the patient had been working out of doors a good deal surveying canals, but had not been exposed to the heat for several days preceding the illness, and the second relapse took place after the patient had been in bed for a few days with synovitis of the knee. The blood was examined during the first attack and during the second relapse, but no spirochœtes were found.

Cases of neurasthenia and influenza also occurred among foreigners.

The hospital of 100 beds has been full, and at times over full, during this summer.

There have been no widespread epidemics. Cases of cholera occurred here and there during July and August. In July there were several cases of bacillary dysentery.

A case of hydrophobia was seen in April, following seven weeks after a dog bite.

An unusual case worth recording was one of acute bulbar paralysis in a man aged thirty-four years. He awoke one night and found that he could not speak clearly or swallow. When I saw him five days later he was suffering from complete inability to swallow, paralysis of both sides of the soft palate, of the right side of the face and of the right side of the tongue. Both vocal cords were freely movable. Temperature 102° F. Pulse 108. He was fed with the stomach-tube and given small doses of strychnine. About a month after the onset the facial paralysis began to show signs of improvement, and a fortnight later he was able to swallow a little fluid. Four or five days later the stomach tube was no longer necessary. About two months after the onset the palate began to move on phonation and a week later he was able to speak with hardly any nasal sound. Although the quick recovery suggests hysteria, the evident great distress of the patient when first seen, the high temperature, and quick pulse which continued for three days and for which there was nothing else to account, point against its being of that nature. No personal history of syphilis could be elicited, but his wife had had one miscarriage and no children during their three years of married life.

China, Imperial Maritime Customs, Medical Reports
(1916—1917)

THE

China Medical Journal

PUBLISHED BY

The China Medical Missionary Association

VOLUME XXXI

1917

SHANGHAI:
PRINTED BY THE PRESBYTERIAN MISSION PRESS
1917

Chinese Customs Service Medical Reports.

PUBLIC HEALTH OF WENCHOW, 1916-1917.

E. T. A. Stedeford, M.B., B. Ch., D. T. M. (Lond.).

The health of the foreign residents has, on the whole, been good during this period. There was one death, that of a child aged 18 months, from acute bacillary dysentery in July. A case of sun traumatism occurred in August in a man of 35; it left no injurious effects.

In February, 1917, the same patient, after suffering from vague abdominal pains for a few weeks, had one night a very sharp attack of pain below the right costal margin which passed off in ten minutes or so leaving some tenderness. A few days later two other attacks occurred on successive evenings. I was then called to see him. Tenderness was present very definitely in the region of the gall bladder but there were no other signs. Patient's appetite had become very poor, he felt languid and complained of pain in the right shoulder but beyond that there were no other symptoms. He said that he had had no fever and none was present then. He had not vomited. Gall stones seemed the most probable diagnosis. After rest in bed for a few days on light diet the patient felt a little better and the tenderness over the gall bladder was less, but the pain in the shoulder persisted with occasional twinges in the gall bladder region. What progress there was, was slow and the possibility of operation was talked of. Then on two nights following he had a drenching sweat, preceded, he thought, by slight fever. These sweatings suggested the possibility of liver abscess and daily injections of emetine (1 gr.) were begun. From that time improvement was rapid and he was able to return to work in a week. Seven injections were given. There was no history of dysentery. When the patient had been back at work for about a month the pain in the shoulder began to return and a few days later he had another sharp attack of pain in the liver region. When I saw him, there was tenderness below the right costal margin in the anterior axillary line. Emetine was again begun and followed again by rapid improvement. The injections are at present being continued.

There have been two confinements during the year: one was normal; the other was a case of placenta prævia in which the child did not survive.

There have been no epidemics among the Chinese.

Diphtheria was prevalent in the city during November and December, coinciding with a time of great drought.

Small-pox was frequent during January and February, especially in the eastern suburb of the city.

China, Imperial Maritime Customs, Medical Reports
(1917—1918)

THE

China Medical Journal

PUBLISHED BY

The China Medical Missionary Association

VOLUME XXXII

1918

SHANGHAI:
PRINTED BY THE PRESBYTERIAN MISSION PRESS
1918

Medical Reports of Chinese Customs Service.

Public Health of Wenchow, 1917-1918.

E. T. A. STEDEFORD, M.B., Ch.B., Customs Medical Officer.

During the year the small foreign community, of some thirty persons, has had more sickness than for some years. Among the children, there have been cases of whooping cough, rubella, broncho-pneumonia, and trachoma; among the adults, rheumatism, sciatica, paratyphoid fever (September), colitis, chronic dysentery (July), gonorrhœa, soft sore followed by buboes, incipient sprue (October-November), general debility, and anæmia. There is nothing of interest to remark about these cases, except that of chronic dysentery which exhibited emetine poisoning. It was a case of frequent relapses during three or four years. Since it had always yielded to emetine previously, that drug was again used though amœbæ could not be found in the stools. At the end of the first week the case showed decided improvement, then, owing to a typhoon, it was impossible to give the injections for two days and the patient relapsed to his original condition. The injections were again begun accompanied by enemata; the dysentery slowly improved. The injections were continued altogether for a month, during which time 22 grains of emetine were administered. The patient then left the port nearly well as far as the dysentery was concerned, but, as I learned from his later medical attendant, soon afterwards he was affected by a general paresis of the voluntary muscles, chiefly affecting the muscles of the neck, shoulder, and arm and the muscles of mastication. The sphincter ani was also involved. The condition improved slowly under strychnine injections.

Among the Chinese there have been no epidemics. Enteric fever was rather prevalent during the autumn and several cases of diphtheria occurred during the winter. Almost no visiting of Chinese sick in their homes has been done, so that it is impossible to form any sufficiently definite idea of the minor fevers from which they suffer, as such cases are rarely brought to the hospital.

During the year, 25,548 out-patients have been seen at the Blyth Hospital and 1,418 treated as in-patients. The number of operations under chloroform was 297. Abdominal operations are a new feature of the surgical work here. Previously it was impossible to get any patient to consent to an abdominal operation, but in the autumn of 1916 one woman was bold enough to have an ovarian (dermoid) tumour removed and since then we have performed 10 abdominal operations; 7 of these were for ovarian tumours, 6 of which were successfully removed, the remaining one being too adherent in the pelvis for safe removal; of the others, one was an omentopexy for cirrhosis of the liver (a very common complaint here) in a woman. She returned to the hospital about six months after the operation, still with fluid in the abdomen (perhaps about ⅓ as much as when she came first), but the processes of exudation and absorption had apparently reached an equilibrium as the quantity of fluid had been stationary for three or four months. She was greatly improved in health and had put on flesh, but the original fascial opening had enlarged and allowed a hernial protrusion. It was decided to cut down and reduce the opening. The day after the operation she seemed to have stood it well, but on the third day she became restless and began to vomit. Unfortunately she got worse, became drowsy, then comatose, and died on the fifth day. Apparently it was a case of delayed chloroform poisoning, favoured by too little liver tissue. This was the only fatality of the series.

Leprosy is a rare phenomenon here, but occasional cases do occur and the majority come from the Jui-an district, half a day's journey to the south. I have seen one case of the anæsthetic variety in a young man during the year. There were pale patches of anæsthetic skin on the back, chest, and arms. The ulnar and extreme popliteal nerves were perhaps slightly thickened.

China, Imperial Maritime Customs, Medical Reports
(1918—1919)

THE

China Medical Journal

PUBLISHED BY

The China Medical ~~~~ onary Association

VOLUME XXXIII

1919

SHANGHAI:
PRINTED BY THE PRESBYTERIAN MISSION PRESS
1919

Public Health of Wenchow, 1918-1919.

E. T. A. STEDEFORD, M.B., Ch.B.

METEOROLOGICAL REPORT.

Monthly temperature :—

	1918, Apr.	May	Jun.	July	Aug.	Sep.	Oct.	Nov.	Dec.	1919, Jan.	Feb.	Mar.
Mean	60.5	68.4	75.1	83.8	82.6	77.9	69.8	57.8	52.8	49.9	44.8	55.7
Mean Max.	66	74	80	90	89	85	76	62	57	52	50	61
Mean Min.	55	62	70	77	77	71	63	53	49	40	39	50

Rainfall :—

5.54 8.66 23.2 9.56 9.18 4.50 1.70 5.46 2.82 3.53 3.65 4.40 inches

MEDICAL REPORT.—The native population of the city of Wenchow is about 100,000.

The foreign community of about 30 persons, as a whole, has been comparatively healthy during the year. Dysentery, malaria, influenza, gonorrhea, bronchitis, rheumatoid arthritis, aortic disease, have been responsible for what sickness there has been.

INFLUENZA AMONG THE CHINESE.

As for epidemics, the most marked feature of the year has been influenza. It began in May. In that month here and there all over the city cases of fever arose accompanied by headache and listlessness; catarrhal symptoms were not prominent then. The fever lasted four or five days and often left the patient very weak. The mortality was practically nil. The number of cases diminished as the summer advanced. Early in September, however, rather suddenly, cases became more numerous and more severe, being generally accompanied by bronchial or pulmonary symptoms, sometimes with bæmoptysis, and often ending in broncho-pneumonia. All places of the district were not affected alike, some being almost untouched. The scourge fell more heavily upon the country districts than upon the towns. In the latter only a few per cent were attacked, except in schools where 50% or 60% suffered, but happily with no mortality, with the exception of one school where one student died. In many country districts, on the other hand, a heavy toll was exacted. Generally speaking, judging from reports, in the affected areas at least one half of the inhabitants of the villages were attacked, the disease appearing in such a severe form that many places lost 10% of their inhabitants by death. Areas in which three-fourths of a family were carried off were not uncommon. The disease often did its work with dramatic swiftness: one day, or even less, often sufficing to bring about a mortal issue.

Three or four members of a household might all contract the disease and succumb in the space of two days. Towards the end of October the terror had fairly well spent itself. Since that time sporadic cases have occurred, but as a rule they have been of a mild form.

Beri-beri is not a common disease in Wenchow, but in the spring of 1918 it broke out among the soldiers who had been stationed here. About a dozen cases occurred, all of the dry form. There were no fatalities.

No other epidemics have occurred.

Neosalvarsan is becoming very popular with the better classes of the Chinese.

EMETINE IN LIVER ABSCESS.

The great value of emetine in the treatment of liver abscess has been experienced again and again. Cases which in former days would surely have had to be operated upon are now apparently quite cured by emetine injection alone, even where the abscess seems within measurable distance of bursting through the skin.

ENLARGEMENT OF PITUITARY BODY.

The following case of enlargement of the pituitary body of long duration is of special interest. The patient, a man of 36, came complaining of blindness in the left eye and partial loss of sight in the right eye, giddiness and loss of strength. Eight years ago the field of the left eye began to contract from the temporal side and gradually progressed until about two years ago he could only see a little "across his nose" as he expressed it." Soon after that the eye became totally blind. About eight years ago also, the field of the right eye began to contract, similarly from the temporal side, but progressed more slowly. At present just half the field is blind. On exertion vision becomes

Medical and Surgical Progress—Internal Medicine.

indistinct (temporary hyperæmia and swelling of the pituitary?). Five or six years ago he became stout. Four or five years ago he began to experience giddiness on walking, which is rather better now than it used to be. No headache, except for a day two years ago. No vomiting.

On admission the subcutaneous fat was much more abundant on the body generally than is usual for a person of his age; it was especially plentiful on the abdomen. There was total blindness of the left eye and temporal hemianopsia of the right, as already described. The light reflex of the left eye was absent ; the consensual reflex was present. The left optic disc was paler than the right. No sugar in the urine. No improvement or alteration of the condition followed the exhibition of potassium iodide for a month.

图书在版编目（CIP）数据

近代温州疾病及医疗概况：瓯海关《医报》译编 /
温州市档案局（馆）译编. -- 北京：社会科学文献出版
社，2018.11
　ISBN 978 - 7 - 5201 - 3460 - 6

　Ⅰ.①近… 　Ⅱ.①温… 　Ⅲ.①疾病 - 史料 - 温州 - 近
代 ②医疗保健事业 - 史料 - 温州 - 近代 　Ⅳ.①R - 092
②R199.2

　中国版本图书馆 CIP 数据核字（2018）第 210110 号

近代温州疾病及医疗概况
　　——瓯海关《医报》译编

译　　编 / 温州市档案局（馆）

出 版 人 / 谢寿光
项目统筹 / 王玉敏
责任编辑 / 王玉敏　赵怀英　张文静

出　　版 / 社会科学文献出版社·独立编辑工作室（010）59367153
　　　　　地址：北京市北三环中路甲 29 号院华龙大厦　邮编：100029
　　　　　网址：www. ssap. com. cn
发　　行 / 市场营销中心（010）59367081　59367083
印　　装 / 三河市东方印刷有限公司

规　　格 / 开　本：787mm × 1092mm　1/16
　　　　　印　张：23.75　字　数：389 千字
版　　次 / 2018 年 11 月第 1 版　2018 年 11 月第 1 次印刷
书　　号 / ISBN 978 - 7 - 5201 - 3460 - 6
定　　价 / 139.00 元